Trauma in Facial Plastic Surgery

Editor

KRIS S. MOE

FACIAL PLASTIC SURGERY CLINICS OF NORTH AMERICA

www.facialplastic.theclinics.com

Consulting Editor
J. REGAN THOMAS

November 2017 • Volume 25 • Number 4

ELSEVIER

1600 John F. Kennedy Boulevard • Suite 1800 • Philadelphia, Pennsylvania, 19103-2899

http://www.theclinics.com

FACIAL PLASTIC SURGERY CLINICS OF NORTH AMERICA Volume 25, Number 4
November 2017 ISSN 1064-7406, ISBN-13: 978-0-323-54877-9

Editor: Jessica McCool
Developmental Editor: Meredith Madeira

Facial Plastic Surgery Clinics of North America (ISSN 1064-7406) is published quarterly by Elsevier Inc., 360 Park Avenue South, New York, NY 10010-1710. Months of issue are February, May, August, and November. Business and Editorial Offices: 1600 John F. Kennedy Blvd., Suite 1800, Philadelphia, PA 19103-2899. Periodicals postage paid at New York, NY, and additional mailing offices. Subscription prices are $390.00 per year (US individuals), $592.00 per year (US institutions), $445.00 per year (Canadian individuals), $737.00 per year (Canadian institutions), $535.00 per year (foreign individuals), $737.00 per year (foreign institutions), $100.00 per year (US students), and $255.00 per year (foreign students). Foreign air speed delivery is included in all *Clinics* subscription prices. All prices are subject to change without notice. POSTMASTER: Send address changes to *Facial Plastic Surgery Clinics*, Elsevier Health Sciences Division, Subscription Customer Service, 3251 Riverport Lane, Maryland Heights, MO 63043. **Customer service: 1-800-654-2452 (US and Canada); 1-314-447-8871 (outside US and Canada); Fax: 314-447-8029; E-mail: journalscustomerservice-usa@elsevier.com (for print support); journalsonline support-usa@elsevier.com (for online support).**

Reprints. For copies of 100 or more of articles in this publication, please contact the Commercial Reprints Department, Elsevier Inc., 360 Park Avenue South, New York, NY 10010-1710. Tel.: 212-633-3874; Fax: 212-633-3820; E-mail: reprints@elsevier.com.

Facial Plastic Surgery Clinics of North America is covered in *MEDLINE/PubMed (Index Medicus)*.

Contributors

CONSULTING EDITOR

J. REGAN THOMAS, MD, FACS
Mansueto Professor and Chairman,
Department of Otolaryngology–Head & Neck
Surgery, University of Illinois at Chicago,
Chicago, Illinois

EDITOR

KRIS S. MOE, MD, FACS
Professor and Chief, Division of Facial Plastic
and Reconstructive Surgery, Departments of
Otolaryngology–Head and Neck Surgery and
Neurological Surgery, University of
Washington School of Medicine, Seattle,
Washington

AUTHORS

MELISSA AMUNDSON, DDS
Attending OMS, Department of Surgery,
Trauma Service, Legacy Emanuel Medical
Center, Head & Neck Surgical Associates,
Portland, Oregon

R. BRYAN BELL, MD, DDS, FACS, FACD
Attending OMS, Department of Surgery,
Trauma Service, Legacy Emanuel
Medical Center, Consultant, Head & Neck
Surgical Associates, Medical Director,
Providence Oral, Head and Neck Cancer
Program and Clinic, Investigator, The
Robert W. Franz Cancer Research Center,
Earle A. Chiles Research Institute,
Providence Health & Sciences, Portland,
Oregon

RONALD BERGMAN, DO
Private Practice, Department of
Plastic and Reconstructive Surgery,
Bergman Folkers Plastic Surgery,
Des Moines, Iowa

SCOTT E. BEVANS, MD
Chief of Facial Trauma Surgery, Department
of Otolaryngology, Major, Medical Corps,
US Army, San Antonio Military Medical
Center, San Antonio, Texas; Assistant
Professor, Department of Surgery,
Uniformed Services University, Bethesda,
Maryland

KOFI D. BOAHENE, MD
Associate Professor, Facial Plastic and
Reconstructive Surgery, The Johns Hopkins
University School of Medicine, Baltimore,
Maryland

JOSEPH BRENNAN, MD
Department of Otolaryngology–Head & Neck
Surgery, San Antonio Uniformed Services
Health Education Consortium, San Antonio,
Texas

TUAN BUI, MD, DDS
Director, Oral and Maxillofacial Pathology,
Sanford Health, Fargo, North Dakota

PATRICK J. BYRNE, MD, FACS, MBA
Professor, Director, Facial Plastic and
Reconstructive Surgery, Departments of
Otolaryngology–Head & Neck Surgery and
Dermatology, Co-Medical Director, Greater
Baltimore Cleft Lip and Palate Team,
The Johns Hopkins University School of
Medicine, Baltimore, Maryland

**SRINIVASA R. CHANDRA, MD, BDS,
FDSRCS**
Assistant Professor, Oral Maxillofacial–Head
and Neck Oncologic Microvascular
Reconstructive Surgery, University of
Washington, Seattle, Washington

ALLEN CHENG, MD, DMD
Attending OMS, Department of Surgery,
Trauma Service, Legacy Emanuel Medical
Center, Consultant, Head & Neck Surgical
Associates, Director, Head and Neck Cancer
Program, Legacy Good Samaritan Medical
Center, Portland, Oregon

RANDALL MATTHER CHESNUT, MD
Professor, Department of Neurological
Surgery, University of Washington, Harborview
Medical Center, University of Washington
School of Medicine, Seattle, Washington

JOHN JARED CHRISTOPHEL, MD
Associate Professor, Department of
Otolaryngology–Head & Neck Surgery,
Division of Facial Plastic and Reconstructive
Surgery, University of Virginia, Charlottesville,
Virginia

ERIC J. DIERKS, MD, DMD, FACS, FACD
Director of Maxillofacial Trauma,
Department of Surgery, Trauma Service,
Legacy Emanuel Medical Center, Consultant,
Head & Neck Surgical Associates, Portland,
Oregon

WILLIAM M. DOUGHERTY, MD
Resident, Department of Otolaryngology–Head
& Neck Surgery, Division of Facial Plastic and
Reconstructive Surgery, University of Virginia,
Charlottesville, Virginia

CELESTE GARY, MD
Clinical Assistant Professor, Department of
Otolaryngology, LSU Health New Orleans,
New Orleans, Louisiana

SAVANNAH GELESKO, MD, DDS
Former Resident, Head & Neck Surgical
Associates, Portland, Oregon

**G. RICHARD HOLT, MD, MSE, MPH, MABE,
D Bioethics**
Department of Otolaryngology–Head & Neck
Surgery, San Antonio Uniformed Services
Health Education Consortium, Department of
Otolaryngology–Head & Neck Surgery,
The University of Texas Health Science Center
at San Antonio, San Antonio, Texas

CLINTON D. HUMPHREY, MD
Associate Professor, Department of
Otolaryngology–Head & Neck Surgery,
University of Kansas Medical Center, Kansas
City, Kansas

ROBERT M. KELLMAN, MD
Chairman, Department of Otolaryngology and
Communication Sciences, SUNY Upstate
Medical University, Syracuse, New York

BABER KHATIB, MD, DDS
Fellow, Advanced Craniomaxillofacial and
Trauma Surgery/Head and Neck Oncologic
and Microvascular Reconstructive Surgery,
Department of Surgery, Legacy Emanuel
Medical Center, Providence Portland Hospital,
Head & Neck Surgical Associates, Portland,
Oregon

DON O. KIKKAWA, MD, FACS
Professor and Chief, Division of Oculofacial
Plastic and Reconstructive Surgery, Vice Chair,
University of California, San Diego,
Department of Ophthalmology,
Professor, Division of Plastic Surgery,
University of California, San Diego, Department
of Surgery, Shiley Eye Institute, La Jolla,
California

IRENE A. KIM, MD
Fellow, Facial Plastic and Reconstructive
Surgery, The Johns Hopkins University School
of Medicine, Baltimore, Maryland

AUDREY C. KO, MD
Clinical Instructor, Division of Oculofacial
Plastic and Reconstructive Surgery, University
of California, San Diego, Department of
Ophthalmology, Shiley Eye Institute, La Jolla,
California

CODY A. KOCH, MD, PhD
Private Practice, Department of Plastic
and Reconstructive Surgery, Koch
Facial Plastic Surgery & Spa, West Des
Moines, Iowa

BOBBY S. KORN, MD, PhD, FACS
Associate Professor, Division of
Oculofacial Plastic and Reconstructive
Surgery, University of California, San Diego,
Department of Ophthalmology, Division of
Plastic Surgery, University of California, San
Diego, Department of Surgery, Shiley Eye
Institute, La Jolla, California

J. DAVID KRIET, MD
Professor, Director, Division of Facial Plastic
and Reconstructive Surgery, Department of
Otolaryngology–Head & Neck Surgery,
University of Kansas Medical Center, Kansas
City, Kansas

G. NINA LU, MD
Resident Physician, Department of
Otolaryngology–Head & Neck Surgery,
University of Kansas Medical Center, Kansas
City, Kansas

JACOB S. MAJORS, MD
Department of Otolaryngology–Head & Neck
Surgery, San Antonio Uniformed Services
Health Education Consortium, San Antonio,
Texas

MELISSA MARKS, DO
Department of Plastic and Reconstructive
Surgery, Mercy Medical Center, Des Moines,
Iowa

KRIS S. MOE, MD, FACS
Professor and Chief, Division of Facial Plastic
and Reconstructive Surgery, Departments of
Otolaryngology–Head & Neck Surgery and
Neurological Surgery, University of
Washington School of Medicine, Seattle,
Washington

J. STUART NELSON, MD, PhD
Beckman Laser Institute and Medical
Clinic, University of California, Irvine,
Department of Biomedical Engineering,
University of California, Irvine, Irvine,
California

ROBERT GLENN OXFORD, MD
Resident, Department of Neurological
Surgery, University of Washington,
Harborview Medical Center, University of
Washington School of Medicine, Seattle,
Washington

STEPHEN S. PARK, MD
Professor, Vice Chair, Department of
Otolaryngology–Head & Neck Surgery,
Director, Division of Facial Plastic and
Reconstructive Surgery, University of Virginia,
Charlottesville, Virginia

ASHISH PATEL, MD, DDS
Attending OMS, Department of Surgery,
Trauma Service, Legacy Emanuel Medical
Center, Consultant, Attending Head and
Neck/Microvascular Surgeon, Head & Neck
Surgical Associates, Consultant, Providence
Oral, Head and Neck Cancer Program and
Clinic, Providence Health & Sciences, Portland,
Oregon

DEREK POLECRITTI, DO
Department of Plastic and Reconstructive
Surgery, Mercy Medical Center, Des Moines,
Iowa

KELLIE R. SATTERFIELD, MD
Physician, Division of Oculofacial Plastic and
Reconstructive Surgery, University of
California, San Diego, Department of
Ophthalmology, Shiley Eye Institute, La Jolla,
California

ALEXIS M. STROHL, MD
Fellow in Facial Plastic and
Reconstructive Surgery, Department
of Otolaryngology and Communication
Sciences, SUNY Upstate Medical University,
Syracuse, New York

E. BRADLEY STRONG, MD
Professor, Department of Otolaryngology,
UC Davis School of Medicine, Sacramento,
California

PREM B. TRIPATHI, MD, MPH
Beckman Laser Institute and Medical Clinic,
University of California, Irvine, Irvine, California;
Division of Facial Plastic Surgery, Department
of Otolaryngology–Head & Neck Surgery,
University of California, Irvine, Orange,
California

BRIAN J. WONG, MD, PhD
Beckman Laser Institute and Medical Clinic,
Department of Biomedical Engineering,
University of California, Irvine, Irvine, California;
Division of Facial Plastic Surgery, Department of
Otolaryngology–Head & Neck Surgery,
University of California, Irvine, Orange, California

KAREN S. ZEMPLENYI, MD, DDS
Resident, Department of Oral Maxillofacial
Surgery, University of Washington, Seattle,
Washington

Contents

Spinal and traumatic brain injuries (TBIs) often accompany craniofacial trauma. Neurosurgical considerations can range from initial emergent surgery to conservative management of closed head injuries in patients with craniofacial injuries. This article discusses the most common disorders managed by neurosurgeons in the setting of craniofacial trauma and reviews the usual timing and setting for various treatments that patients with TBI encounter throughout the course of treatment. It also highlights the consequences of TBI on the timing and planning of craniofacial repairs and the importance of multidisciplinary cooperation to provide comprehensive care to survivors of trauma.

Trauma centers must prepare to manage high-velocity injuries resulting from mass casualty incidents as global terrorism becomes a greater concern and an increasing risk. The most recent conflicts in Iraq and Afghanistan have significantly improved the understanding of battlefield trauma and how to appropriately address these injures. This article applies combat surgery experience to civilian situations, outlines the physiology and kinetics of high-velocity injuries, and reviews applicable triage and management strategies.

The optimal management of frontal sinus fractures remains controversial. Fortunately, the severity of these injuries has diminished with more stringent auto-safety regulations, changing the treatment paradigms used to repair these injuries. Appropriate patient selection and close follow-up may allow for conservative management strategies when dealing with frontal sinus fractures, largely replacing the more morbid and invasive techniques that have been the mainstay for years. Because acute and delayed sequelae can arise after the initial injury, patients should be thoroughly counseled about the importance of follow-up and the need to seek medical care if they develop any concerning signs or symptoms.

Orbital reconstruction is one of the most challenging tasks for surgeons who treat craniofacial trauma. Suboptimal outcomes carry a high level of morbidity, with functional, emotional, and aesthetic implications. However, advances in reconstruction techniques, including the use of orbital endoscopy, computer-guided navigation, and mirror image overlay techniques, have been shown to provide significant improvements in outcomes. This article provides practical advice for applying these techniques to orbital reconstruction following trauma.

Nasal bones are the most frequently fractured facial bone, and these fractures are caused by blunt facial trauma, resulting in a significant number of patients seeking treatment. Proper evaluation and treatment in the acute setting can minimize secondary surgeries, lower overall health care costs, and increase patient satisfaction. Nasal fracture management, however, varies widely between surgeons. The open treatment of isolated nasal fractures is a particularly controversial subject. This review seeks to describe the existing literature in isolated nasal fracture management.

Zygomaticomaxillary fractures account for approximately 25% of all facial fractures. They can be grouped into high-velocity and low-velocity injuries. A complete head and neck examination is critical for accurate clinical diagnosis. A thin-cut axial computed tomographic scan with sagittal, coronal, and 3-D reconstruction is important for accurate diagnosis and treatment planning. A thorough understanding of the bony tetrapod anatomy and fracture mechanics is critical to treatment planning. Treatment options include closed and open reduction with internal fixation. Computer-aided applications can reduce the need for open reduction and improve the accuracy of both closed and open repairs.

This article includes updates in the management of mandibular trauma and reconstruction as they relate to maxillomandibular fixation screws, custom hardware, virtual surgical planning, and protocols for use of computer-aided surgery and navigation when managing composite defects from gunshot injuries to the face.

Treatment of subcondylar fractures has been the subject of debate for many years. Options for treatment include physical therapy, elastic maxillomandibular fixation, and open repair. Proper imaging and clinical evaluation are imperative when deciding on the best management option. In the past, most subcondylar fractures were treated with a closed approach. Recent data support open repair, when feasible. Studies show increased interincisal opening, lateral excursion, and protrusion with less mandibular shortening, jaw deviation, and pain. There are serious side effects that may be associated with open repair. The surgical technique for endoscopic repair is outlined in detail.

Pediatric maxillofacial fractures are rare owing to anatomic differences between juvenile and adult skulls. Children's bone is less calcified, allowing for "greenstick fractures." The overall ratio of cranial to facial volume decreases with age. In children, tooth buds comprise the majority of mandibular volume. The most common pediatric craniomaxillofacial fractures for children ages 0 to 18 years are mandible, nasal bone, and maxilla and zygoma. Growth potential must be considered when addressing pediatric trauma and often a less-is-more approach is best when considering open versus closed treatment. Regardless of treatment, pediatric trauma cases must be followed through skeletal maturity.

Emergency personnel, surgeons, and ancillary health care providers frequently encounter soft tissue injuries in facial trauma. Appropriate evaluation and management is essential to achieve optimal functional and aesthetic outcomes.

Facial trauma often involves injuries to the eyelid and periorbital region. Management of these injuries can be challenging because of the involvement of multiple complex anatomic structures that are in close proximity. Restoration of normal anatomic relationships of the eyelids and periocular structures is essential for optimum functional and aesthetic outcome after trauma. This review provides an overview of the current literature involving soft tissue trauma of the eyelid and periorbital tissue and highlights key steps in patient evaluation and management with various types of injuries.

Laser treatment for posttraumatic injury offers the clinician the unique opportunity for early intervention in mediating early scar formation or for reducing the appearance of scars after maturation. In this review, the authors focus on the mechanisms by which lasers exert their therapeutic effects, highlighting several popular lasers and dosimetry used, and underscoring the power of combined surgical scar revision in managing posttraumatic facial scars.

This article provides the reader with a comprehensive review of high-level evidence-based medicine in facial trauma and highlights areas devoid of high-level evidence. The article is organized in the order one might approach a clinical problem: starting with the workup, followed by treatment considerations, operative decisions, and postoperative treatments. Individual injuries are discussed within each section, with an overview of the available high-level clinical evidence. This article not only provides a quick reference for the facial traumatologist but also allows the reader to identify areas that lack high-level evidence, perhaps motivating future endeavors.

FACIAL PLASTIC SURGERY CLINICS OF NORTH AMERICA

RELATED INTEREST

Surgical Clinics, October 2017 (Vol. 97, No. 5)
Trauma
Oscar Guillamondegui and Bradley Dennis, *Editors*
Available at: http://www.surgical.theclinics.com/

THE CLINICS ARE AVAILABLE ONLINE!
Access your subscription at:
www.theclinics.com

Preface
Advances in Craniofacial Trauma

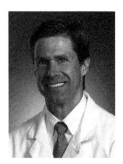

Kris S. Moe, MD, FACS
Editor

The epidemiology of craniofacial injury has changed significantly due to influences such as the advent of airbags and an increase in the sophistication of civilian weaponization. The emergency management of severe trauma has also evolved, leading to the survival of injuries that would have previously proved fatal. Together, these forces have had a notable impact on the challenges that surgeons treating craniofacial trauma now face.

Fortunately, there have been advances in technologies and techniques to treat these increasingly complex injuries. Surgical techniques have become less disruptive. Endoscopic procedures provide improved lighting and visualization. Implants are available with improved contouring and diminished profile. New technologies have been created for surgical planning and intraoperative guidance. All of these innovations provide significant benefit in restoring premorbid function and appearance.

Given the increase in severity of trauma that we are now seeing, along with advances in the variety and complexity of procedures and technology that are now available, a review of the current state-of-the-art of care for these injuries is needed. The goal of this issue of *Facial Plastic Surgery Clinics of North America* is thus to provide the surgeon who treats craniofacial trauma with a multidisciplinary perspective and reference on critical issues

in the treatment of these patients. This includes the full range of injuries resulting from civilian, terrorist, and military events, as well as the broad spectrum of organ damage that may occur involving the brain, eyes, upper respiratory structures, dentition, craniofacial skeleton, and associated soft tissue.

Even the most experienced trauma surgeon will continue to be faced with new problems and unanticipated or controversial issues. We hope the exciting topics covered in this issue will provide a basic foundation of learning as well as a description of current evidence-based medicine, latest surgical techniques, and the unique challenges and frontiers of this rapidly evolving field.

Kris S. Moe, MD, FACS
Division of Facial Plastic and
Reconstructive Surgery
Departments of Otolaryngology–
Head & Neck Surgery
and Neurological Surgery
University of Washington School
of Medicine
Box 356515
Health Sciences Building, Suite BB1165
Seattle, WA 98195-6515, USA

E-mail address:
krismoe@uw.edu

http://dx.doi.org/10.1016/j.fsc.2017.08.001
1064-7406/17/© 2017 Published by Elsevier Inc.

facialplastic.theclinics.com

Neurosurgical Considerations in Craniofacial Trauma

Robert Glenn Oxford, MD, Randall Matther Chesnut, MD*

KEYWORDS

- Craniofacial trauma • Traumatic brain injury (TBI) • Critical care of TBI
- Medical home for TBI • Medical home for craniofacial trauma

KEY POINTS

- Craniofacial trauma is often accompanied by traumatic brain injuries (TBIs). Proper stratification of all of the patient's injuries is crucial in avoiding complications and optimizing outcomes.
- A coordinated multidisciplinary approach is ideal in each medical setting: emergency department, operative theater, intensive care, acute care, rehabilitation, and outpatient clinics.
- Hypotension and hypoxia invite deleterious effects on patients with TBI. If cerebral autoregulation is disrupted, fluctuations in mean arterial pressure or intracranial pressure caused by anesthetics can result in secondary insults and further injury.

INTRODUCTION

Every important hospital should have on its resident staff of surgeons at least one who is well and able to deal with any emergency that may arise.
— *William S. Halstead, MD[1]*

If we were to start all over again and there were no surgical specialties, the ideal would be to create a single society of head and neck surgery to include everything above the clavicles with the exception probably of the eye and brain.
— *Joel J Pressman, MD[2]*

Although Halstead and Pressman[2] were well intentioned, most trauma centers in the United States offer comprehensive craniofacial trauma care through consultations of multiple subspecialties: neurologic surgery, otolaryngology–head and neck surgery (HNS), ophthalmology, general surgery, oral-maxillofacial surgery, plastic surgery, critical care medicine, anesthesia, interventional radiology, and physical medicine and rehabilitation. In this setting of multiple specialties, optimal care for patients with complex craniofacial injuries requires coordination, understanding of the complications each specialty encounters, and stratification of the severity of each injury by its implications for morbidity and mortality. Traumatic brain injury (TBI) is a common and often life-threatening comorbidity in the setting of craniofacial trauma. This article discusses TBI and the role of neurosurgery in the setting of craniofacial trauma and the effects of TBI on the overall care of patients.

CAUSE OF TRAUMATIC BRAIN INJURY IN CRANIOFACIAL TRAUMA

TBI is a leading cause of death and permanent disability for patients. Of all patients with

Disclosure: Dr R.M. Chesnut serves as the Integra Foundation Endowed Professor in Neurotrauma at the University of Washington. Dr R.G. Oxford has nothing to disclose.
Department of Neurological Surgery, University of Washington, Harborview Medical Center, UW Medicine, Box 359924, 325 Ninth Avenue, Seattle, WA 98104-2499, USA
* Corresponding author.
E-mail address: chesnutr@neurosurgery.washington.edu

Facial Plast Surg Clin N Am 25 (2017) 479–491
http://dx.doi.org/10.1016/j.fsc.2017.06.002
1064-7406/17/© 2017 Elsevier Inc. All rights reserved.

trauma, nearly half of all deaths are associated with TBI.[3] Although trauma has been globally associated with young adults, in economically wealthy countries, elderly patients have the highest mortality associated with TBI and the incidence of hospital admissions for TBI in elderly patients continues to increase.[4] Motor vehicle crashes (MVCs) and assaults have always been associated with TBI and craniofacial trauma but, with the increase in elderly patients, falls are becoming a more frequent mechanism of injury.

TBI can be broadly classified by mechanism of injury: blunt force trauma, penetrating trauma, or a combination of both. Although blunt trauma–associated TBI is more prevalent, almost half of the approximately 50,000 annual TBI-related deaths are associated with gunshot wounds to the head (GSWH).[4] MVCs (particularly high-impact crashes) are the most common source of blunt TBI in the United States in all patients, and GSWH are the most common penetrating TBI managed at our institution. For elderly patients, falls have become the most common cause of TBI. In all cases, the precipitating event often results in maxillofacial trauma to accompany the TBI. For neurosurgeons, each mechanism portends unique complications and challenges. The blast or impact associated with penetrating trauma can also cause injuries seen in blunt trauma, but penetrating objects such as bullets, knives, or shrapnel can also inflict harm through disruption of brain by the path of the object and cavitation forces related to high-velocity missiles.

GSWH are particularly serious injuries. In the state of Maryland, 786 GSWH were recorded over a 2-year period. Of those, 594 (75.6%) of the injured died at the scene. Patients with GSWH admitted to trauma centers experienced a 61.5% mortality. Of those admitted to the hospital, 18.4% of GSWH had an orbital or facial point of entry with associated craniofacial trauma. Of the patients who survived to hospital discharge, 59.5% died within the 2-year follow-up, but 35.7% of discharged patients had Glasgow Outcome Scale scores of 4 or 5 (**Table 1**). The strongest predictors of death or a debilitating outcome include Glasgow Coma Scale (GCS) less than 8 and absent pupillary light reflex on admission; bullet trajectory that crosses beyond the x, y, and z planes; intraventricular hemorrhage; and effacement of the basal cisterns were also associated predictors of poor outcomes.[5,6]

Besides the devastating initial injury from GSWH or other penetrating injuries, delayed infections leading to abscess, meningitis, and ventriculitis often preclude any chance of meaningful recovery. In the setting of GSWH, prophylactic antibiotic use

Table 1 Glasgow Outcome Scale	
Score	**Description**
1	Death
2	Persistent vegetative state Patient exhibits no obvious cortical function.
3	Severe disability Conscious but disabled. Patient depends on others for daily support.
4	Moderate disability Disabled but independent. Patient is independent as far as daily life. Disabilities include varying degrees of dysphasia, hemiparesis, or ataxia as well as intellectual and memory deficits and personality changes.
5	Good recovery Resumption of normal activities even though there may be minor neurologic or psychological deficits.

Data from Jennett B, Snoek J, Bond MR, et al. Disability after severe head injury: observations on the use of the Glasgow Outcome Scale. J Neurol Neurosurg Psychiatry 1981;44(4):285–93.

to prevent meningitis and/or abscess has not been studied in a controlled manner. An association between postoperative antibiotic use and a decreased infection rate in military GSWH case series was recognized. The Guidelines for the Management of Penetrating Brain Injury recommend postoperative antibiotic administration, although neither the type nor duration of antibiotics could be specified.[7] Broad-spectrum antibiotic coverage for 48 to 72 hours is the current practice at our institution.

PATHOPHYSIOLOGY OF TRAUMATIC BRAIN INJURY IN CRANIOFACIAL TRAUMA

TBI with craniofacial trauma has a variety of causes, the most common of which include MVCs, ground-level falls, and assaults. Subdural, epidural, and intraparenchymal hematomas displace normal brain, with midline shift being the most common result. Without intervention, a large enough hematoma will cause herniation of a lobe or region of the brain from its native intracranial compartment into a non-native intracranial compartment or an extracranial space, resulting in physical tissue injury and stroke caused by interruption of cerebral blood flow. Edema from intraparenchymal hemorrhages, ischemic injury (stroke), or venous injuries can also result in mass effect. Subfalcine and uncal herniations are the most common life-threatening mass effects that require surgical intervention. In the case of subfalcine herniation, the anterior carotid arteries can be occluded or injured. The posterior carotid artery is at risk in uncal herniation.

The Monroe-Kellie hypothesis dictates that the cranium serves as a closed vault with a set volume containing brain (1200–1600 mL), cerebrospinal fluid (CSF) (100–150 mL), and blood (100–150 mL). These 3 components are in steady state. Any volumetric additions (eg, clot, edema) first result in compensatory displacement of the other contents. CSF is displaced first. Second, blood volume is decreased by extracranial displacement, primarily of the venous component (assuming patency of venous outflow channels). Third, brain parenchyma is displaced, through herniation. When the rate of volume expansion exceeds that of compensation, the intracranial pressure increases. This increase becomes precipitous when the compensatory mechanisms become exhausted.

INTRACRANIAL HEMATOMAS
Epidural Hematoma

The classic epidural hematoma (EDH) is associated with laceration of the middle meningeal artery, usually as a result from a skull fracture, but EDHs can also arise from fracture bleeding or from large veins (**Fig. 1**). Although a lucid interval is classically associated with EDH, in the setting of severe craniofacial injuries the patient is often obtunded from the moment of injury.

Subdural Hematoma

Lacerations to the cortical surface or vessels within a sulcus are frequent causes of subdural hematoma (SDH), although they may also arise from a severed cortical bridging vein (**Fig. 2**). In contrast with EDH, in which the mass is the only threat, the outcome from SDH is usually largely related to the underlying brain injury. Extrapolation of the International Classification of Diseases, Ninth Revision (ICD-9) diagnosis codes from a large retrospective study estimates the incidence of traumatic acute SDHs in the United States to be 14.7 per 100,000.[8]

Intraparenchymal Hemorrhage and Diffuse Axonal Injury

Intraparenchymal hemorrhages (cerebral contusions) can be some of the most challenging injuries to manage (**Fig. 3**). Contusions can often "blossom" over time, and those lesions that do not require immediate surgery still require rigorous intensive care unit (ICU) monitoring because of the risk of delayed deterioration. Contusions may be numerous or the injury may be diffuse, as seen in diffuse axonal injury.

Deep bifrontal contusions are unique injuries. Patients with these injuries are prone to late deterioration despite a reassuring initial neurologic examination. The usual cause is progressive development of edema around the contusions, a phenomenon that is much less common in older patients. One study found that 54% of patients with severe deep frontal contusions (hematoma volume >30 cm³) and a GCS greater than

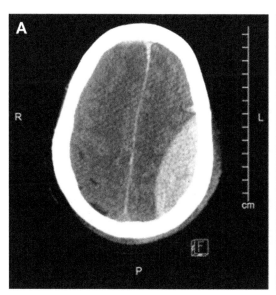
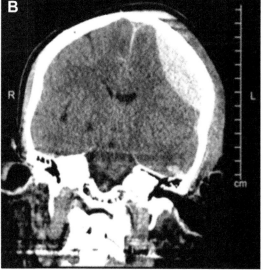

Fig. 1. (*A, B*) An epidural hematoma.

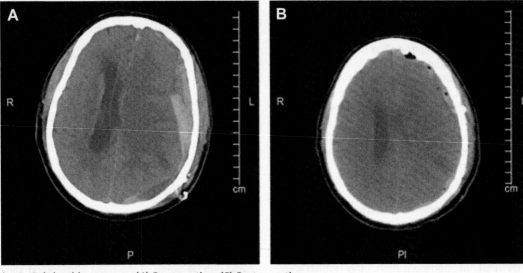

Fig. 2. Subdural hematoma. (*A*) Preoperative. (*B*) Postoperative.

13 acutely deteriorated at a mean of 4.5 days after injury.[9] Rapid surgical decompression of those deteriorated patients preserved good functional outcomes. The natural history of such severe bifrontal contusions and the ability to prevent devastating neurologic outcomes with surgical intervention indicates that these patients should be closely observed in an ICU setting for 5 days. The authors recommend delaying major nonemergent surgical procedures requiring general anesthesia until at least the 5 days of ICU monitoring have been completed.

HOSPITAL COURSE OF TRAUMATIC BRAIN INJURY IN CRANIOFACIAL TRAUMA
Emergency Department

In most TBI settings, patients are initially evaluated in the emergency department. A history and physical is obtained: for severely injured intubated or noncommunicative patients, the history is gathered from witnesses or first responders. The mechanism of injury is determined. The primary survey includes determination of the pupillary response and the level of consciousness, whereas the secondary survey examines the

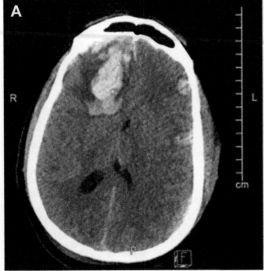
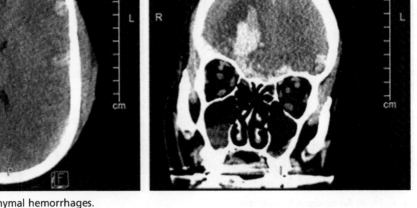

Fig. 3. (*A, B*) Intraparenchymal hemorrhages.

motor, sensory, and reflex systems; the rectal sphincter tone; and reassesses the level of consciousness. The most common acceptable consciousness assessment tool is the GCS score[10] (**Table 2**[11]).

The GCS and pupillary light reflex examination are the most predictive of outcome (although the GCS may be influenced by drugs, hypothermia, and so forth). A noncontrast head computed tomography (CT) scan is performed as soon as possible. The head CT may reveal a focal mass lesion (extra-axial or intraparenchymal hemorrhage or diffuse severe injury) that warrant immediate surgical intervention. Unless a patient can reliably follow commands and report neck pain in the absence of distracting injuries, and has a symmetric examination without deficits, the spine cannot be cleared without imaging. All patients with TBI unable to follow commands require additional imaging of the spine to detect injuries, with noncontrast CT of the cervical spine (C-spine) being the most useful. If the CT C-spine is unremarkable and the patient's neurologic examination (including deep tendon reflexes) is symmetric (eg, not suggestive of neurologic dysfunction not explained by the TBI), the spine can be cleared. If a patient needs emergent surgery before evaluation of the spine, full spine precautions should be observed until the work-up can be obtained. Patients requiring emergent surgery may have a delay in diagnosis or delineation of the extent of maxillofacial trauma.

Some patients have a combination of neurologic examination and imaging consistent with injuries that are best managed nonoperatively in the intensive care setting with repeated imaging and sequential neurologic examinations to ensure that the intracranial injuries are not worsening. A subset of these patients with a poor neurologic examination (GCS 9 or less) require some type of invasive monitor for intracranial pressure (ICP) monitoring; either an extraventricular drain (EVD)

and separate brain tissue oxygen partial pressure (Pbo_2) monitor or a combination fiber optic ICP monitor (Camino) and Pbo_2 monitor. The authors prefer the combination Camino and Pbo_2 monitor as the first line in invasive monitoring. We place EVDs when traditional medical interventions for increased ICP (increased sedation, positioning, hyperosmotic therapy) have failed. Placement of monitors or EVDs can be complicated by fractures or soft tissue trauma overlying the planned insertion sites.

Operating Theater for Blunt Trauma

Most patients requiring surgery for TBI are transported to the operative theater directly from the emergency department. Craniectomy or craniotomy for evacuation or decompression for a focal clot is first-line therapy when mass effect (midline shift or herniation) is present. The role for decompression for diffuse injuries or increased ICP without a focal lesion is not as well understood and is discussed further later in this article. Patients requiring emergent craniectomy for evacuation of a focal mass lesion or for decompression are ideally cared for by an anesthesia team familiar and accomplished with neuroanesthesia. Although the typical unilateral decompressive craniectomy can be performed in less than an hour, approaches and techniques are tailored to successfully treat epidural, subdural, and/or intraparenchymal hematomas.

For large SDHs with significant mass effect, a frontotemporoparietal craniotomy or craniectomy is performed. Larger craniectomy prevents injury to the brain by minimizing herniation or mushrooming of the brain through the bone defect. To achieve a large enough craniotomy, a standard Falconer incision is made, starting just anterior to the root of the helix of the pinna to access the root of the zygoma. The inferior point of the incision can compromise the superficial temporal

Table 2					
GCS					
Eye Opening		**Best Verbal Response**		**Best Motor Response**	
Spontaneous	4	Orientated	5	Obey commands	6
To Sound	3	Confused	4	Localise	5
To Pain	2	Inappropriate	3	Flexion: normal	4
Never	1	Incomprehensible	2	Flexion: abnormal	3
		None	1	Extension	2
				Nil	1

Courtesy of Teasdale, Murray, Parker, and Jennett; and *Data from* Teasdale G, Murray G, Parker L, et al. Adding up the Glasgow Coma Score. Acta Neurochir Suppl (Wien) 1979;28(1):13–6; with permission.

artery, and, if it is placed too far anteriorly, it could sever the temporal and zygomatic branches of the facial nerve. The superior portion of the incision should go to the midline or just beyond. The incision usually ends just posterior to the hairline. Having a broad myocutaneous flap facilitates access to the superior sagittal sinus if it is a source of bleeding, preserves the anterior blood supply from the supratrochlear and supraorbital arteries, and prevents violation of the 1:3 ratio of width to length to avoid compromise of random blood flow to the edges of the flap. For a holohemispheric lesion, the superior osteotomy of the bone flap is taken to within 3 cm of the midline. The inferior osteotomy extends to the floor of the middle fossa. The posterior extent of the osteotomy is made to offer access to the lesion, but exposing the transverse sinus is unnecessary and should be avoided. The inferioanterior edge of the craniectomy is usually completed by rongeuring away the temporal bone until the skull base and the temporal pole are visualized. Removing this portion of the temporal bone addresses potential uncal herniation, which is often the primary goal of the surgery. It also requires reconstruction on replacement of the craniotomy bone flap or synthetic cranioplasty. If open reduction and internal fixation (ORIF) of the lateral orbital wall or zygomatic arch fractures (as seen in tripod fractures) is required, the risk of injury to nearby and exposed temporal lobe is significantly increased.

In general, SDHs large enough to warrant surgical decompression require duraplasty. Typically, the authors fashion an on-lay duraplasty with DuraGen (Integra Life Sciences Inc, Plainsboro, NJ), but a sutured patch using DuraMatrix (Stryker, Kalamazoo, MI), or AlloDerm (LifeCell, Bridgewater, NJ) can be used. Depending on underlying brain injuries or edema, the surgeon must decide whether the bone flap will be replaced or if it will be stored, either sterilely in a $-80°$ C freezer or in the abdomen, superficial to the rectus sheath. Delayed cranioplasty timing depends on the recovery of the patient, resolution of brain edema, and the status of the wound. The ideal of completing a cranioplasty in a combined procedure with maxillofacial repairs is complicated by the increased rate of infection with cranioplasty performed earlier than 2 weeks after injury. Most fractures are repaired in a time frame of 7 to 10 days to facilitate ORIF with reduced edema but without scarring or fractures fusing in malalignment. In this situation, we discuss with patients or family whether the convenience and benefits of a combined ORIF of facial fractures with early cranioplasty outweigh the increased risk of infection.

Craniotomy for evacuation of EDH is planned based on the location and size of the lesion. Very large clots are best treated with a holohemispheric craniotomy through a Falconer incision in a fashion similar to the incision described for SDH. Smaller EDHs are treated with a craniotomy tailored to size of the lesion, and the myocutaneous flap is planned to preserve local blood supply from named axial arteries (superficial temporal arteries or occipital artery). The source of epidural bleeding is identified and controlled, usually with bipolar cautery. To prevent recurrence of the epidural hematoma or expansion of the epidural hematoma, circumferential and central tack-up sutures are placed between the dura and the bone. Imaging can be deceiving, and small SDHs may have been obscured by compression from the epidural clot. Therefore, the dura is carefully inspected and, if it is tense or discolored by underlying clot, the dura is opened and the subdural clot is evacuated. If no evidence of underlying clot is identified, the dura may be left intact. In the absence of injury to the underlying brain, the bone flap is replaced with central tack-up sutures. These tack-up sutures should be kept in mind if the bone flap has to be removed in future repairs or revisions. The sutures must be cut before elevating the bone flap to prevent inadvertent durotomies.

Severe frontal injuries may necessitate emergent decompression. As noted previously, they may also progress to delayed deterioration related to edema formation, particularly if bilateral. Access is via a bicoronal (Sutar) incision, followed by a unilateral or bilateral craniotomy. Bilateral approaches involve excision of both frontal and temporal bones. At our institution, we prefer several modifications to the classic Kjellberg bifrontal technique. The classic Kjellberg technique unroofs the superior sagittal sinus, following which the falx is transected at the frontal floor to let the brain raise and expand. Depending on the height of the frontal paranasal sinuses, this can result in a bone defect that precludes leaving the anterior bony support for the helmet that will be required to mobilize the patient before cranioplasty. If the bone over the superior sagittal sinus must be removed, an anterior midline wedge of frontal bone is excluded from the craniectomy to provide a resting point for the helmet. However, in most cases, we do not unroof the superior sagittal sinus. Instead, we perform 2 independent frontotemporoparietal craniectomies leaving a midline sagittal strip of bone in place (Harborview Bonehawk). This technique offers several advantages. First, iatrogenic injuries to the underlying sinus are avoided. Second, bleeding from venous lakes or from the sinus can be controlled with Gelfoam packing, using the midline strip of bone as a buttress for packing. Third, the bone facilitates easier fitting of a helmet. Fourth, a semicircular peninsula of bone reaching 4 cm lateral to the midline can be left in place as an anchor point for ICP monitors, Pbo_2 monitors, and EVDs. In addition, the eventual cranioplasty is facilitated, because the patient's forehead does not collapse as the brain swelling dissipates, so scalp contraction is lessened.

When dealing with a large scalp or forehead laceration, we try to operate through this laceration, or incorporate it into a larger incision if possible. Stellate fractures are particularly challenging if an underlying craniectomy is required. In this setting, we try to plan out flaps that do not disrupt major arteries, and advancement flaps may be required in this setting to achieve optimal results. Such an approach exemplifies an important general consideration, which is to plan skin incisions to maximize flap perfusion and accommodate both the immediate surgical exposure and any anticipated future needs. In many instances, this requires preoperative consultation between the various services that might be involved in the care of the patient's craniofacial injuries.

Following craniotomy, if the patient is hemodynamically unstable or continues to have intracranial hypertension, the patient is taken immediately to the ICU for further resuscitation or other interventions. If the patient is stable, the timing of the craniofacial repair is contemplated. Often, the face is too edematous to easily facilitate ORIF of midface or orbital fractures at this time. In general, more severe facial swelling is seen with severe TBI, and these patients are often too unstable for extending general anesthetic for immediate repair. Other patients with less significant TBI may significantly benefit from immediate repair. The common trauma flap (Falconer flap) can offer excellent access to zygoma fractures or orbital fractures that may have otherwise been addressed through a Gilles incision. Severe mandible fractures that compromise the patient's ability to protect the airway are a special concern. Intubation interferes with the patient's neurologic examination because assessment of language and mentation is limited without speech. Also, delaying repair of open fractures can result in infection and increased rates of nonunion. Therefore, in severe mandibular fractures every attempt is made to facilitate an early repair, because early ORIF of mandible fractures can facilitate earlier extubation,[12] which can reduce invasive ICP monitoring duration and minimize the complications of treatment in addition to reducing the rate of ventilator-associated pneumonias. In some cases, severe edema from maxillofacial trauma is the main obstacle to extubation, and in this setting tracheotomy may be necessary because of concern for airway compromise in a patient who would be better managed without endotracheal intubation.

Depressed or comminuted fractures involving the frontal sinus may be repaired through the exposure from decompressive craniectomies performed via a coronal incision. For many patients, the coronal incision is cosmetically superior to an incision through a forehead rhytid or the classic gull-wing incision associated with a Lynch procedure. Immediate repair can avoid the unintended durotomies and potential CSF leaks that can occur because of scarring to the dura in a delayed repair. It can also facilitate a pedicled pericranial flap for cranialization of the frontal sinus or repair of the anterior skull base. If the frontal sinus will be obliterated, the inner table of the craniectomy bone flap can serve as an ideal source of autologous bone. In delayed repairs, the pericranium may be scarred from the original surgery or compromised by the initial incision used in decompression. The definitive repair for frontal sinus fractures is simplified by an initial coronal incision. Increasing the neurosurgeon's awareness of this issue may ensure that a coronal incision is used in the rare setting of severe frontal sinus fractures and unilateral intracranial injury. Ultimately, coordination and communication between craniofacial surgeons and neurosurgeons are the keys to superior holistic care, but in many cases this coordination requires early consultation of the craniofacial service by the emergency medicine team.

Operative Theater for Penetrating Trauma

As mentioned in relation to the cause of TBI, penetrating injuries can be devastating. For patients with a chance of survival, surgical interventions are tailored relative to the extent of injury. In the absence of surgical intracranial mass lesions (eg, hematomas), small slugs or penetrating particles through a small entrance site are treated with local wound care, meticulous skin closure, and antibiotic administration. More extensive injuries are treated with superficial debridement and watertight closure of galea and skin. In some cases, local advancement flaps may be required for a tension-free closure. Severe penetrating injuries (usually GSWH) with uncontrollable intracranial hypertension require decompressive craniectomy with continued ICP monitoring. Obvious contamination (or a delayed abscess or empyema along the tract of the projectile) requires irrigation and debridement. However, there is no indication for extensive exploration toward removing all foreign bodies, because this does not seem to change the risk of epilepsy or infection and may cause further injury.[13,14] Only those immediately available should be removed. Lower velocity projectiles, such as nails or debris from MVCs that penetrate the skull, have a higher risk of infection than GSWH (**Fig. 4**).

Intensive care unit setting

Institutions vary in organization of their critical care services. At our institution, a dedicated neurologic critical care service cares for patients with isolated head or spine injuries or those same patients with concomitant maxillofacial trauma. Patients with such injuries plus trauma involving the thorax and abdomen, or extremity fractures requiring operative repair, are managed by a trauma critical care service. In either case, coordination between services regarding treatment parameters and clearance for surgery is required. Neurosurgeons often find themselves in the position of being the service that declines clearance for the operative theater. Once the primary injury from TBI has been identified and addressed through either surgery or medical management, minimizing or avoiding secondary injury from hypoxia or hypotension becomes the focal goal of treatment. It then becomes feasible to allow nonemergent procedures as long as these secondary brain insults can be avoided by surgical and anesthetic teams. Doing so requires some understanding of the physiology underlying cerebral perfusion.

Cerebral blood flow of 50 mL/100 g/min is required for normal brain function. At a cerebral blood flow of 18 mL/100 g/min electrical failure occurs (loss of electroencephalogram and somatosensory evoked potential monitoring). At a cerebral blood flow of 10 mL/100 g/min, ischemia can develop and metabolic dysfunction and cell death will occur with a persistent cerebral blood flow of 10 mL/100 g/min or less. Cell death leads to edema, and that edema can result in increased ICPs, which further compound the compromised cerebral blood flow.

When discussing the brain, the concept of cerebral perfusion pressure (CPP) is substituted for mean arterial pressure (MAP). CPP is calculated by subtracting the ICP from the MAP, so that CPP = MAP – ICP. Cerebral perfusion autoregulation refers to the maintenance of fairly constant cerebral blood flow over a range of CPP values between approximately 50 mm Hg and 150 mm Hg (**Fig. 5**).

Autoregulation may be compromised following TBI, resulting in disruption of the so-called plateau range wherein cerebral blood flow is kept fairly constant despite variations in arterial pressure. The result is cerebral blood flow being passively proportional to CPP. This relationship is likely a key to understanding why hypotension is so strongly linked to worse outcomes in TBI.[15] Essentially, hypotension in the presence of disrupted autoregulation can easily result in brain ischemia. In the acute setting, elective surgeries should be delayed until intact autoregulation can be proved through static autoregulation testing or until ICP and CPP are stable and satisfactory without interventions.[16] This schedule can help to avoid any secondary insults from hypotension that can occur with general anesthetic. If there is emergent extracranial surgery, it is critical that anesthesia staff carefully monitor and maintain CPP, with an absolute intraoperative lower threshold of 60 mm Hg.

For patients with a reliable neurologic examination (GCS 10 or higher), or intubated patients able to follow commands (GCS 8T or better), hourly neurologic examinations can be followed. For patients with GCS 9 or less and intubated patients not following commands, ICP monitors are placed.

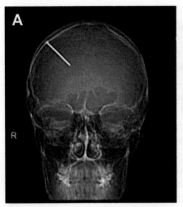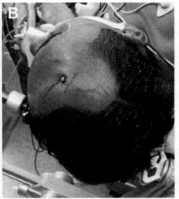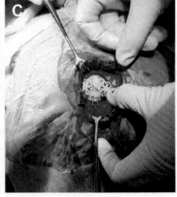

Fig. 4. Intracranial penetrating trauma. (*A*) Head CT with coronal scout reformat of right frontal nail. (*B*) Planned incision for craniotomy to remove nail. (*C*) Replating of craniotomy bone flap.

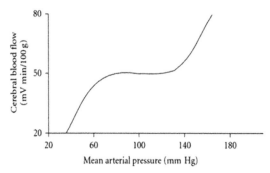

Fig. 5. Idealized curve showing cerebral pressure autoregulation. (*Data from* Peterson EC, Wang Z, Britz G. Regulation of cerebral blood flow. Int J Vasc Med 2011;2011:823525.)

At our institution, we simultaneously place ICP and Pbo_2 monitors (**Fig. 6**). An EVD can be used as an ICP monitor that can also drain CSF. Our preference is to use EVDs as a second-line therapy when we think intermittent CSF drainage can assist with management. ICP transduction through an EVD requires a closed system, and therefore an EVD cannot measure ICP if it is actively draining. When the measurement restrictions and lack of Pbo_2 monitoring are combined with the higher complication rate of EVD placement compared with intraparenchymal devices, we think that EVDs are best used as a step between an intraparenchymal ICP and Pbo_2 monitoring combination and decompressive craniectomy.

Decompression versus medical management for diffuse injury

The role of decompressive craniectomy versus medical management of increased ICP refractory to medical treatment is being rigorously studied. The DECRA (Decompressive Craniectomy) and RescueICP (Randomized Evaluation of Surgery with Craniectomy for Uncontrolled Elevation of IntraCranial Pressure) trials were both designed to offer insight into this management dilemma.[17,18] The DECRA trial revealed that early decompression resulted in fewer interventions for increased ICP and shorter ICU stays, but it also resulted in more unfavorable outcomes compared with second-line medical therapies.[17] In the RescueICP trial, early decompression resulted in a 30.4% mortality compared with a 52.0% mortality in the medically treated group, but rates of moderate disability and good recovery at 1 year following the injury were similar between surgical intervention and medical management (22.2% vs 20.1% and 9.8 vs 8.4% respectively). The major effect of surgery was shifting the outcome of these severely injured patients from mortality primarily to the upper-severe level of recovery. Surgical decompression was associated with a higher rate of complications (16.3% vs 9.2%) and a higher rate of vegetative state (6.2 vs 1.7%).[18] The authors have incorporated these trials into our counseling, education, and consent processes for families of patients with severe TBI. Our concern for severe disability and persistent vegetative states has led to increased preference for aggressive second-line medical therapy as opposed to rapid decompression, given that the RescueICP trail's survival advantage seems to result in severe disability.

Delayed complications of traumatic brain injury and maxillofacial trauma

Skull fractures Skull fractures can be classified as open or closed. In each group, the fracture may be comminuted or not, and depressed or not. Fractures of the cranium require operative intervention in a variety of settings: an open contaminated fracture requiring irrigation and debridement, a depressed skull fracture resulting in neurologic deficit (often over the rolandic cortex), a fracture restricting venous outflow by compressing the venous sinuses (sagittal or transverse), or a fracture with an

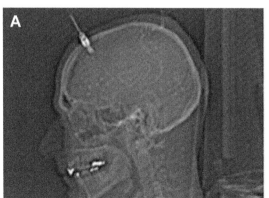
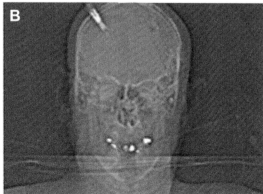

Fig. 6. Example of (*A*) ICP and (*B*) Pbo_2 monitors being used simultaneously.

unacceptable cosmetic defect. These fractures are often repaired in an emergent or urgent time frame, but the authors have found that complications can often present in a delayed fashion. Fractures of the anterior skull base, including the frontal, ethmoid, and sphenoid sinuses in addition to the orbital roof, can result in CSF leak, mucoceles, or meningoencephaloceles. Often these complications require surgical repair. In addition to these criteria and delayed complications, skull fractures in infants are unique because of the risk of growing skull fracture, which is essentially a meningoencephalocele protruding through the splayed fracture because of the normal rapid growth of the brain. Infants with skull fractures are followed to monitor for a growing skull fracture requiring intervention.

Skull fractures can also injure the cerebral venous sinuses, possibly resulting in increased ICP, hydrocephalus, watershed infarcts, and ultimately arterial distribution ischemic stroke without corrective measures. Operative repair can be complicated and treacherous. Excessive blood loss can be life threatening. The repair can lead to thrombosis of the sinus, and the standard therapy of anticoagulation with heparin increases the risk of exacerbating other intracranial hemorrhage in addition to complicating any additional emergent surgical procedures.

Temporal bone fractures are subdivided into squamosal and petrosal variants. Petrosal fractures are further categorized as transverse or longitudinal. Transverse fractures are associated with a greater chance of inner ear violation and subsequent insult to hearing or vestibular function. In general, otolaryngology-HNS is consulted for temporal bone fractures. The initial work-up in communicative patients includes Weber and Rinne tests. Conductive hearing loss can be followed with reassurance and a follow-up audiogram and otology evaluation in 6 to 12 weeks. Sensorineural hearing loss should be treated with prednisone 60 mg daily for 10 days and an early audiogram. Facial nerve weakness in the setting of temporal bone fracture can be based on the physical examination in awake cooperative patients, but in unconscious patients, electroneurography after 72 hours can offer diagnosis and prognosis for facial nerve function. In awake patients, delayed loss of initially present function is most likely the result of edema and can be observed and treated with a course of steroids. Immediate loss of function at the time of injury is suggestive of a severed nerve and may warrant early exploration for attempted anastomosis.

Cerebrospinal fluid leak Violations of the dura can result in CSF leak. The route of the fistula may be through the wound in open skull fractures, or the CSF may find egress through communication with the paranasal sinuses or the temporal bone. Rarely, CSF may communicate through the middle ear and the eustachian tube to cause CSF rhinorrhea, but most CSF rhinorrhea cases are secondary to fractures of the skull base and the paranasal sinuses, including the ethmoid, frontal, or sphenoid sinuses. CSF leaks can occur with disruption of the orbit and rarely communicate with the maxillary sinus.

Acute CSF leaks may resolve with elevation of the head. Lying supine results in $\sim 15°$ of rotation of the brain away from the skull base, and, in these cases, closing the potential space between the undersurface of the brain and skull base helps to reduce the flow of CSF.[19] Historically, our threshold for observation has been 48 to 72 hours; if the leak continues at that point, a lumbar drain was placed to divert CSF. Once placed, we typically drained for 3 days before clamping. More recently, with the advent of endoscopic techniques, we have become increasingly focused on early exploration, with direct patching so that early consultation with otolaryngology is now routine.

Supratentorial mass lesions (hemorrhage or edema) or, more rarely, cerebellar lesions are relative contraindications to lumbar drains because of the risk of midbrain herniation caused by the exacerbation of the pressure gradient between the cranium and the drain. When midbrain or tonsillar herniation is a concern, an EVD is a safer and likely more effective choice for CSF diversion. For CSF leaks involving the temporal bone, a Pope Oto-Wick can confound the clinical examination. Although the Oto-Wick is often necessary to prevent stenosis of the external auditory canal (EAC), it can in theory tapenade the flow of CSF. Therefore, the authors remove and replace the wick at the 48-hour mark to facilitate an examination of the EAC and tympanic membrane.

Prophylactic antibiotics are not indicated and are associated with increased incidence of multidrug-resistant infections. In a randomized study of 170 patients with traumatic CSF leaks, antibiotic prophylaxis resulted in a 5-fold relative risk of meningitis compared with avoiding antibiotics unless an active infection is diagnosed.[20] The investigators speculated that antibiotic prophylaxis alters the natural bacterial flora of the paranasal sinuses, but this hypothesis has not been tested to our knowledge. At our institution, catheters used for CSF diversion are rifampin impregnated. Patients with EVDs or lumbar drains receive 24 hours of perioperative antibiotics following placement. The authors have found no increase in catheter-associated infections and our rates of *Clostridium difficile* infections have been dramatically decreased once the practice of continuous antibiotics for indwelling catheters was discontinued.[21]

Tension pneumocephalus can be a devastating complication of CSF leaks. Conservative management with 100% fraction of inspired oxygen (Fio$_2$) for intubated patients or with nonrebreathers and Fio$_2$ of 100% for extubated patients can be attempted, but, if the mass effect is great enough, the patient will require decompression. In such cases, excessive positive pressure ventilation can cause or complicate tension pneumocephalus, including during bag-valve-mask (BVM) preoxygenation before intubation. Therefore, the most experienced airway expert (usually anesthesia or otolaryngology-HNS) should manage the airway. These airways are not appropriate teaching scenarios, and the team should consider the neurologic complications that may result. In some cases, a surgical airway may be more appropriate than repeated attempts at intubation requiring extensive BVM and positive pressure ventilation.

Late complications of sinus injuries/CSF leaks can include encephaloceles, mucoceles, CSF leak recurrence, and meningitis.

Cranioplasty Craniectomized patients ultimately require cranioplasty to restore the skull after the patient's acute injuries have been treated, the intracranial disorder has stabilized, and the scalp/brain contour is favorable to reconstruction. Craniectomized patients require a helmet when out of bed until the cranium can be restored. At our center, bone flaps are stored in a −80°C freezer for up to 1 year from the time of banking. In facilities lacking a frozen-bone bank, the autologous bone flap (ABF) can be stored in the abdomen above the rectus fascia. Storage in the abdomen can be advantageous if the patient will be transferred to another facility for the cranioplasty. ABFs are used whenever possible, but the ABF is frequently unable to be salvaged because of either open contamination or severely comminuted fractures that would ultimately lead to reabsorption of the flap. Such situations require a cranial prosthesis.

A recent study of 754 cranioplasties performed at the University of Washington led to several observations regarding infection and timing. First, the results of bacterial culture swabs of ABFs without obvious gross contamination at the time of craniectomy were not predictive of infection following cranioplasty. Second, the only statistically significant predictor of postcranioplasty infection was performing the operation sooner

than 14 days after the craniectomy. Based on this study, we have discontinued bacterial cultures for bone flaps when no sign of infection is present, and we do not perform cranioplasties sooner than 14 days following craniectomies.[22] Although we attempt to perform cranioplasty as soon as possible, persistent cerebral edema must resolve before reconstruction. Because this process can be protracted, most craniofacial fractures requiring operative fixation have to be repaired earlier than the cranioplasty.

Temporal wasting is the most common cosmetic issue following cranioplasty after decompression. Techniques to minimize wasting include elevation of the temporalis muscle in an inferior-to-superior fashion during the decompression (so that it remains intact with the myocutaneous flap) and reconstruction of defects from piecemeal removal of the squamous temporal bone with titanium plates during cranioplasty. However, in some patients, the cosmetic results are unsatisfactory. In such cases, a prefabricated porous high-density polyethylene temporal implant (Porex Surgical Inc, College Park, GA) can be used in similar fashion to reconstruction of the donor site following temporalis myofascial flaps. Alternatively, fat grafting can be performed either with an open approach or by percutaneous fat injections with the advantage of a softer, more physiologic texture. It has been our preference to proceed with cranioplasty and perform a delayed correction only if the end result is unsatisfactory.

Hydrocephalus Hydrocephalus can develop following TBI, primarily because of interference with CSF resorption or occlusion of flow pathways. In cases of craniectomy, it may also develop in response to the lack of a solid barrier to intracranial volume expansion, in which it may manifest as panventricular dilatation or the formation of a new CSF collection under the scalp flap (so-called fifth ventricle). It may also manifest after a delayed cranioplasty when the increased capacitance afforded by the original craniectomy is eliminated. Patients with hydrocephalus may have craniofacial trauma without a closed head injury or TBI. Hydrocephalus is broadly divided into communicating and noncommunicating hydrocephalus. Almost all posttraumatic hydrocephalus cases are communicating hydrocephalus. CSF diversion in the form of a shunt is the mainstay of hydrocephalus treatment. The proximal portion of the shunt can be placed into the ventricle or the lumbar thecal sac. The peritoneum, right atrium, and pleural space are the preferred locations for the distal catheter. Much less common sites include the bladder or gallbladder. Lumboperitoneal shunts fail at a much higher rate because of the increased mechanical wear on the system. The preferred ventriculoperitoneal shunts can be placed through either a frontal approach or parietoccipital approach for the ventricular catheter. Frontal catheters are easier to place and associated with fewer complications. The parietoccipital catheter requires a longer intracranial trajectory but, once it is reliably placed, it functions in the same manner as the frontal catheter. The catheters and valve are located deep to the galea plane postauricularly into the neck, over the clavicle and chest, and the abdomen before being placed into the peritoneum.

Shunt placement poses a significant risk of infection. If the hardware is infected, the shunt must be externalized or explanted and replaced with an EVD or lumbar drain until the infection has been cleared. In the setting of craniofacial trauma, shunting can be complicated by the need for alternative distal catheter routes caused by injury to the soft tissues of the scalp or neck overlying the preferred tract, but the most common complicating scenario is failing to account for shunt hardware that may be exposed during revision surgeries.

The prevalence of hydrocephalus is estimated to be approximately 0.5% of the population of the United States,[23] and it may result from causes such as congenital causes, prior trauma, subarachnoid hemorrhage, or infection. Any concerns about involvement of the shunt during surgery should prompt the involvement of a neurosurgeon to be present or available to assist with any alterations to the shunt hardware. The shunt hardware configuration should be clearly delineated. The type of catheters and valves should be identified if any component requires replacement. A head CT and a plain film shunt series that shows the entire system in continuity to detect any kinks or breaks in the system is usually sufficient to understand the shunt configuration. In some cases, consideration may be given to rerouting shunt hardware to an alternative configuration such as a parietoccipital ventricular catheter or a distal catheter that is tunneled contralaterally for distal insertion. When operating on a patient with a previously placed shunt, exposing, prepping, and draping the entire course of the shunt from scalp to abdomen as a precaution prevents the inconvenience of having to reposition, prep, and drape if a complete shunt revision is required. Inadvertent exposure of shunt hardware mandates intraoperative neurosurgery consultation and may result in externalization of the distal hardware with eventual replacement of the entire system.

Rehabilitation Although most recovery in patients with TBI is made within the first 3 months, patients may continue to improve on average 18 months after the initial injury. Discovery of malocclusion, diplopia, or other deficits from maxillofacial trauma may develop as the patients improve. A medical home for these patients can be instrumental in facilitating timely referrals and treatment. In many cases, a patient's primary care provider may not be familiar with all of the consulting services. At our institution, the physical medicine and rehabilitation service offers a TBI clinic that is ideal for the optimal prolonged care for these patients, and we have found our physiatrist colleagues' expertise invaluable.

SUMMARY

Neurosurgical considerations can significantly affect patients with craniofacial trauma. In the acute setting, immediate management of fractures and complex soft tissue injuries may be delayed because of untenable ICPs, cardiovascular instability, or to determine whether the patient will survive potentially devastating head injuries. Ideally, surgeries can be coordinated between services to reduce trips to the operating room, repeat intubations, and to prevent confusion and complications. Some patients continue to deal with hydrocephalus or functional deficits that require neurosurgical management long after their initial injury. Ideally, an outpatient multispecialty clinic can serve as a medical home for these patients until all of their craniofacial and neurosurgical injuries have been resolved. With attention to providing coordinated care, the outcomes can be significantly improved for patients with craniofacial trauma and their families.

REFERENCES

1. Halstead WS. The training of a surgeon. Bull John Hopkins Hosp 1904;15:267–75.
2. Pressman JJ. Atlas of head and neck surgery-otolaryngology. In: Bailey BJ, editor. Atlas of head and neck Surgery—otoaryngology, volume 2. Philadelphia: Lippincott Williams & Wilkins; 2001. p. 1018.
3. Maas AI, Stocchetti N, Bullock R. Moderate and severe traumatic brain injury in adults. Lancet Neurol 2008;7(8):728–41.
4. Coronado VG, Xu L, Basavaraju SV, et al. Surveillance for traumatic brain injury-related deaths–United States, 1997-2007. MMWR Surveill Summ 2011;60(5):1–32.
5. Aarabi B, Tofighi B, Kufera JA, et al. Predictors of outcome in civilian gunshot wounds to the head. J Neurosurg 2014;120(5):1138–46.

6. Jennett B, Snoek J, Bond MR, et al. Disability after severe head injury: observations on the use of the Glasgow Outcome Scale. J Neurol Neurosurg Psychiatry 1981;44(4):285–93.

7. Aarabi B, Pruitt BA. Guidelines for the management of penetrating brain injury: antibiotic prophylaxis of penetrating brain injury. J Trauma 2001; 51(2 Suppl):S34–40.

8. Kalanithi P, Schubert RD, Lad SP, et al. Hospital costs, incidence, and inhospital mortality rates of traumatic subdural hematoma in the United States. J Neurosurg 2011;115(5):1013–8.

9. Peterson EC, Chesnut RM. Talk and die revisited: bifrontal contusions and late deterioration. J Trauma 2011;71(6):1588–92.

10. Teasdale G, Jennett B. Assessment of coma and impaired consciousness. A practical scale. Lancet 1974;2(7872):81–4.

11. Teasdale G, Murray G, Parker L, et al. Adding up the Glasgow Coma Score. Acta Neurochir Suppl (Wien) 1979;28(1):13–6.

12. Kellman RM, Losquadro WD. Comprehensive airway management of patients with maxillofacial trauma. Craniomaxillofac Trauma Reconstr 2008;1(1):39–47.

13. Part 1: Guidelines for the management of penetrating brain injury. Introduction and methodology. J Trauma 2001;51(2 Suppl):S3–6.

14. Peterson EC, Wang Z, Britz G. Regulation of cerebral blood flow. Int J Vasc Med 2011;2011: 823525.

15. Chesnut RM. Avoidance of hypotension: conditio sine qua non of successful severe head-injury management. J Trauma 1997;42(5 Suppl):S4–9.

16. Tiecks FP, Lam AM, Aaslid R, et al. Comparison of static and dynamic cerebral autoregulation measurements. Stroke 1995;26(6):1014–9.

17. Cooper DJ, Rosenfeld JV, Murray L, et al. Decompressive craniectomy in diffuse traumatic brain injury. N Engl J Med 2011;364(16):1493–502.

18. Hutchinson PJ, Kolias AG, Timofeev IS, et al. Trial of decompressive craniectomy for traumatic intracranial hypertension. N Engl J Med 2016;375(12): 1119–30.

19. Moe KS, Bergeron CM, Ellenbogen RG. Transorbital neuroendoscopic surgery. Neurosurgery 2010;67(3 Suppl Operative):16–28.

20. Choi D, Spann R. Traumatic cerebrospinal fluid leakage: risk factors and the use of prophylactic antibiotics. Br J Neurosurg 1996;10(6):571–5.

21. Dellit TH, Chan JD, Fulton C, et al. Reduction in Clostridium difficile infections among neurosurgical patients associated with discontinuation of antimicrobial prophylaxis for the duration of external ventricular drain placement. Infect Control Hosp Epidemiol 2014;35(5):589–90.

22. Morton RP, Abecassis IJ, Hanson JF, et al. Predictors of infection after 754 cranioplasty operations and the value of intraoperative cultures for cryopreserved bone flaps. J Neurosurg 2016;125(3): 766–70.

23. Lemire RJ. Neural tube defects. JAMA 1988;259(4): 558–62.

Management of High-Velocity Injuries of the Head and Neck

Jacob S. Majors, MD[a],*, Joseph Brennan, MD[a],
G. Richard Holt, MD, MSE, MPH, MABE, D Bioethics[a,b]

KEYWORDS

- High-velocity injury • Mass casualty incident • Head and neck surgery

KEY POINTS

- The most recent conflicts in Iraq and Afghanistan have significantly improved understanding of battlefield trauma and how to appropriately address these injures.
- Blast injuries causing primary, secondary, tertiary, and quaternary injuries require a thorough evaluation of each of those systems to which they can cause injury. These types of injuries can be among the most devastating soft and hard tissue trauma to the human body.
- Triage is the first step in determination of patient stability and identification of the need for airway or surgical intervention. Understanding triage principals allows the surgeon to provide the most benefit to the most patients in the event of a mass casualty situation.
- The primary goals during the initial surgery for high-velocity injuries are to reapproximate wound edges and to achieve soft tissue coverage of plates and exposed bone. Revision surgery can be considered after initial wounds heal and the surrounding temporary cavity injury resolves.
- As the incidence of high-velocity injuries increases in the civilian sector, so must the understanding of these injuries by community and academic head and neck, facial plastic, and reconstructive surgeons.

INTRODUCTION

High-velocity projectiles from improvised explosive devices (IEDs) and assault rifles on the battlefield result in unique head and neck injuries and injury patterns far different than those caused by civilian low-velocity projectiles. Although few surgeons will have the experience of treating injuries sustained in the combat theater, the rise of global and domestic terrorism and injuries caused by high-velocity weapons highlight the importance and application of these wartime principals to the civilian sector.

From 2006 to 2015, more than 77,000 incidents related to terrorism were reported globally. The United States alone experienced more than 170

The authors have nothing to disclose.

The views expressed herein are those of the authors and do not reflect the official policy or position of Brooke Army Medical Center, the US Army Medical Department, the US Army Office of the Surgeon General, the Department of the Army, Department of Defense, or the US Government.

[a] Department of Otolaryngology–Head and Neck Surgery, San Antonio Uniformed Services Health Education Consortium, Brooke Army Medical Center, 3551 Roger Brooke Drive, JBSA, Fort Sam Houston, TX 78234-6200, USA; [b] Department of Otolaryngology–Head and Neck Surgery, University of Texas Health Science Center at San Antonio, 325 East Sonterra Boulevard, Suite 210, San Antonio, TX 78258, USA

* Corresponding author. Department of Otolaryngology–Head and Neck Surgery, MCHE-SDT-Otolaryngology, 3551 Roger Brooke Drive, Fort Sam Houston, TX 78234-4504.

E-mail address: jacobscottmajors@hotmail.com

facialplastic.theclinics.com

incidents, leading to hundreds of injuries and fatalities.[1] The mass shooting in Orlando on June 12, 2016, lead to 49 fatalities with 53 injured.[2] Six months before the Orlando shooting, 14 people were killed and 21 wounded in a terrorist attack in San Bernardino, California.[3] However, gunshot wounds are not the only types of injuries sustained at the hands of terrorists in the United States. On April 15, 2013, 2 IEDs were detonated near the finish line of the 117th Boston Marathon, killing 3 people and injuring 264 others. At least 10% of the injuries sustained from the bombing resulted in high-velocity injuries to the head and neck.[4]

Most trauma centers have experience with managing head and neck injuries sustained by low-velocity weapons. However, the management of high-velocity injuries caused by IEDs or other weapons is rarely performed outside the battlefield. Preparing to manage these high-velocity injuries resulting from a mass casualty incident (MCI) is becoming more integral to health care teams as global terrorism becomes a greater concern and an increasing risk. The most recent conflicts in Iraq and Afghanistan have significantly improved understanding of battlefield trauma and how to appropriately address these injures.

INJURY PATTERNS OF RECENT CONFLICTS

Historically, head and neck surgeons, including facial plastic and reconstructive surgeons, have been essential members of multispecialty head and neck surgical teams involved in treating injuries sustained during combat. The modern specialty of plastic surgery developed largely due to advancements in the treatment of injuries sustained during World War I.[5] Although the lethality of weapons has increased with a significantly higher percentage of lethal explosive injuries (IEDs) in modern warfare, soldiers have a significantly higher rate of survival compared with previous conflicts.[6] This increase in survival can be explained by multiple factors, including rapid mobilization of the wounded to higher echelons of care, improved access to immediate and urgent medical care, and improvements in body armor.[7] Injuries to the chest, abdomen, and pelvis that previously proved to be fatal have dramatically decreased with technical advancements in body armor. Although body armor has a negligible effect on the incidence of head and neck injuries, a higher percentage of wounded are presenting with survivable head and neck trauma due to this decreased incidence chest, abdomen, or pelvic trauma.[8] Consequently, the percentage of head and neck injuries treated in modern combat has significantly increased, making the role of the head and neck or facial plastic surgeon paramount in treating these high-velocity injuries.[8]

During the Operation Iraqi Freedom (OIF) and Operation Enduring Freedom (OEF), conflicts, more than 43,000 US military personnel were injured, 25% to 40% of which sustained injuries involving the head, face, and/or neck.[9–11] The most commonly performed head and neck procedures were repair of facial lacerations, tracheotomy, neck exploration for penetrating neck trauma (PNT), arch bars or intermaxillary fixation, and open reduction or internal fixation of facial fractures.[8,12,13]

Essential to the understanding of the treatment of high-velocity head, neck, and facial injuries is a basic knowledge of the physiology and kinetics of modern battlefield trauma. Although the type of head, neck, and facial procedures performed during OIF and OEF are not uncommonly performed in civilian trauma centers, the physiology and presentation of these high-velocity injuries differs significantly from the typical low-velocity injuries. Understanding these differences is essential to appropriate preoperative and postoperative planning and care. As the incidence of high-velocity injuries increases in the civilian sector, so must the understanding of these injuries by community and academic head and neck, facial plastic, and reconstructive surgeons.

PHYSIOLOGY AND KINETICS OF HIGH-VELOCITY INJURIES

The mechanism of injury of different weapons or projectiles and the amount of energy transferred to tissues is directly related to the size and velocity of the projectile.[14] Measuring the kinetic energy of a projectile, allows one to more accurately predict the type and degree of tissue injury. Kinetic energy is calculated by the following equation:

$$KE = \frac{1}{2}m\ (V1 - V2)^2$$

in which KE is kinetic injury, m is missile mass, V1 is entry or impact velocity, and V2 is exiting velocity of the projectile.[14,15] The most lethal projectiles are those that enter the target tissue with a high entering velocity, then dissipate all their energy into the tissue without exiting the target (V2 = 0).[14,15]

Advancements in modern warfare have led to the development of high-velocity weapons that are able to transfer maximal energy to vital structures. A high-velocity weapon is able to fire a projectile at a velocity of greater than 610 m/s.[14,15] Handguns generally have a muzzle velocity between 210 and 600 m/s, defining them as low-velocity weapons, whereas the muzzle velocity of a rifle exceeds 610 m/s, which is the definition of a high-velocity weapon.[14] Close-range shotguns (<5m) generate high-velocity projectiles, whereas at longer range (>5m) the projectiles become low-velocity.[15] Mortars or rockets, grenades, and IEDs are missile or projectile weapons that cause high-velocity injury.[15] The behavior of high-velocity projectiles in tissue is very different from that of low-velocity projectiles and must be considered when facing injuries of this nature.

As a projectile of sufficient velocity tears through tissue, it imparts its kinetic energy to the surrounding soft tissues, causing them to compress radially away from the projectile tract.[14] A temporary or compression cavity is produced that may be 30 times as large as the cross-section of the projectile.[14] Within 5 to 10 ms after generation of the compression cavity, it contracts, leaving a permanent cavity 3 to 4 times the size of the cross-section of the projectile.[14] The disruption and damage sustained by the tissues in the temporary cavity closely resembles that of severe blunt trauma and extend significantly beyond the tract of the permanent cavity.[14] Tissues that are within the permanent cavity tract are either compressed into the surrounding structures and/or ejected through the entrance and exit wounds.[14]

For lower velocity injuries, the temporary cavity is much smaller and most the damage is localized to those tissues directly affected or compressed by the projectile.[14] Because of the lower velocity at which the projectile enters the tissue, its path may be altered, deviating the course of the projectile around important structures such as vessels, nerves, and muscle, causing its point of termination to be distant from that which would be expected by looking at the entrance wound.[14] If the projectile is not seen in the entry region (ie, neck) on imaging studies, then the rest of the body should be evaluated for the projectile's final resting place. Although both the temporary and permanent cavities are smaller for lower velocity projectiles, injuries to important structures occur if they are encountered along the permanent tract and if the properties of the tissue do not allow its displacement from this tract.[14]

The undulating temporary cavity produced by high-velocity missiles causes significantly more distant tissue injury than that caused by low-velocity projectiles.[14] Disrupted tissue, ruptured blood vessels and nerves, and fractured bones are more commonly encountered despite their distance from the tract or permanent cavity of the missile.[14] Dense structures such as muscle may swell significantly as they absorb great amounts of energy, resulting in vascular and tissue fluid extravasation. Those important structures directly in the path of the missile are severely disrupted or severed because the high-velocity projectile is less likely to deviate from its course. A bone in the direct path of a missile may produce multiple fragments that may act as secondary projectiles with their own devastating effects (**Figs. 1–3**).[14]

IEDs act as multiple high-velocity weapons and are now the most common mechanism of battlefield injury, accounting for as many as 76% of combat injuries in Iraq and Afghanistan.[16,17] Injuries sustained from IED explosions are separated into primary, secondary, tertiary, and quaternary injuries.[18] The severity of injury depends on the distance of the victim from the nucleus of the blast, as well as the projectiles thrown from the device on activation.[19]

Primary injuries occur due to the barotrauma sustained during the initial high pressure blast wave and from the subsequent drop in pressure. The changes in pressure during this phase result in injury to gas-filled organs such as the lungs, the middle ear, and, rarely, the bowel.[19] Injuries to the ear, including tympanic membrane rupture, ossicular fractures, and dislocations, are very common in blast victims and must be looked for in any patient exposed to this type of injury.[19–22] Secondary blast injuries cause most of the injuries encountered in blast victims.[19,23] They result from

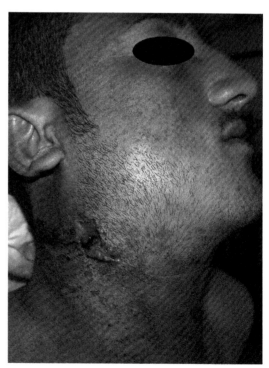

Fig. 1. Entry wound on a National Guard soldier shot with an AK-47 round.

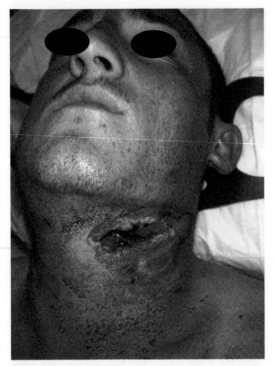

Fig. 2. Bullet tract transverses the neck just above the thyroid cartilage and exits the contralateral neck.

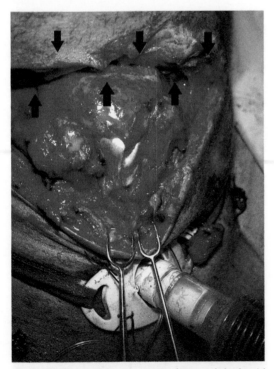

Fig. 3. The large temporary cavity shattered the hyoid cartilage, which was 2 to 3 cm from the bullet tract (*arrows* point to permanent cavity), into 3 fragments.

the high-velocity debris or projectiles carried by the blast wind and cause a similar pattern of injury (see previous discussion) (**Figs. 4** and **5**). In contrast to primary blast injuries, which occur within tens of meters from the blast site, projectiles during the secondary blast can cause human trauma hundreds or even thousands of meters from the blast site.[19] Tertiary blast injuries are caused when the victim is physically displaced by the blast wave and sustains blunt or penetrating trauma on impact with immovable objects such as cars or walls.[19] These injuries are similar to those that would be experienced during a fall or when a pedestrian is struck by a moving vehicle.[19] Quaternary injuries result in burns, inhalational injuries, and even asphyxiation from the heat, flames, gas, and smoke caused by the explosive device.[18]

An understanding of the physiology and kinetics of high-velocity missile injuries is important for any head, neck, and facial plastic reconstructive surgeon. With high-velocity injuries, the surgeon must thoroughly evaluate all structures and surrounding tissue, as well as the entire body, because the damage will likely extend beyond the trajectory of the projectile. Blast injuries causing primary, secondary, tertiary, and quaternary injuries require a thorough evaluation of each of those systems to which they can cause injury. These types of injuries can be among the most devastating soft and hard tissue trauma to the human body.

MASS CASUALTY, TRIAGE, AND MANAGEMENT OF MEDICAL ASSETS

A MCI is any incident in which emergency medical services are overwhelmed by the number and or

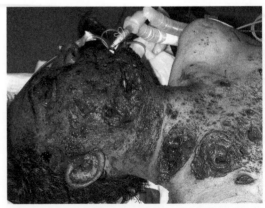

Fig. 4. A US contractor hit with an IED sustained devastating soft tissue injuries, including extensive foreign body implantation.

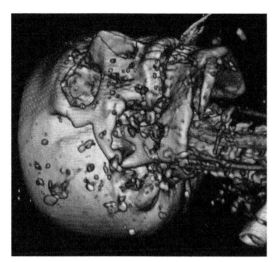

Fig. 5. Computed tomography (CT) scan showing multiple foreign bodies throughout the head and neck. Operations included extensive irrigation and removal of foreign bodies with soft tissue closure, and open reduction and internal fixation of mandible fractures.

severity of the casualties. It is not defined by a specific number of patients seen in a certain period of time but as a situation in which the need for emergency care exceeds medical resources such as equipment and personnel. There is significant concern about the readiness of the United States to respond to MCIs as evidenced by the 2014 Report Card on America's Emergency Care Environment score of C minus for disaster preparedness.[24] Much of what is known and practiced today regarding the management of MCIs in the civilian emergency or trauma setting has been learned on the battlefield.

IEDs have become the predominant cause of military causalities, accounting for as high as 76% of combat injuries in Iraq and Afghanistan.[17] Despite the lethality of high-velocity weapons used in modern wartime conflict, service members injured during mass casualty events are surviving at higher rates. The survival rate for PNT in Iraq and Afghanistan was 97%, despite that 70% of these would were caused by high-velocity weapons.[25] The survival rates for soldiers with PNT in previous conflicts was 86%, 93%, and 93% to 96% in World War I, World War II, and in the Vietnam War, respectively.[26–28] This increase in survival is due to multiple factors, including rapid mobilization of the wounded to higher echelons of care, improved access to immediate and urgent medical care, and improvements in body armor.[7] According to data from the Israeli National Trauma Registry, explosives used in terror attacks are 3 times more deadly than those used in war because

civilians do not have body armor, the victims span a wider range of age and health, and because preparedness tends to be less systematic.[29] With MCIs caused by high-velocity projectiles becoming more common in terrorist attacks against civilians, it is important that civilian medical facilities are ready for MCIs of this nature.

The obligation of a surgeon during an MCI is to care for patients in a manner that will provide the most benefit to the most patients.[30] When medical resources are overwhelmed, triage is essential to the appropriate prioritization of time, equipment, supplies, personnel, and evacuation capabilities. The principles of triage, as described in *Emergency War Surgery*,[31] are as follows:

- Injury priority or severity (from highest to lowest: airway, breathing, circulation, and neurologic changes)
- Salvageability
- Available resources or personnel
- Treatment time, distance, or environment (aeroevacuation capability or availability).[31]

The military uses the following triage categories to help prioritize care for those patients with the most acute care needs while preserving resources for patients with the best chance of survival:

- Immediate (red)
- Delayed (yellow)
- Minimal (green)
- Expectant (black).[31]

Patients in the immediate category require immediate life-saving measures and should have a high chance of survival.[31] Patients in this category include those with acute traumatic airway obstruction, tension pneumothorax, or internal hemorrhage. The delayed category represents patients who require definitive treatment but whose conditions allow a delay in treatment without endangering their life.[31] Examples in this category include those with panfacial fractures who have a controlled airway, those with extremity fractures, or those with a laceration in which the hemorrhage is currently controlled. The minimal category includes those patients with minor injuries, are ambulatory, and can seek care for themselves or be helped by nonmedical personnel.[31] The expectant are those patients with lethal injuries who will likely die despite treatment even with the benefit of massive medical resources.[31] These patients should be cared for with comfort measures and in a setting removed from other patients and personnel.

The role of the head and neck surgeon during an MCI is airway and hemorrhage control. The 3 leading causes of death on the battlefield include airway compromise, compressible hemorrhage, and tension pneumothorax.[8,32] Because 75% of the injuries in OIF involved penetrating face and neck trauma, traumatic airway control and evaluation of large vessel injury to the neck was essential to the initial management of those patients.[33]

Injuries from IEDs and other high-velocity weapons can result in acute hemorrhage, tissue prolapse, and massive edema that may result in significant airway obstruction, necessitating emergent airway control.[8] The best method to initially assess for airway patency during the primary trauma survey is to ask the patient to speak.[33] The ability of the patient to give an intelligible and appropriate reply implies a patent airway, adequate ventilation to vibrate the vocal cords and generate voice, and a Glasgow Coma Scale score of 8, indicating adequate brain perfusion.[33] In the initial patient evaluation, the surgeon should also assess the tract of the projectile to gain clues regarding the possibility of swelling leading to airway compromise. Patients with impending airway compromise and active head and neck bleeding should be managed with an awake tracheotomy rather than attempting a difficult oral or nasal intubation that can cause additional airway edema and bleeding, necessitating an emergent cricothyroidotomy for a failed airway.[33] In OIF, 10% of patients with high-velocity head and neck injuries required immediate intubation or emergent cricothyroidotomy or tracheostomy by a head and neck surgeon after initial attempts at airway management failed.[33] At the onset of any MCI, the head and neck surgeon must recognize that the necessary rate of emergent airway control is 3 times higher in high-velocity injuries than in low-velocity injuries of the head and neck.[34–36]

The leading cause of death in penetrating neck injuries is hemorrhage from cervical vascular injury.[37] Management of PNT is usually divided into 3 anatomic zones of injury.[38] Zone I defines the region between the clavicle inferiorly, and superiorly by the inferior border of the cricoid cartilage. Significant vascular structures in this zone include the large vessels of the thoracic inlet, such as the subclavian and innominate vessels; the common carotid; and the internal jugular vein. Zone II lies between the inferior border of the cricoid cartilage and the angle of the mandible superiorly. Major vascular structures in this region include the internal and external carotid arteries and the internal jugular vein. Zone II is the area most commonly involved in penetrating injuries (60%–75%).[26] Zone III is the space extending

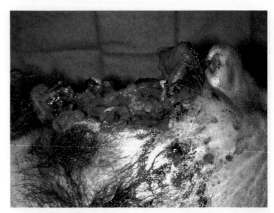

Fig. 6. Lateral view of Afghani National Guard solider hit by an IED, which caused moderate midface and mandible injury.

from the angle of the mandible superiorly to the base of skull. Critical vascular structures in this zone are the internal and external carotid, the internal jugular vein, and the vertebral artery.

Physical examination should not be relied on as the sole diagnostic evaluation of a patient with a penetrating neck injury. Studies in both combat and civilian literature show that with both a negative physical examination and appropriate

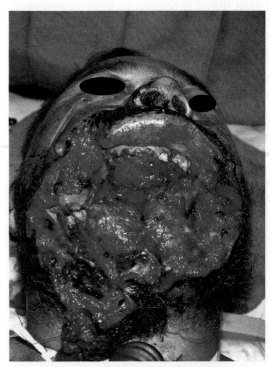

Fig. 7. Frontal view of patient showing extensive injury that required emergent airway control.

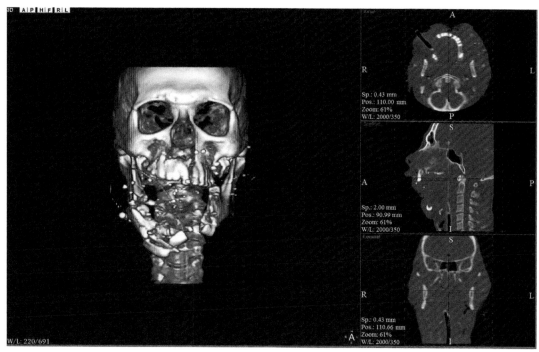

Fig. 8. CT and 3-dimensional (3D) reconstruction showing mandible and midface fractures sustained as a result of the IED effects.

negative diagnostic imaging, the sensitivity and specificity is greater than 95% that the patient is without vascular injury.[39,40] The use of computed tomography angiography (CTA) is advocated in evaluating stable zone I and zone III injuries in many civilian trauma centers.[41] The accuracy of CTA (98.5%), as well as its use for both diagnostic and therapeutic intervention through endovascular

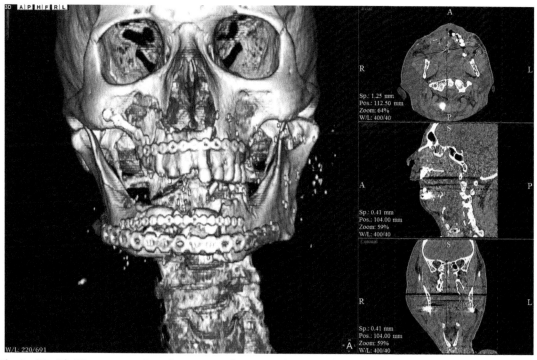

Fig. 9. CT with 3D reconstruction after open reduction and internal fixation.

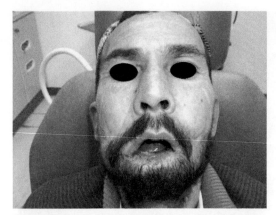

Fig. 10. Patient approximately 3 months after open reduction and internal fixation and soft tissue repair.

techniques, has made it the gold standard of care.[42] Formal angiography is reserved for those patients in whom CTA is equivocal or nondiagnostic. Neck exploration is indicated for symptomatic patients with hard signs of PNT and for asymptomatic patients (no hard signs of PNT) with positive diagnostic studies (CTA, panendoscopy, or swallow study) showing significant injury.[38,43] In the absence of radiographic or endovascular capabilities, neck exploration should be considered for all PNTs.

Initial emergency management in an MCI should follow the principals of advanced trauma life support, with identification of immediate life-threatening injuries and a focus on airway, breathing, and circulation. Triage is the first step in determination of patient stability and identification of the need for airway or surgical intervention. Understanding and applying the principles as previously outlined allows the surgeon to provide the most benefit to the most patients in the event of a mass casualty situation.

SPECIAL CONSIDERATIONS IN RECONSTRUCTION OF HIGH-VELOCITY INJURIES

As previously discussed, the injury patterns seen from high-velocity gunshot and blast injuries are unique from injuries sustained from the blunt, low-velocity trauma commonly seen in the civilian trauma setting. The large concussive wave created by the high kinetic energy of the projectile disrupts tissue, ruptures blood vessels and nerves, and fractures bones despite their distance from the tract or permanent cavity of the missile.[14] This secondary area of injury has important implications regarding the timing and nature of repair of these devastating injuries.

Despite the great vascular supply to the face, doing too much too soon with extensive soft tissue undermining and flap rotation may result in dead tissue.[44] The gross contamination, marginal viability of residual soft tissue, and underlying osseous trauma characteristic of these injuries necessitates staged protocols.[45] The soft tissue should be closed immediately after extensive irrigation and conservative debridement with only grossly contaminated and devitalized tissue being removed.[44] The primary goals during the initial surgery are to reapproximate the wound edges with primary closure and to achieve soft tissue coverage of the plates and exposed bone.[44] Revision surgery can be considered after the initial wounds heal and the surrounding temporary cavity injury resolves. The surgical results in Afghanistan, with only 1.7% (2/215) of plates requiring removal due to loss of overlying sift tissue coverage after 51 facial or mandibular fracture repairs, support this recommendation (**Figs. 6–10**).[44]

SUMMARY

During the past decade in the Iraq and Afghanistan, more than 30,000 head and neck injuries have been treated at American medical facilities in both war zones.[9] The experience of head and neck, facial plastic, and reconstructive surgeons on the battlefield has significantly improved understanding concerning the appropriate evaluation and management of high-velocity injuries. As injuries of this nature become more frequent off the battlefield due to terrorist attacks and availability of high-velocity weapons, this understanding will help lead to improved patient care, decreased morbidity and improved survival.

REFERENCES

1. National Consortium for the Study of Terrorism and Responses to Terrorism (START). 2016. Global Terrorism Database [Data Set]. Available at: https://www.start.umd.edu/gtd. Accessed August 1, 2016.
2. Tsukayama H, Berman M, Markon J. Gunman who killed 49 in Orlando nightclub had pledged allegiance to ISIS. The Washington Post. 2016. Available at: https://www.washingtonpost.com/news/post-nation/wp/2016/06/12/orlando-nightclub-shooting-about-20-dead-in-domestic-terror-incident-at-gay-club/?utm_term=.3e21bbe161f2. Accessed November 20, 2016.
3. Botelho G, Ellis R. San Bernardino shooting investigated as 'act of terrorism'. CNN. 2015. http://www.cnn.com/2015/12/04/us/san-bernardino-shooting/index.html. Accessed November 20, 2016.

4. Singh AK, Buch K, Sung E, et al. Head and neck injuries from the Boston Marathon bombing at four hospitals. Emerg Radiol 2015;22:527–32.

5. Chambers JA, Ray PD. Achieving growth and excellence in medicine: the case history of armed conflict and modern reconstructive surgery. Ann Plast Surg 2009;63(5):473–8.

6. Gawande A. Casualties of war – Military care for the wounded from Iraq and Afghanistan. N Engl J Med 2004;351:2471–5.

7. Lopez MA, Arnholt JL. Safety of definitive in-theater repair of facial fractures. Arch Facial Plast Surg 2007;9(6):400–5.

8. Brennan J. Experience of first deployed otolaryngology team in Operation Iraqi Freedom: the changing face of combat injuries. Otolaryngol Head Neck Surg 2006;134(1):100–5.

9. Feldt BA, Salinas NL, Rasmussen TE, et al. The joint facial and invasive neck trauma (J-FAINT) project, Iraq and Afghanistan 2003-2011. Otolaryngol Head Neck Surg 2013;148(3):403–8.

10. Owen BD, Kragh JK, Wenke JC, et al. Combat wounds in Operation Iraqi Freedom and Operations Enduring Freedom. J Trauma 2008;64:295–9.

11. Lew TA, Walker JA, Wenke JC, et al. Characterization of craniofacial battle injuries sustained by United States service members in the current conflicts in Iraq and Afghanistan. J Oral Maxillofac Surg 2010;68:3–7.

12. Power DB. Distribution of civilian and military maxillofacial surgical procedure performed in an Air Force theatre hospital: implications for training and readiness. J R Army Med Corps 2010;156(2):117–21.

13. Rajguru R. Role of ENT surgeons in managing battle trauma during deployment. Indian J Otolaryngol Head Neck Surg 2013;65(1):89–94.

14. Holt GR, Kostohryz G Jr. Wound ballistics of gunshot injuries to the head and neck. Arch Otolaryngol 1983;109:313–8.

15. Brennan JA. Pathophysiology of head and neck injuries. Textbooks of military medicine otolaryngology/ head and neck surgery combat casualty care in Operation Iraqi Freedom and Operation Enduring Freedom. Fort Sam Houston (TX): Department of Defense (DOD), The Borden Institute 2015. p. 105–6.

16. Champion HR, Bellamy RF, Roberts P, et al. A profile of combat injury. J Trauma 2003;54(5):S13–9.

17. Kelly JF, Ritenour AE, McLaughlin DF, et al. Injury severity and causes of death from Operation Iraqi Freedom and Operation Enduring Freedom: 2003-2004 versus 2006. J Trauma 2008;64:S21–7.

18. Champion HR, Holcomb JB, Young LA. Injuries from explosions: physics, biophysics, pathology, and required research focus. J Trauma 2009;66(5):1468–77.

19. Sign AK, Ditkofsky NG, York JD, et al. Blast Injuries: From Improvised Explosive Device Blasts to the Boston Marathon Bombing. Radiographics 2016;36(1):295–307.

20. Cho SI, Gao SS, Xia A, et al. Mechanisms of hearing loss after blast injury to the ear. PLoS One 2013;8(7):e67618.

21. Hong SM, Lee JH, Park CH, et al. Transverse fracture of the stapes anterior crus caused by the blast pressure from a land mine explosion. Korean J Audiol 2014;18(3):137–40.

22. Patterson JH Jr, Hamernik RP. Blast overpressure inducted structural and functional changes in the auditory system. Toxicology 1997;121(1):29–40.

23. Popivanov G, Mutafchiyski VM, Belokonski EI, et al. A modern combat trauma. J R Army Med Corps 2014;160(1):52–5.

24. America's Emergency Care Environment: A State-by-State Report Card. 2014. Available at: http://www.emreportcard.org/. Accessed November 20, 2016.

25. Brennan J, Lopez M, Gibbons MD, et al. Penetrating neck trauma in Operation Iraqi Freedom. Otolaryngol Head Neck Surg 2011;144:180–5.

26. Obeid FN, Haddad GS, Host HM, et al. A critical reappraisal of a mandatory policy for penetrating wounds of the neck. Surg Gynecol Obstet 1985;160:517–22.

27. Narrod JA, Moore EE. Selective management of penetrating neck injuries: a prospective study. Arch Surg 1984;119:574–8.

28. Brennan J, Meyers AD, Jafek BJ. Penetrating neck trauma: a 5-year review of the literature, 1983 to 1988. Am J Otol 1990;11:191–7.

29. Gawande A. Why Boston's hospitals were ready. The New Yorker. 2013. http://www.newyorker.com/news/news-desk/why-bostons-hospitals-were-ready. Accessed November 20, 2016.

30. Holt GR. Making difficult ethical decisions in patient care during natural disasters and other mass casualty events. Otolaryngol Head Neck Surg 2008;139:181–6.

31. Cubano MA, editor. Emergency war surgery, third United States revision. Washington, DC: Department of the Army, Office of the Surgeon General, Borden Institute; 2004.

32. Bellamy R. How people die in ground combat. Presented at: the Joint Health Services Support Vision 2010 Working Group. September 1996.

33. Brennan J, Gibbons MD, Lopez M, et al. Traumatic airway management in Operation Iraqi Freedom. Otolaryngol Head Neck Surg 2011;144:376–80.

34. Kellman RM, Losquadro WD. Comprehensive airway management of patients with maxillofacial trauma. Craniomaxillofac Trauma Reconstru 2008;1:39–48.

35. Tung TC, Tseng WS, Chen CT, et al. Acute life-threatening injuries in facial fractures patients: a review of 1,025 patients. J Trauma 2000;49:420–4.

36. Taicher S, Givol N, Peleg M, et al. Changing indications for tracheostomy in maxillofacial trauma. J Oral Maxillofac Surg 1996;54:292–5.

37. Hong S, Klem C. Hemorrhage management and vascular control. Textbooks of military medicine otolaryngology/head and neck surgery combat casualty care in Operation Iraqi Freedom and Operation Enduring Freedom. Fort Sam Houston (TX): Department of Defense (DOD), The Borden Institute; 2015. p. 147.

38. Roon AJ, Christensen N. Evaluation and treatment of penetrating cervical injuries. J Trauma 1979;19: 391–7.

39. Meghoo CA, Dennis JW, Tuman C, et al. Diagnosis and management of evacuate casualties with cervical vascular injuries resulting from combat-related explosive blast. J Vasc Surg 2012;55:1329–37.

40. Osborn TM, Bell RB, Qaisi W, et al. Computed tomographic angiography as an aid to clinical decision making in the selective management of penetrating injuries to the neck: a reduction in the need for operative exploration. J Trauma 2008;64:1466–71.

41. Driscoll IR, Fuenfer MM, Shriver CD, et al. High velocity penetrating wounds to the neck: lesion learned from the battlefields in Afghanistan and Iraq. J Am Coll Surg 2007;205:S67.

42. Miller RH, Duplechain JK. Penetrating wounds of the neck. Otolaryngol Clin North Am 1991;24:15–29.

43. O'Brien PJ, Cox MW. A modern approach to cervical vascular trauma. Perspect Vasc Surg Endovasc Ther 2011;23(2):90–7.

44. Brennan J. Head and neck surgery in Iraq and Afghanistan: different war, different surgery, lessons learned. Laryngoscope 2013;123:2411–7.

45. Sheean AJ, Scott TM, Rhee PC. Soft tissue and wound management of blast injuries. Curr Rev Musculoskelet Med 2015;8(3):265–71.

Trauma in Facial Plastic Surgery: Frontal Sinus Fractures

Irene A. Kim, MD[a],*, Kofi D. Boahene, MD[a], Patrick J. Byrne, MD, FACS, MBA[b,c]

KEYWORDS

- Frontal • Sinus • Fracture • Trauma • Obliteration • Cranialization

KEY POINTS

- Frontal sinus fractures represent 5% to 15% of all maxillofacial fractures; their location near the brain and orbit can predispose them to several extracranial and intracranial complications.
- Management of frontal sinus fractures is controversial, especially with regard to fractures of the frontal sinus outflow tract. Recently, there has been a trend from aggressive surgical management to more conservative therapies.
- The most important goal of frontal sinus fracture management is to create a safe sinus by (1) reestablishing frontal bone contour, (2) restoring patency of the drainage system, (3) obliterating or cranializing the sinus cavity if a patent drainage system cannot be reestablished, and (4) creating a watertight barrier between the intracranial system and nose to prevent infectious complications.
- Lifelong follow-up and heightened awareness for symptoms/signs of infection or mucocoele are imperative in the management of frontal sinus fractures.

INTRODUCTION

Frontal bar and sinus fractures constitute approximately 5% to 15% of maxillofacial fractures and typically result from high-energy collisions associated with motor vehicle accidents, assaults, and sporting injuries.[1–6] Considerable force is required to cause these fractures, and thus patients usually have other associated injuries, which should prompt a thorough initial survey and examination. To place into perspective the amount of energy required to cause frontal sinus fractures, 2.4 kN to 4 kN are required for mandibular fractures, 0.7 kN to 1.3 kN for alveolar ridge fractures, 0.9 kN to 2.9 kN for malar fractures, and 3.6 kN to 7.1 kN for frontal bar/sinus fractures[7] (**Fig. 1**).

The goals of frontal sinus fracture repair are multifold: (1) avoidance of short-term and long-term complications, (2) return of normal sinus function, and (3) reconstruction of the frontal bar to obtain premorbid aesthetics.[1] In the pursuit of these endeavors, there has been a paradigm shift from aggressive surgery toward more conservative approaches with close patient follow-up.

ANATOMY

The frontal sinus is a cavity located anterior to the frontal lobes and superior to the bony orbits. It has been thought to play a protective role for the ocular globes and brain.[8] The sinus is bounded anteriorly by a thick table that provides the

Disclosure Statement: The authors have nothing to disclose.
[a] Facial Plastic and Reconstructive Surgery, Johns Hopkins University School of Medicine, 601 North Caroline Street 6th Floor, Baltimore, MD 21287-0910, USA; [b] Facial Plastic and Reconstructive Surgery, Department of Otolaryngology Head and Neck Surgery, Greater Baltimore Cleft Lip and Palate Team, Johns Hopkins University School of Medicine, 6701 N Charles Street, Baltimore, MD 21204, USA; [c] Department of Dermatology, Johns Hopkins University School of Medicine, 601 North Caroline Street 6th Floor, Baltimore, MD 21287-0910, USA
* Corresponding author.
E-mail address: irenekim415@gmail.com

Facial Plast Surg Clin N Am 25 (2017) 503–511
http://dx.doi.org/10.1016/j.fsc.2017.06.004

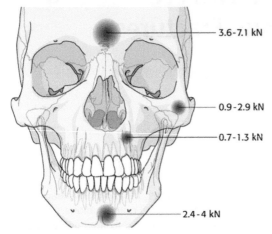

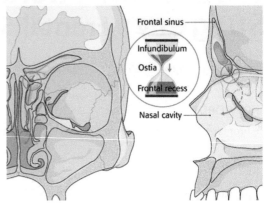

Fig. 1. Frontal bone anatomy. The anterior wall of the frontal sinus is thick and resistant to injury. It requires greater force to fracture this bone than any other facial bone. (*From* AO surgery reference cranial vault & skull base. Available at: www.aosurgery.org; with permission. Copyright by AO Foundation.)

Fig. 3. Frontal sinus drainage. The frontal sinus drainage pathway has an hourglass configuration with the infundibulum above the ostia and the frontal recess below. The sinus drains via a small outflow tract into the ethmoid sinus/nasal cavity. The outflow tract is hour-glass shaped with the true ostium (3–4 mm) at the narrowest portion. (*From* AO surgery reference cranial vault & skull base. Available at: www.aosurgery. org; with permission. Copyright by AO Foundation.)

forehead with its contour. The posterior table forms the anterior wall of the anterior cranial fossa. The frontal bone surrounds the sinuses superiorly and laterally, with the frontal outflow tract located medially[2] (**Fig. 2**). The sinus infundibulum rests above the ostia and the recess lies below it; because it is the only outflow tract for the frontal sinus, frontal recess patency is imperative[5,9] (**Fig. 3**).

Given its unique location, injury to the frontal bone and sinus may be associated with potentially catastrophic consequences.[4,10–12] Mismanagement of frontal sinus fractures or unpredictable

scarring during healing could result in a range of complications from sinus outflow obstruction to meningitis, encephalitis, and even brain abscesses.

DIAGNOSIS
Physical Examination

Given the relatively higher force required to cause frontal bar and sinus fractures, patients should be carefully examined for accompanying injuries. Cerebrospinal fluid (CSF) rhinorrhea, orbital trauma, and neurologic abnormalities should be evaluated for.[5,6]

Imaging

Thin-cut (1.5-mm) CT scans are typically obtained to help diagnose frontal sinus fractures. The axial, coronal, and sagittal images provide detailed information regarding the state of the anterior and posterior tables, the orbital roof and sinus floor, and the patency of the frontal recess, respectively. Additionally, reconstructed 3-D images are invaluable in providing a more comprehensive view of the nature and extent of frontal sinus injury.[1,3,12]

Evaluation for Cerebrospinal Fluid Leak

Patients who are stable and awake can be evaluated for salty-tasting postnasal drainage and CSF rhinorrhea. Collected fluid can initially be placed onto filter paper to assess for a halo sign and sent to a laboratory for a beta-2 transferrin

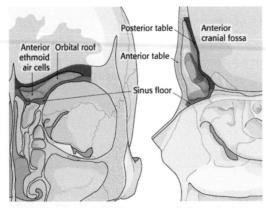

Fig. 2. Frontal sinus anatomy. The anterior table provides the forehead contour and is thicker than the posterior table. The sinus floor constitutes a portion of the orbital roof. The posterior table lies anterior to the anterior cranial fossa. (*From* AO surgery reference cranial vault & skull base. Available at: www.aosurgery. org; with permission. Copyright by AO Foundation.)

assay.[1] Intraoperatively, nasofrontal outflow tract patency can be evaluated by saline, dye, and contrast studies; however, these tests may not always accurately diagnose a CSF leak because evaluation can be complicated by mucosal edema or obstructive bony debris.[6,8,11]

TYPES OF FRONTAL BONE/SINUS FRACTURES

Frontal sinus fractures can be classified by the evaluation of 4 anatomic parameters: (1) anterior table, (2) posterior table, (3) nasofrontal recess, and (4) dural violation with or without CSF leak.[1,5,8] The extent and involvement of each of these parameters can be used to design the appropriate treatment strategy for repair. Fractures can further be characterized based on the level of displacement and comminution.

Although the treatment algorithm for mild to moderately displaced anterior table fractures is straightforward and focuses on improving the forehead contour, reconstructive strategies of posterior table and frontal recess fractures are more controversial. Complex fractures that involve the posterior table and sinus outflow tract (as well as attempts to repair them) carry risks of CSF leak, mucocele formation, meningitis, and intracranial infections or injuries.[3]

TREATMENT

The most important goal of frontal sinus fracture repair is to create a safe sinus,[12,13] using 4 basic guidelines:

1. Reestablish frontal bone contour.
2. Restore patency of the drainage system (if feasible).
3. Obliterate the sinus cavity if a patent drainage system cannot be reestablished.
4. Create a watertight barrier between the intracranial system and nose to prevent infectious complications.[12]

In general, the frontal sinus treatment algorithm usually follows one of the following approaches: observation, endoscopic repair, open reduction and internal fixation, sinus obliteration, or sinus cranialization.[5] Antibiotic prophylaxis is recommended for complex frontal sinus fractures given the potential for intracranial infections.[6]

Approaches

Preexisting lacerations

If a patient has a preexisting laceration over the glabella or forehead, this can be used to access the anterior table. Care should be taken not to extend the laceration.

- Advantages: there is no need for a secondary incision, and there is less soft tissue dissection to obtain exposure.
- Disadvantages: if the laceration proves limited or located in a suboptimal position to obtain adequate exposure, secondary incisions (discussed later) may be required.

Endoscopic

The endoscopic approach uses similar incisions used in an endoscopic brow lift surgery and is best suited for mildly depressed fractures located at or above the orbital rim.[2,3] A subperiosteal dissection is typically undertaken to the level of the fractures, at which time a percutaneous incision is made over the fracture site to introduce an elevator, which can reduce the depressed fragments. Various biocompatible materials like porous polyethylene[14] can be inserted through the working incision and screwed into place to camouflage the defect.[3,15]

- Advantages: endoscopic repair reduces patient morbidity, operative time, hospital stay, and cost.[3,14] There is also a reduced risk of larger scars, alopecia, paresthesia, and the need for extensive soft tissue dissection.
- Disadvantages: steep learning curve, requirement of specialized equipment and monitor towers, and need for a surgical assistant.[3] Acute repair of fractures using the endoscopic approach is ideal if the fragments can be easily reduced and not require alloplastic implants to maintain their reduction. If interfragmentary resistance is high, however, fracture repair can be extremely challenging or even impossible, requiring conversion to an open approach.[3,14]

Direct brow incision

Although the direct brow incision approach offers direct access to the fracture, it has largely been replaced by other less morbid procedures like the extended superior lid incision, which dissects the upper lid in the supratarsal plane and reaches the anterior frontal bone (**Fig. 4**).[16] Direct brow incisions, however, are still used in patients with deep horizontal forehead rhytids or in men with male-pattern baldness.[2]

- Advantages: less soft tissue dissection, quick and direct access to fracture
- Disadvantages: unfavorable scar in patients without deep forehead rhytids

Bicoronal incision

Coronal incisions are more extensive and are reserved for frontal bar and sinus fractures that cannot be managed expectantly or endoscopically.

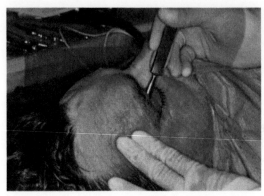

Fig. 4. A suprasupratarsal lid incision is performed here. A lateral segment of the anterior table is temporarily removed to allow a blunt elevator to be introduced into the sinus and reduce the fracture. Microplates are used to achieve osteosynthesis. (*From* Gassner HG, Schwan F, Schebesch KM. Transorbital approaches: minimally invasive access to the anterior skull base. Chapter 6. Boahene KD, editor. Minimal access skull base surgery. Philadelphia: Jaypee; 2016. p. 64; with permission.)

To avoid facial nerve injury, dissection in the temporal region should be carried through the temporoparietal fascia and onto the deep temporal fascia, just above the temporalis muscle. The integrity of the temporoparietal fascia should be maintained as flap elevation continues, because the frontal branch resides in this layer. The temporal flap is then joined with the central dissection, sharply cutting the fibers along the temporal lines bilaterally.[5]

- Advantages: optimal exposure and ability to harvest pericranium, muscle, split calvarial bone grafts, and temporalis fascia[12]
- Disadvantages: large scar, dense paresthesias, headache, facial nerve (temporal branch) injury, temporal wasting, and alopecia[1,14,15]

Anterior table fractures

Isolated, nondisplaced anterior table fractures Isolated anterior table fractures are the most common type of frontal sinus fracture.[15] Fractures that are nondisplaced (0–2 mm) are usually managed nonoperatively, because they pose a low risk of contour deformity or sinus complications.[2,5,8] Medical treatment includes nasal decongestants and sinonasal toilet.[12]

Comminuted, depressed fractures Fractures with 2 mm to 6 mm of displacement are associated with increased risk of forehead contour deformity, and either acute reduction or delayed camouflage is recommended. In general, fracture repair occurs in a bimodal pattern; it can either be repaired acutely within 1 day to 10 days or at approximately 2 months to 4 months after the injury.[3] The latter approach allows the complete resolution of forehead edema, allowing for a more accurate evaluation of the resultant contour deformity.[5]

Comminuted, depressed fractures can result in irregularities (especially in patients with thin skin) and should be considered for reduction.[2] If a fracture is not severely comminuted or impacted, an endoscopic approach may be used to reduce the bone fragments and restore contour with mesh. More severely comminuted fractures typically require a more invasive approach like a bicoronal incision to obtain optimal exposure. Prior to reapproximating the bone fragments, it is important to remove any trapped sinus mucosa between the segments, because this could lead to mucocele formation.[2]

Severely impacted fractures or those that have begun to heal can be challenging to reduce. During the course of trauma to the frontal region, the frontal bone goes through a compression phase before becoming concave; the fragments need to be pulled back through the compression phrase before reduction can be achieved.[5] In situations where the fragments are unable to be elevated adequately, postage-stamp perforations can be drilled along the edges of bone, releasing the tension and reducing the interfragmentary resistance. A bone hook can then be placed between the fragments to help with elevation.[5] This particular technique was used in a patient of the authors' who suffered a head-on collision with another individual during a soccer match and developed an isolated, impacted anterior table fracture (**Fig. 5**A, B). The patient presented 2.5 weeks after his injury and was taken to the operating room 5 days afterward. A bicoronal incision was used to gain exposure, and the anterior table fractures were found severely impacted (see **Fig. 5**C). A drill was uses to perforate the edges of the fractures (see **Fig. 5**D), and a hook was used to elevate the central bone segment; this allowed a freer elevator to be placed within the sinus cavity and elevate the other fragments, which were then fixated with mesh. A thin layer of hydroxyapatite cement was pasted over the mesh, providing a smooth contour. This technique allowed direct visualization of the sinus cavity, specifically of the posterior table and the frontal outflow tract, both of which appeared grossly intact. Five weeks after his surgery, the patient has no palpable irregularities, and the premorbid convex contour has been restored (see **Fig. 5**E).

In cases of severe comminution, attempted reduction of fragments may lead to large bone gaps that need to be replaced with split bone grafts, usually from the calvarium.[8] Sinus obliteration is typically reserved for cases in which severe

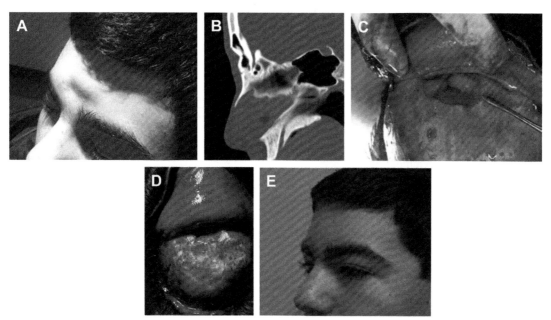

Fig. 5. (*A*) This is a 15-year-old boy who was involved in head-on collision with another player during a soccer match. He immediately noticed (visually and tactilely) a convex deformity in the lower central aspect of his forehead. (*B*) CT, sagittal view of the frontal bone illustrates a comminuted, impacted anterior frontal table fracture. (*C*) A bicoronal approach was used to access the fracture. There was significant interfragmentary resistance between the fracture segments, and a hook could not be placed in between the fragments to elevate the bone. (*D*) A drill was used to create postage-stamp perforations along the fragment edges centrally; this allowed a window through which an elevator was used to reduce the fragments. This maneuver allowed for inspection of the frontal sinus cavity, evaluation of the sinus outflow tract (which appeared patent), and extraction of bony debris and blood clots. (*E*) A 5-week postoperative photo shows smooth, premorbid forehead contour with restored convexity.

fractures of the anterior and/or posterior table render the frontal sinus nonfunctional. During the procedure, there must be complete removal of the sinus mucosa, especially of the scalloped areas above the orbits and laterally at the periphery of the sinus. The frontal sinus infundibulum mucosa is elevated and inverted inferiorly to occlude the ostium, a plug of temporalis muscle is placed atop this, and the sinus cavity is obliterated with one of many autologous materials (abdominal fat, pericranium, cancellous bone, and/or muscle). Complete removal of the sinus mucosa is imperative for successful outcomes, because residual mucosa can lead to chronic sinusitis, mucoceles, and pain, which can require secondary interventions.[5] On removing the sinus mucosa, the inner bony cortex is burred, because this ensures a clean cavity as well as the potential for vascularization of the fat graft used for obliteration.[15]

Delayed presentation In patients who present for treatment many weeks or months after their injury, forehead edema has largely resolved, and contour deformity may be better assessed. Certainly, fully healed fractures are not amenable to traditional

open reduction.[3] If the aesthetic deformity remains obvious, the defect can be camouflaged. Through an endoscopic or coronal incision, biocompatible materials that are malleable and stable over time (titanium mesh, hydroxyapatite cement, methyl methacrylate, and polyether ether ketone implants) can be used to improve forehead contour.[2,17]

Posterior table fractures Treatment recommendations for posterior table fractures are complex and controversial, because they are usually associated with the anterior table, fovea ethmoidalis, and cribiform plate as well.[15] Because the anterior table can withstand up to 998 kg of force, it serves to protect the posterior table and brain parenchyma; thus, if the posterior table is indeed fractured, there is a higher likelihood of other severe injuries (central nervous system, truncal, and extremity).[8,10,15,18] Although some surgeons use the thickness of the posterior table (approximately 2 mm) as a metric for determining the acceptable posterior wall displacement for nonsurgical therapy,[5] others believe that all posterior table fractures warrant surgical exploration to rule out dural tears and frontal sinus recess injury.[8,12]

Comminuted posterior table fractures with CSF leaks and nasofrontal ostia involvement have traditionally led to surgical exploration because of the risk of long-term complications.[12,13,18]

Many investigators believe that the amount of displacement of the posterior table is not the main factor in determining whether surgical intervention is required; rather, the presence or absence of a CSF leak and the presence of absence of frontal outflow tract injury are key determinants in making treatment decisions.[18]

Minimally displaced fractures plus cerebrospinal fluid leak plus no frontal outflow tract injury Patients with minimally displaced posterior table fractures and no apparent frontal outflow tract injury may be observed. If a CSF leak is apparent at the time of examination, conservative therapy (stool softener, head of bed elevation, and sneezing through open mouth) for 1 week is indicated. A lumbar drain can be considered to lessen the pressure at the level of the dural tear. If there is no spontaneous resolution within 1 week to 2 weeks, exploration with possible dural repair and/or sinus obliteration is recommended. The incidence of posttraumatic meningitis can range anywhere from 3% to 50%, but it increases when the leak persists beyond 7 days.[5,15,18] Dural repair can be performed with several biocompatible materials as well as native tissue like temporalis fascia, after which it may be reinforced with a pericranial flap to provide additional vascularized tissue.[12]

Gassner and colleagues[16] describe a minimally invasive transorbital approach to sealing dural defects (eg, for subdural air) after posterior table fractures. Through a suprasupratarsal incision, the fractured posterior table is encountered, and sealing material (autologous tissues or sponge, like fibrin sealant patch) can be used to seal the defect (**Fig. 6**).

Moderately to severely displaced fractures plus cerebrospinal fluid leak plus frontal outflow tract injury More severely displaced and fractured posterior tables are associated with frontal outflow tract injury and dural violation.[18] In cases of severely comminuted fractures with CSF leak or if the injury or repair causes disruption of greater than 25% to 30% of the posterior table, sinus cranialization has traditionally been the recommended treatment modality.[5,15]

During sinus cranialization, a pericranial flap should be carefully elevated and harvested for use as a barrier to separate the anterior skull base from the nasal cavity.[6] Bone fragments from both the anterior and posterior tables are removed, and the dura is carefully separated from the remnant posterior table. The sinus mucosa is completely stripped, and the remaining bone is burred to remove mucosal lining invaginations along the channels of Bréchet.[10,12] The frontal recess is occluded, and the anterior table is reconstructed after the anterior lobe is allowed to expand into the space previously held by the frontal sinus. Some surgeons prefer to use a pericranial flap with fibrin glue to occlude the ducts.[12,13] In instances of severe fractures where the anterior wall, posterior wall, and dura are missing or severely injured, free tissue transfer is used to close the wound.[12]

Recently, changing guidelines that reflect recent trends (mechanism and severity of injury) have encouraged conservative management of injuries

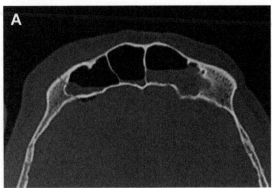
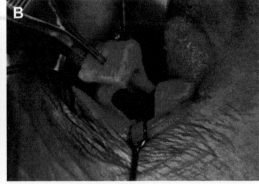

Fig. 6. (*A*) This CT scan is of a 55-year-old man who presented with a fractured posterior frontal table as well as subdural air on the right side. (*B*) A suprasupratarsal incision was used to expose the comminuted anterior table and gain access to the lateral posterior table fracture with subsequent placement of fibrin sealant patch to seal the subdural air. (*From* Gassner HG, Schwan F, Schebesch KM. Transorbital approaches: minimally invasive access to the anterior skull base. Chapter 6. Boahene KD, editor. Minimal access skull base surgery. Philadelphia: Jaypee; 2016. p. 69; with permission.)

that may have previously met the criteria for cranialization.[15] In 1 study, for example, 7 of 59 patients who met the criteria for cranialization were instead observed; no complications were seen at 92 days, but these data are limited by the paucity of long-term follow-up.[15]

Frontal sinus recess/frontal sinus outflow tract injury Combined fractures of the anterior and posterior tables are usually accompanied by injuries to the frontal outflow tract[6] (**Fig. 7**). Patency of the tract is essential in preventing serious early and late complications,[15] but the decision to treat these injuries is a challenging one, because high rates of postoperative stenosis have been associated with recanalizing the nasofrontal ostia with mucosal flaps and stents.[12,18]

Typically, sinus obliteration is indicated when there is a high likelihood that the sinus will be nonfunctional as a sequela of the sinus fractures. Obliteration requires (1) complete removal of sinus mucosa, (2) removal of the inner sinus bone cortex with a burr, (3) occlusion of nasal frontal recess, and (4) filling of the sinus cavity.[8] If the posterior table fracture is significantly comminuted or there is dural injury, cranialization may need to be performed, as previously described.

In the setting of traumatic injury (as opposed to cases of chronic frontal sinusitis), effective obliteration is usually more challenging to achieve secondary to comminution of bone, difficulties with effectively removing all of the sinus mucosa, and inherent issues with bone fragment devascularization and their subsequent resorption.[6,9] If the

adipose fat graft used for obliteration does not have an adequate vascular bed, it too can resorb and undergo necrosis, ultimately forcing the sinus to undergo an incomplete process of auto-obliteration.[9]

In light of these challenges, studies have recently come forth examining the role of conservative management in cases of frontal outflow tract injury. A recent study by DeConde and colleagues[4] reviewed 19 patients with frontal sinus fractures; 8 of them had injuries, which also involved the frontal recess, and 7 of these patients were managed conservatively. Interval CT imaging (mean: 73.9 ± 49.6 weeks) showed spontaneous clearance of sinus opacification. Only 1 of the 8 patients continued to have radiographic sinus opacification and ocular symptoms, but that patient's injury involved the naso-orbitoethmoid complex and had significant comminution of the orbital walls. The investigators extend their findings, suggesting that most patients with frontal sinus fractures (involving the frontal recess) without significant medial wall blowouts and obstruction may be offered conservative management and close follow up.

This study as well as others suggest that in patients with frontal sinus fractures with frontal recess involvement and concomitant naso-orbitoethmoid fractures, there should be stronger consideration to surgically intervene, because obstruction of the frontal recess by orbital contents may impede ventilation.[4,9] The superior margin of the nasal bones is above the frontal sinus floor, and, therefore, displaced fractures involve the frontal outflow tract and potentially disrupt the outflow tract into the ethmoid sinuses.[13]

Smith and colleagues[9] propose the following treatment protocol in patients with anterior frontal sinus wall fractures with frontal outflow tract injury: (1) assessment of the outflow tract with CT, (2) restoration of the anterior table fragments with rigid fixation, (3) postoperative broad-spectrum antibiotics for 4 weeks, and (4) serial postoperative CT scans to check for ventilation. After conservative management, in patients whom frontal sinus obstruction persists, endoscopic frontal sinusotomy or an endoscopic Lothrop procedure is also a viable option to reestablish mucociliary clearance.

These results certainly depend on patient follow-up, and this is a clear limitation—especially in the cohort of patients who suffer facial trauma in the first place.[15] Although the basic tenet of frontal sinus obliteration for the treatment of frontal outflow tract injuries still stands, the more conservative regimen with close follow-up is becoming

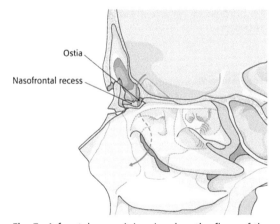

Fig. 7. A frontal recess injury involves the floor of the frontal sinus and the outflow tract. The green *arrow* delineates the frontal sinus drainage pathway. It may also involve the anterior skull base. (*From* AO surgery reference cranial vault & skull base. Available at: www.aosurgery.org; with permission. Copyright by AO Foundation, Switzerland.)

Ostia

Nasofrontal recess

more mainstream for all types of frontal sinus fractures. Prospective studies with long-term follow-up data need to be analyzed, but there is certainly a current shift in trends.[15]

COMPLICATIONS

The intimate location of the frontal bone and sinus with the brain and orbit plays a significant factor in the potentially catastrophic consequences that injury to this area can cause. Frontal sinus outflow obstruction can lead to problems like chronic sinusitis, chronic pain, chronic osteomyelitis, Pott puffy tumor, mucoceles, and mucopyoceles many years after the initial injury.[1,5,6] Other associated problems like meningitis, encephalitis, and brain abscesses may develop as well.

Treatment of fractures, depending on the approach, certainly carries risks. These include bleeding, pain, hematoma, infection, mesh extrusion, infection of biocompatible products, alopecia, scar, paresthesia, frontal nerve injury, and persistent forehead contour deformity. Sometimes, the approach taken to improve the contour deformity may lead to adverse effects on their own. Frontal recess stenting in the acute setting can cause restenosis, and frontoethmoidectomy at the time of exploration can result in anosmia.[9] Cranialization requires a craniotomy, and it is a morbid procedure associated with complications like abscesses or increased intracranial pressure requiring decompression.[10,13]

In patients with poor compliance, serial examinations and radiographic imaging may not be feasible; in these situations, aggressive management with osteoplastic obliteration at the time of acute injury is favored.[9] Complications are normally easier to prevent than to treat, so careful surveillance with serial imaging, diligent follow-up, and vigilance on the patient end are imperative.

CONTROVERSIES

The management of frontal sinus fractures has remained debated and will evolve further with time. Typically, anterior table fractures with forehead contour deformity likely necessitate intervention to improve aesthetics. What is not as clearly delineated is the need for surgical intervention in managing the injured posterior table and frontal outflow tract in the absence of persistent CSF leaks or excessive debris.[9] Frontal sinus fracture treatment paradigms were largely established before modern endoscopic and imaging techniques were born and, therefore, may not accurately reflect current trends. Moreover, present-day frontal sinus fracture patterns may

not represent the conclusions of previous studies, because airbag safety systems and improved seatbelt compliance have slowly changed the mechanisms of frontal sinus fractures from high-impact injuries to lower ones associated with interpersonal violence and sports.[4,6,9,15] An obvious trend is the movement away from trephination, frontal outflow tract stenting, and frontal sinus ablation for fracture management.[11]

SUMMARY

The optimal management of frontal sinus fractures remains controversial, even among several surgical specialties.[5,6] Fortunately, the severity of these injuries has diminished with increased seatbelt compliance and with more stringent auto-safety regulations. This, then has changed the treatment paradigms used to repair these injuries. Appropriate patient selection and close follow-up may allow for conservative management strategies when dealing with frontal sinus fractures, largely replacing the more morbid and invasive techniques that have been the mainstay for years. Lengthier follow-up data are required to make any conclusions about these approaches, however.[11]

Acute and delayed sequelae, like mucocele formation, sinusitis, contour deformity, and chronic sinusitis, can occur immediately or years after the initial injury. Therefore, patients should be thoroughly counseled about the importance of follow-up and the need to seek medical care if they develop any concerning signs or symptoms, such as frontal headaches, symptoms consistent with chronic or recurrent sinusitis, and swelling/tenderness.

REFERENCES

1. Strong BE. Frontal sinus fractures. Oper Tech Otolaryngol 2008;19:151–60.
2. Delaney SW. Treatment strategies for frontal sinus anterior table fractures and contour deformities. J Plast Reconstr Aesthet Surg 2016;69:1037–45.
3. Strong EB. Endoscopic repair of anterior table frontal sinus fractures. Facial Plast Surg 2009;25:43–8.
4. Jafari A, Nuyen BA, Salinas CR, et al. Spontaneous ventilation of the frontal sinus after fractures involving the frontal recess. Am J Otolaryngol 2015;36(6):837–42.
5. Strong EB, Johnson JT, Rosen CA. Bailey's Head and Neck Surgery–Otolaryngology. 5th edition. Baltimore (MD): Lippincott Williams & Wilkins; 2014. p. 3279–328. Chapter 84, Frontal sinus fractures.

6. Metzinger SE, Metzinger RC. Complications of frontal sinus fractures. Craniomaxillofac Trauma Reconstr 2009;2:27–34.

7. Diagnosis: frontal sinus fractures. Available at: http://www2.aofoundation.org/wps/portal/surgerymobile?contentUrl=/srg/93/01-Diagnosis/frontal_sinus.jsp&soloState=precomp&title=&Language=en&bone=CMF&segment=Cranium. Accessed December 1, 2016.

8. Prein J. Manual of internal fixation in the cranio-facial skeleton. Berlin: Springer; 1998. p. 148–54.

9. Smith T, Han JK, Loehrl TA, et al. Endoscopic management of the frontal recess in frontal sinus fractures: a shift in the paradigm? Laryngoscope 2002; 112:784–90.

10. Choi M, Li Y, Shapiro SA, et al. A 10-year review of frontal sinus fractures: clinical outcomes of conservative management of posterior table fractures. Plast Reconstr Surg 2012;130(2):399–406.

11. Gossman DG, Archer SM, Arosarena O. Management of frontal sinus fracture: a review of 96 cases. Laryngoscope 2006;116(8):1357–62.

12. Metzinger SE, Guerra AB, Garcia RE. Frontal sinus fractures: management guidelines. Facial Plast Surg 2005;21(3):199–206.

13. Chegini S, Gallighan N, Mcleod N, et al. Outcomes of treatment of fractures of the frontal sinus: review from a tertiary multispecialty craniofacial trauma service. Br J Oral Maxillofac Surg 2016; 54:801–5.

14. Kim KK, Mueller R, Huang F, et al. Endoscopic repair of anterior table: frontal sinus fractures with a Medpor implant. Otolaryngol Head Neck Surg 2007; 136:568–72.

15. Weathers WM, Wolfswinkel EK, Hatef DA, et al. Frontal sinus fractures: a conservative shift. Craniomaxillofac Trauma Reconstr 2013;6:155–60.

16. Gassner HG, Schwan F, Schebesch KM, et al. Minimal access skull base surgery: open and endoscopic assisted approaches. In: Transorbital approaches: minimally invasive. Access to the anterior skull base. Chapter 6. New Delhi (India): Jaypee Brothers Medical Publishers; 2016. p. 69.

17. Tieghi R, Consorti G, Clauser LC. Contouring of the forehead irregularities (Washboard Effect) with bone biomaterial. J Craniofac Surg 2012;23(3):932–4.

18. Chen KT, Chen CT, Mardini S, et al. Frontal sinus fractures: a treatment algorithm and assessment of outcomes based on 78 clinical cases. Plast Reconstr Surg 2006;118:457–68.

Advances in the Reconstruction of Orbital Fractures

Scott E. Bevans, MD[a,b], Kris S. Moe, MD[c],*

KEYWORDS

- Orbit fracture • Navigation • Mirror image • Computer • Preoperative planning • Endoscopic
- Outcomes

KEY POINTS

- Repair of orbital fractures should be carried out to restore premorbid orbital contours with the greatest possible precision.
- Reconstruction should be performed after resolution of edema from the injury.
- Exophthalmometry is important in the decision to operate, intraoperative measurements, and postoperative outcome evaluation.
- Orbital endoscopy improves ability to visualize the entire extent of the fracture with increased illumination and magnification while reducing retraction of orbital contents.
- Surgical navigation with mirror-image overlay guidance provides a template for reconstruction when normal anatomic landmarks have been damaged and, when used with an endoscopic technique, leads to significant improvement in multiple surgical outcome metrics.

INTRODUCTION

Orbital reconstruction is one of the most challenging tasks of the surgeon who treats craniofacial trauma. Suboptimal outcomes may lead to debilitating morbidity with significant emotional, functional, and occupational deficits. These deficits can include diminished visual acuity, diplopia, loss of depth perception, chronic or severe pain, as well as depression and impaired mobility. Given that the orbital region is perceived as the greatest determinant of beauty, failure to restore preoperative appearance in this highly visible and difficult-to-camouflage location often creates significant emotional distress.

In addition to the high functional and emotional impact of these injuries, repair of orbital fractures is challenging because of the complexity and variability of the anatomy. Reconstructive landmarks are often obscured by the trauma; the contralateral structure cannot be exposed for comparison; and the orbital contents are often markedly displaced

Disclosure Statement: S.E. Bevans is a member of the United States Army. The views expressed here are those of the authors and do not reflect the official policy or position of the Department of the Army, Department of Defense, or the U.S. Government. Additionally, reference herein to any specific commercial products, process, or service by trade name, trademark, manufacturer, or otherwise, does not necessarily constitute or imply its endorsement, recommendation, or favoring by the United States Government. K.S. Moe is the Founder of SPI Surgical, Inc but has no conflicts of interest.

[a] Department of Otolaryngology, Medical Corps, US Army, San Antonio Military Medical Center, 3551 Roger Brooke Drive, San Antonio, TX 78234, USA; [b] Department of Surgery, Uniformed Services University, 4301 Jones Bridge Road, Bethesda, MD 20814, USA; [c] Division of Facial Plastic and Reconstructive Surgery, Departments of Otolaryngology and Neurological Surgery, University of Washington School of Medicine, 325 9th Avenue, Seattle, WA 98104, USA
* Corresponding author.
E-mail address: krismoe@uw.edu

1064-7406/17/© 2017 Elsevier Inc. All rights reserved.

into adjacent anatomic regions. Furthermore, even minor inaccuracy in repair of the fracture can cause functional and esthetic disturbances postoperatively, as can the edges of a fracture or entrapment of orbital contents under the implant.

Orbital fractures are frequent injuries, with a nationwide incidence exceeding more than 100,000 patients per year in the United States.[1] The cause of orbital injuries is shifting in the United States and other developed countries; motor vehicle accidents have overtaken assault as the most common cause. An increasing rate of falls make this the third most common cause of orbital fracture, followed by sports and industrial injuries. In all reports, the most frequently injured subgroup is men between 21 and 35 years of age; however, injuries to women, adolescents, and the elderly are also common.[2,3] Domestic violence remains an important cause of midface or isolated orbital injury among women.

Brain injury occurs in 38% to 61% of patients with orbital injuries, and the incidence of multiple facial fractures and brain injury increases with higher-impact injuries.[4] The rate of ocular injury ranges from 14% to 40% of patients with facial fractures, highlighting the need for a low threshold for ophthalmologic evaluation.[5] Most fractured orbits are minimal, however, and do not require repair even if other coincident facial fractures require surgical intervention.[2,3,5,6]

A recent biomechanical study validated historical observations regarding the amount of force required to fracture orbital walls, finding only 2 N-m of force was required to fracture the orbital floor relative to more than 4 N-m of force required to fracture the medial orbital wall.[7] Several theories of force transfer have been proposed. The hydraulic theory suggests that force is transferred to the orbital contents, increasing orbital pressure, and, thus, exerting hydraulic pressure on the orbital walls causing a fracture. Alternatively, the buckling theory describes transmission of force from direct contact with the orbital rim, creating a shockwave whereby the weakest area bone succumbs to forces of deformation. Less commonly, direct contact only with the globe results in retropulsion into an orbital wall causing a fracture.[8–10]

Despite the relative frequency with which surgeons will be asked to evaluate and manage patients with orbital fractures, there remains a great deal of controversy about patient selection for operative management and how to achieve optimal results. Specifically, debate remains about how to determine which patients will need operative intervention, timing of surgery, preoperative and postoperative antibiotic use, and a myriad of intraoperative techniques (eg, surgical approach, material used for reconstruction, intraoperative implant positioning confirmation, and so forth). In this article, the authors describe the technique they have developed and currently use at the University of Washington Harborview Medical Center (a level I trauma service) with a summary of recent literature applicable to these controversial topics.

ORBITAL ANATOMY

The orbit is formed by the confluence of 7 bones (**Figs. 1** and **2**). Conceptually, these are categorized into an orbital *exoskeleton* and *endoskeleton*. The exoskeleton is created by the external portions of the maxillary and frontal and zygomatic bones, which form the orbital rims. The endoskeleton, the internal walls of the orbit, are created by the intraorbital portions of these bones with the addition of the lacrimal, palatine, and sphenoid bones.

At the junction of the ethmoid and frontal bones are the ethmoid arteries. It is typically taught that there are 2 vessels, the anterior ethmoid artery located 24 mm posterior to the anterior lacrimal crest and the posterior branch 12 mm further posterior, 6 mm from the optic canal. There is actually significant variability in the number and location of branches of ethmoid arterial system, most often with 3 arteries in unpredictable positions.[11] At the junction of the lateral orbital wall with the orbital floor is the zygomaticofacial neurovascular bundle anteriorly and the zygomaticotemporal neurovascular bundle posteriorly. The superior orbital fissure and adjacent bone contain both sensory and motor nerves as well as the mechanical anchors important to extraocular motion, whereas the inferior orbital fissure contains only minor sensory nerves, which can be sacrificed without notable deficit (see **Fig. 1**).

The orbital floor is the shortest wall of the orbit and comprises the roof of the maxillary sinus. It is 35 to 40 mm in anterior/posterior length and variably concave, with a depression just behind the orbital rim and an upward slope to the orbital apex. The inferior rectus muscle runs in close proximity to the orbital floor for most of its length. The muscle belly is normally oval in appearance on coronal imaging but can become rounded when damaged or inflamed (a sign to evaluate on imaging). Because of the close approximation to the orbital floor, small spicules of bone are often in close approximation to the inferior rectus on coronal imaging.[12] The total orbital volume for an adult is approximately 30 to 35 mL, approximately 7 mL of which is occupied by the globe.[13]

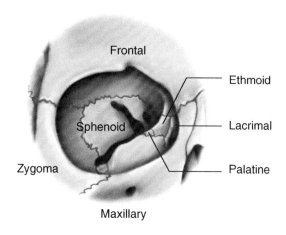

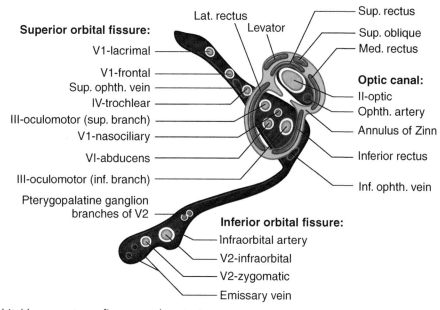

Fig. 1. Orbital bone anatomy, fissures, and contents.

INITIAL EVALUATION AND MANAGEMENT

Any patient with a history of blunt trauma to the orbit should undergo evaluation for orbital fracture. Because of the high frequency of coincident facial or intracranial injury, this should include a full craniofacial trauma evaluation at the time of presentation. After ruling out significant intracranial injury and assuring hemodynamic stability, targeted examinations must rule out damage to the globe, with ophthalmology consultation as indicated. This evaluation should include palpation of the orbit rim and adjacent soft tissue to assess for discontinuity, mobility, or emphysema. Ocular examination should include pupil shape and size, surface examination (for conjunctival edema or

hemorrhage), visual acuity, effortful extraocular motion (for motility status and pain with motion), and color vision status. Evidence of hyphema, decreased visual acuity, loss of color vision, or an afferent pupillary defect can represent damage to the globe or neural pathways, which warrants further specific neuro-ophthalmologic evaluation. These types of injuries will influence both the need for and timing of surgical intervention.

An orbital fracture may be present in up to 7% of patients with a history of periorbital trauma who have no findings on examination.[3] Therefore, a low threshold for obtaining cross-sectional imaging should be maintained. The authors recommend obtaining a maxillofacial computed tomography (CT) scan with 0.625-mm axial slices

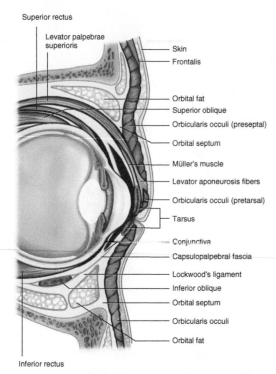

Superior rectus

Levator palpebrae superioris

Skin

Frontalis

Orbital fat

Superior oblique

Orbicularis occuli (preseptal)

Orbital septum

Müller's muscle

Levator aponeurosis fibers

Orbicularis occuli (pretarsal)

Tarsus

Conjunctiva

Capsulopalpebral fascia

Lockwood's ligament

Inferior oblique

Orbital septum

Orbicularis occuli

Orbital fat

Inferior rectus

Fig. 2. Sagittal view of the orbit soft tissues relevant to surgical approach.

from the vertex through the mandible, with navigation protocol. The authors request 3-dimensional (3D) reconstructions be performed on all scans with significant fractures to improve understanding of the fracture geometry.

Actual extraocular muscle entrapment within a fracture is relatively rare, though gaze restriction is common in the setting of orbital fractures. Entrapment is thought to occur when a fracture separates allowing soft tissue herniation, then reduces in green-stick fashion. This entrapment is more likely to occur in the softer bone of the pediatric orbit. True entrapment should be suspected if there is a hard stop during extraocular motion accompanied by nausea, vomiting, and/or bradycardia, even if there is little external evidence of fracture (white eye fracture). Typical CT findings include herniation of an extraocular muscle within a relatively small orbital defect. When actual entrapment occurs in the pediatric population, the fracture should be repaired urgently to prevent permanent muscle damage. A more common presentation is patients with reduced extraocular motion in at least one direction, often with a CT showing an edge of bone near a slightly rounded extraocular muscle without true entrapment. When there is uncertainty regarding entrapment, forced ductions should be considered.

Acute treatment in the absence of muscle entrapment is directed toward decreasing edema. In cases of significant edema, a steroid taper for 4 to 7 days may be considered. The authors counsel patients to ice with saline-soaked gauze or a thinly covered bag of frozen peas for 10 to 20 minutes per hour while awake for the first 72 hours and elevate the head of the bed while sleeping. The authors recommend oxymetazoline nasal spray for a short period after injury as needed for epistaxis and saline nasal spray but no nasal irrigations. Patients should be educated on sinus precautions: most importantly sneezing with an open mouth and avoiding nose blowing. These practices speed the resolution of edema, which improves the ability to assess functional and esthetic deficits, improves intraoperative visualization, and reduces the need for retraction of orbital contents. The use of prophylactic antibiotics does not seem to be indicated.[14,15]

PREOPERATIVE CLINIC MANAGEMENT

Unless there are urgent issues related to the globe, the authors typically delay the first clinic visit until at least 5 days (typically 7–10 days) after injury. This delay allows the edema to resolve, making physical examination more effective and improving the ability to predict what the untreated globe position will be. Furthermore, as the edema decreases, early onset diplopia may resolve. Conversely, diplopia that was not present or identifiable at the initial examination because of edema of the orbital contents may become apparent in a delayed fashion.

At the initial clinic visit, patients are questioned regarding diplopia or other visual disturbances and whether they notice a difference in the position of the eye. A detailed physical examination of the face and eyes is performed. This examination includes visual acuity, a pupil examination, and assessment of extraocular muscle function. The presence of any diplopia (monocular or binocular) is noted, including the approximate location of binocular diplopia measured by degree of deviation from the horizon or midline (eg, 15°, 30°, or 45°). Complete absence of muscle function, such as adduction, suggests injury to a cranial nerve; neuro-ophthalmologic evaluation should be considered.

Function of sensory nerves in the periorbital region is also checked both to determine the extent of injury and to counsel patients before surgery.

The globe position is measured and noted. Hertel exophthalmometry is performed to measure the position of the globe (exophthalmometry value [EV]) relative to the lateral orbital rim (**Fig. 3**). Rather than using this measurement as an

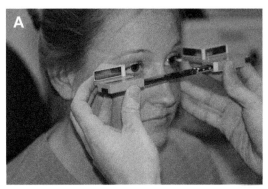
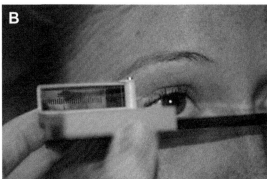

Fig. 3. Hertel exophthalmometry. (*A*) The instrument rests on the lateral orbital rims. (*B*) The farthest projection of the cornea is measured on the grid visible in the prism.

absolute value, the authors compare it with the normal side. The measurement can be confounded by abnormalities in bone or soft tissue overlying the lateral orbit, but it is nevertheless useful as a guide.

The difference in EV should be 2 mm or less between the eyes. If an exophthalmometer is not available, the projection of the eyes can be estimated by viewing from above and below. Any abnormality in eyelid position is documented. The function of the levator muscle and aponeurosis is measured from extreme down gaze to extreme upward gaze, while holding the brow stationary (there should be at least 5 mm of lid excursion).

If not already available, a fine-cut CT scan of the face protocoled for intraoperative navigation is obtained. The scans are reviewed for the location of the fracture, number of walls involved, and degree of herniation of orbital contents into the adjacent ethmoid and maxillary sinuses. Adjacent structures are evaluated for injury with special attention to the skull base and brain; the presence of pneumocephalus is a strong indicator of cerebrospinal fluid (CSF) leak, which would be addressed at the time of orbital surgery if indicated.

It is often suggested that the percentage of the orbital floor that is involved with the fracture should be noted with the recommendation that if it is greater than 50%, patients should undergo repair. As noted later, the authors do not follow this practice: it is not possible to conveniently measure the percentage of the floor that is fractured, as it is not visualized on a single CT image, and many patients with even larger fractures will have no functional compromise. More important than the percentage of the structure that is involved is whether the orbital support structure, particularly the periosteum, is left intact to prevent herniation of the orbital contents.

Photographic documentation is then performed when indicated, including views demonstrating globe projection (basal or superior views).

DECISION TO OPERATE

The decision to recommend surgery is based on the presence of an alteration in form and/or function manifesting as globe malposition or diplopia, respectively. There is no absolute indication for surgery, and the judgment is not made based on CT findings alone. **Fig. 4** demonstrates the CT

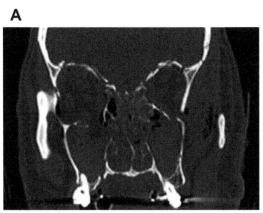
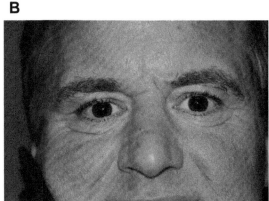

Fig. 4. Severe bilateral 4 wall orbital fractures. (*A*) Coronal CT. (*B*) Photograph demonstrating only mild asymmetry in globe position. The patient declined surgical intervention.

images and photograph of a man who sustained severe bilateral orbital fractures when he was ejected from a vehicle in a high-speed collision. Despite the CT findings of fractures of all the orbital bones and skull base, after resolution of the initial edema, he had only slight asymmetry of globe position with mild enophthalmos and hypoglobus on the right side. His initial diplopia resolved. Because the orbital asymmetry did not bother him, he elected not to undergo surgical reconstruction. Five months after the injury, he remained symptom free.

This example illustrates that increase in orbital volume associated with orbital fractures is variable.

In fact, there have been several attempts to use objective measurements and formulas to calculate the change in orbital volume without success.[16] Several studies have attempted to correlate size of fracture, location of fracture (naso-ethmoidal strut, posterior floor fractures), degree of orbital content displacement, and rounding of inferior rectus to predict the degree of enophthalmos or restriction with varying success.[16–19] Subsequent publications attempted to use computer modeling to calculate increase in orbital volume to predict the degree of enophthalmos. Correlations of volumetric increase relative to enophthalmos varied widely, from 0.4 mm to 0.8 mm of enophthalmos per 1-cm^3 increase in orbital volume.[20–22] Substratisfying the fracture based on location and calculating a ratio of native to increased orbital volume may be more predictive of patients requiring operative intervention but still has an imperfect correlation.[23] Orbital volume estimation becomes dramatically more complex in patients with multi-wall fractures. Despite the significant amount of research in this area, a clear-cut reproducible formula for predicting the degree of enophthalmos has not been accepted.

There are other factors as well to consider in the decision to operate, not the least of which is the occupational impact. For the professional athlete who depends on perfect binocular vision, the authors do not operate to correct globe malposition unless there is also diplopia that is not improving. For a lumberjack who works overhead, a small amount of diplopia in superior gaze might mandate surgical correction that would not be required for an undertaker.

Timing of surgery is important. Several publications have evaluated operating within 14 or 21 days of injury, concerned that rate of complication is higher in patients who have more delayed intervention. Conversely, when possible, the authors delay surgical correction until the edema

from the initial injury has resolved, which can often take 2 or 3 weeks. This delay increases the ability to displace the mobile orbital contents within the finite volume of unfractured orbital bones. This displacement creates a larger optical cavity, making it is easier to see the entire fracture site, retrieve the orbital contents from the paranasal sinuses, and accurately place and shape the implant. Restoration of the final orbital shape and volume is, thus, more accurate.

The presence of bilateral orbital fractures presents a unique challenge. In this situation, the authors' preferred technique of creating a mirror-image overlay (MIO) template (see later discussion) is ineffective for initial repair, given the lack of a normal contralateral bone structure to superimpose over the fracture site. When this is the case, the authors first repair the side with the least damage to critical reconstructive landmarks, such as the apex of the orbital floor and the orbital rims. They use navigation to aid in implant positioning and shaping and occasionally intraoperative CT scan if needed (mobile 3D radiographs can also be used). The authors then let the edema subside and obtain a new CT scan. With the new reference CT, a MIO can be created for reconstruction of the second orbit. In this manner, they are able to achieve postoperative bone symmetry, which, even if the bone position is not in the exact premorbid state, seems to achieve good outcomes in both globe position and resolution of diplopia (**Fig. 5**).

Another critical issue is the presence of other adjacent fractures. As noted earlier, the authors consider the orbital bones as consisting of the internal endoskeleton formed by the walls, floor, and roof and the exoskeleton formed by the orbital rims and nasal bone. It is essential to accurately reconstruct the exoskeleton before repairing the endoskeleton. If the orbital rims and zygomaticomaxillary complex are not in the correct position, the error will be propagated to the orbital bones when they are reconstructed. Because of this, they often elect to repair significant injuries of the exoskeleton first, let the surgical edema resolve, then return to the operating room at a later date to perform the endoskeletal reconstruction when it can be performed more accurately as described earlier. This staged reconstruction avoids issues with navigation error cause by edema or significant movement of the navigation reference points (which decreases the navigation utility during orbital repair). Although this can be overcome by obtaining an intraoperative CT scan and reregistering the navigation, this adds significantly to the time and complexity of the procedure.

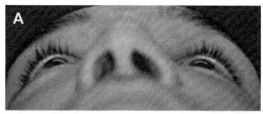

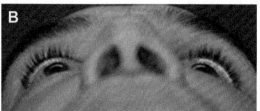

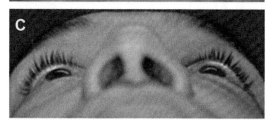

Fig. 5. Bilateral orbit fractures. (*A*) Right orbit has been repaired. Note hyperglobus from residual edema. (*B*) Edema has resolved from right orbit; patient is now ready for repair of left side, which is enophthalmic. (*C*) Left side has been repaired, enophthalmos resolved.

Although there are benefits to waiting to reconstruct the orbital endoskeleton, and there is no set point that is too long to wait (the authors have reconstructed orbits 10 years or more after injury), there can be drawbacks to a long delay in the reconstruction. If there is significant herniation of orbital contents into the adjacent sinus, the orbital fat and periosteum may scar down and adhere to those structures. Repositioning of the orbital contents is more challenging in this situation, and there can be damage and subsequent atrophy of the orbital fat leading to enophthalmos.

Given the complexity of the reconstruction, before proceeding with surgery it is critical to obtain informed consent through a detailed discussion with patients about the details of the procedure as well as its risks. The most common risks of the procedure are persistent temporary or permanent diplopia, persistent globe malposition, eyelid malposition, corneal abrasion, and postoperative retrobulbar hemorrhage that could require revision surgery. Although extremely rare, there is a risk of globe rupture and blindness.

SURGICAL TECHNIQUE

Meticulous surgical technique plays a critical role in the outcome of orbital reconstruction. This point is true in the placement of incisions to gain access to the orbit, in isolating the region of the fracture and reduction of orbital contents back into the orbit, and in the shaping and placement of the implant. Suboptimal performance of any of these tasks may lead to a poor functional and/or esthetic outcome, with a major impact on quality of life (**Figs. 6–9**).

Three technologic advances have had a profound influence on the authors' surgical outcomes:

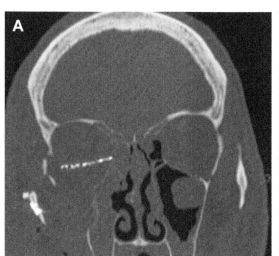

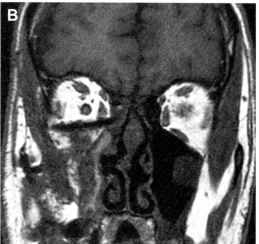

Fig. 6. (*A*) Coronal CT scan showing implant with improper position and shape in the central right orbit. (*B*) MRI demonstrating location of the implant between the inferior rectus muscle and the globe, with damage to the medial rectus muscle. The patient did not regain normal motion after correction of the implant surgery.

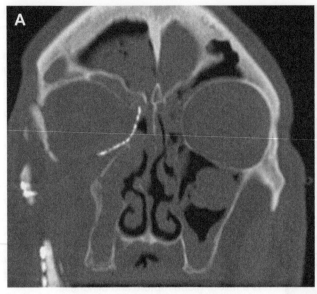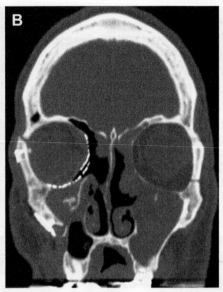

Fig. 7. (*A*) CT of implant that perforated skull base during placement causing CSF rhinorrhea; implant was undersized and placed in a nonanatomic medial position that obstructed frontal outflow tract causing sinusitis. Note pneumocephalus. (*B*) CSF leak repaired; new double implant anatomically placed, spanning the large defect while allowing normal frontal outflow function with clearance of frontal opacification.

A. Orbital endoscopy
B. Virtual surgical planning with mirror-image CT overlay
C. Navigation-guided implant placement and shaping

Orbital Endoscopy

Orbital endoscopy provides several major advantages over standard open approaches.[24] The lighting is improved, with reduced shadowing and blind spots; the image is significantly magnified; display of the image on video monitors allows the entire surgical team to assist more effectively and learn from the case; and less retraction of the orbital contents and eyelids is required (**Figs. 10** and **11**).

Orbital endoscopy is performed with standard sinus endoscopes or with smaller 3-mm diameter endoscopes. The latter allow increased space for instrumentation within the optical cavity. The orbital contents are gently retracted with malleable brain retractors, taking care not to

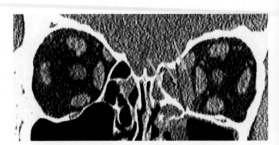

Fig. 8. CT demonstrating an undersized implant placed in an excessively lateral position, with the medial component protruding between the globe and the medial rectus. The implant failed to span the full defect in the medial wall, allowing herniation of orbital contents into the maxillary sinus. This herniation will result in recurrent sinusitis and orbital cellulitis.

Fig. 9. CT scan showing porous polyethylene implant placed to repair a left medial wall fracture more than a decade earlier. The patient developed multiple episodes of sinusitis and orbital cellulitis with persistent diplopia. Medial arrow: medial orbital wall displaced into the ethmoid sinus causing obstruction; center arrow: lucency indicating position of implant; lateral arrow: mucocele within the medial orbit.

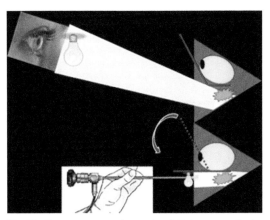

Fig. 10. Open versus endoscopic orbital surgery. Endoscopic approach moves light source from surgeon to orbit, allows reduced optical cavity with improved geometry, improves ability to visualize entire fracture site, and decreases the displacement of orbital content.

place excessive pressure on the globe. The cornea is protected with lubricating ointment, and the pupil is monitored throughout the procedure for enlargement or change in shape that suggests excessive pressure on the globe or ciliary ganglion. If this occurs, the pressure is taken off the globe until normal contours return. Typically, the assistant retracts the eyelid margin with a Ragnell retractor in one hand and the orbital contents with a conformed malleable retractor in the other hand (which is bent to allow decreased fulcrum and holding the retractor further from the incision). Without withdrawing the retractor, pressure on the retractors should be minimized at every opportunity. The surgeon holds the endoscope in one hand and dissects in a subperiosteal plane using a suction Freer elevator in the other

hand. (It is helpful to attach the Freer with a length of silicon rubber (Silastic) tubing, which is more compliant and easier to maneuver than standard suction tubing.) In this fashion, the periorbita is lifted off the orbital bone over the complete anatomic structure that is involved. Once this is achieved, the orbital contents are meticulously dissected out of the fracture site, taking care to preserve as much of the involved periorbita as possible, avoiding damage to the orbital fat and muscles. The excellent lighting and magnification provided by endoscopy are highly beneficial for this (**Fig. 12**).

Virtual Surgical Planning with Mirror-Image Overlay

MIO is another aid that plays a critical role in the authors' method of posttraumatic and oncologic orbital reconstruction[25] that helps by providing virtual anatomic landmarks. With this technique, the CT scan is uploaded in typical fashion into the navigation system. The same scan is then uploaded again but this time in mirror image (left over right). This image is then reduced to the anatomic area of interest, colored to distinguish it from the original, and then superimposed over the original CT (**Figs. 13** and **14**). In the authors' initial report of this technique, they studied 113 consecutive cases and found a significant decrease in postoperative diplopia using this method. This finding was particularly true with more severe fractures. By using this technique for severe 3- and 4-wall fractures, they reduced the need for revision surgery from 20% to 4%. As their experience with this technology has increased, their outcomes have continued to improve. An example of the symmetry that can be obtained with this technique is demonstrated in **Fig. 15**. An additional use of this advanced

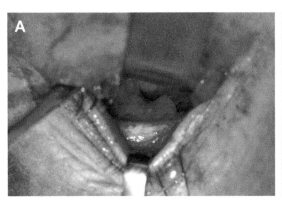
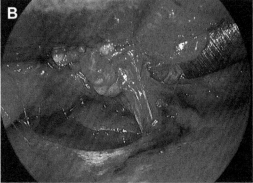

Fig. 11. Open versus endoscopic fracture visualization. (*A*) Open approach. (*B*) Endoscopic approach demonstrating internal lighting, magnification, and panoramic view improving ability to visualize the entire fracture as well as orbital contents entrapped within the floor fracture.

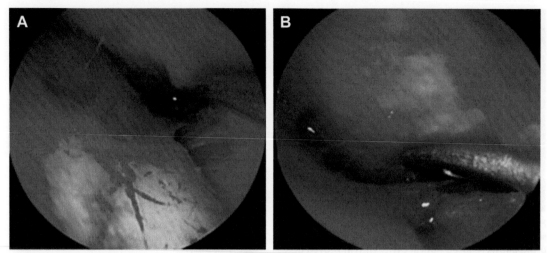

Fig. 12. Lighting, magnification, and exposure achievable with orbital endoscopy. Note fracture of left medial wall and floor. (*A*) Medial wall and floor, suction Freer elevator raising orbital contents. (*B*) Visualization of apex of orbital floor for placement of implant; this region is challenging to view with open approach but critical to repair for an optimal outcome.

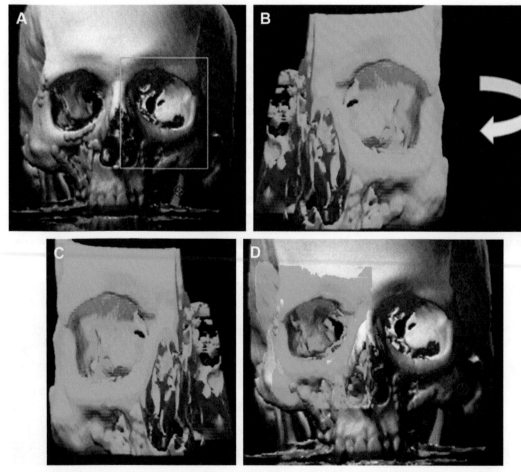

Fig. 13. MIO. (*A*) Navigation-guidance CT for revision surgery, area to be mirrored. (*B*) Mirror area colored and (*C*) reversed in mirror image. (*D*) Mirrored area fused with original scan provides template for reconstruction of the orbital and adjacent bone.

A   B

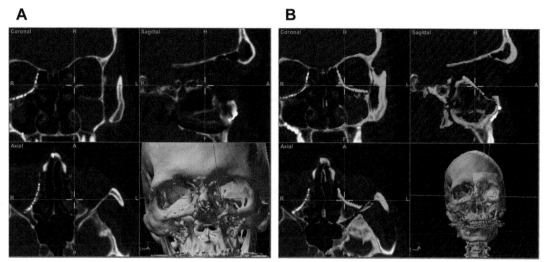

Fig. 14. MIO navigation. Panfacial fractures, with bilateral orbital floor and medial wall fractures. (*A*) The right orbit was repaired earlier and will be used as a template. (*B*) MIO template colored green, superimposed over fractures. Implant is then placed, and navigation is performed on all aspects of its surface to compare it with the contralateral side for shape and position. Crossed lines indicate position of navigation instrument tip. After adjustment, navigation confirms conformity with surgical plan.

technology is for planning approaches. For example, when approaching a fracture in the region adjoining the orbital floor and medial wall, either a medial or inferior approach could be used. The choice of approaches in this case can actually be aided by navigation vector analysis at the beginning of the procedure by using the vector propagation feature built into the manufacturer's software. This feature is particularly useful when treating fractures of the medial wall that approach the optic nerve or for orbital apex or/optic nerve decompression. Fractures of the orbital roof that include injury to the frontal lobe of the brain are another indication for this type of planning and intraoperative navigation, particularly if there is a component of subdural hemorrhage.

Navigation-Guided Implant Placement and Shaping

In addition to the aforementioned benefits of using virtual surgical planning, navigation-guided surgery can also be of significant benefit in improving the accuracy of implant placement and shaping. With moderate to severe fractures, particularly those involving multiple regions, it can be difficult to determine whether the orbital contents have been fully repositioned with the construct, whether the posterior edge of the fracture has been bridged, and whether the implant is a safe distance from the optic nerve. Once an orbital implant is in place, the authors, therefore, navigate along its entire surface to confirm its position. They also note any changes in shape that are

necessary. To adjust the shape, they use a small right-angle instrument similar to a nerve hook (the Browne Hook) to make corrections in situ, without removing the implant, under endoscopic visualization. They then renavigate the implant to confirm that the desired contouring has been achieved.

Although there have been multiple reports that advocate the use of intraoperative imaging to confirm that the orbital implant is in appropriate position, the use of MIO has nearly eliminated the need for intraoperative imaging in the authors' practice.

SURGICAL APPROACH AND REPAIR

The basic steps of orbital reconstruction are similar for each anatomic region of the orbit. The pupils are checked at the beginning of surgery to note their size, shape, and symmetry to allow monitoring for change during the procedure. Asymmetric change in the pupil during surgery suggests increased intraocular pressure or excessive retraction of the orbital contents and mandates temporary removal of instrumentation from the orbit until normalization occurs. A tarsorrhaphy placed at the lateral limbus on the nonoperated eye allows for frequent visual reference of the normal pupil while still keeping the cornea protected. Ophthalmic lubricant is placed and maintained over both corneas. Extraocular motion is checked using forced ductions at the beginning and end of the surgical case.

The authors perform Hertel exophthalmometry with patients under anesthetic at the beginning of

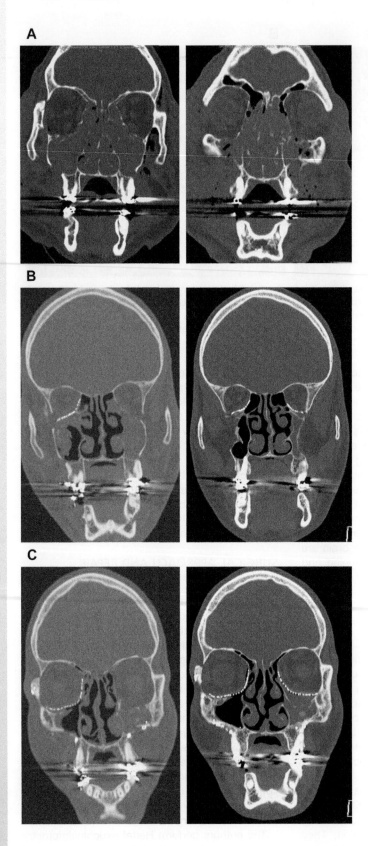

Fig. 15. Outcomes with MIO. (A) Bilateral severe orbital fractures involving the medial and lateral walls and floor. (B) Right orbit has been repaired with navigation guidance. (C) Left orbit has been repaired using MIO (see Fig. 14) of right side over left for reconstruction guide. Note the symmetry between the right and left reconstructions.

the operation to note the degree of asymmetry in globe position and again at the end of the procedure to determine how much the globe has advance and its position relative to the contralateral side. Because of intraoperative (or unresolved preoperative) edema, if the globe is not at least 2 mm proptotic when the reconstruction is complete, there is a significant likelihood that the restoration is not anatomic and postoperative enophthalmos and hypoglobus may result.

The incision and surgical approaches are chosen based on the quadrant of the orbit that is affected. The approaches to the medial and lateral walls and floor are transconjunctival; the approach to the roof is transcutaneous as noted later.

Orbital Roof Fractures

To access the orbital roof, the authors use a blepharoplasty approach through an incision in the upper lid crease.[26,27] A preseptal dissection is performed, raising a skin-orbicularis muscle flap to the orbital rim. Care is taken to preserve the supraorbital and supratrochlear neurovascular pedicles as they course inferior to or through the rim (**Fig. 16**).

At the superior orbital rim, the periosteum is incised and the dissection continues onto the orbital roof, elevating the plane between the bone and periorbita. Once the dissection has proceeded several millimeters into the orbit, endoscopic visualization is begun and dissection is performed with a suction Freer elevator. Dissection proceeds around the bone fragments to

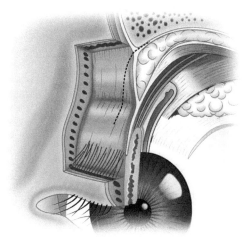

Fig. 16. Upper eyelid, skin, and orbicularis muscle removed. Dotted line demonstrates dissection plane to orbital rim, where the periosteum is incised and the plane between the orbital roof and periorbita is dissected.

visualize the adjacent bone. The fragments are then repositioned or removed depending on the degree of fragmentation and ability to maintain the bone in its repositioned site without fixation. If removed, care must be taken to dissect the dura from the superior surface of the bone. If the bone is removed, the dura is repositioned and devitalized brain is gently debrided as needed. The area is then resurfaced with allogenic dermis or dura substitute as desired (**Fig. 17**). Rigid reconstruction of this region is not required, and the authors typically avoid its use to prevent pressure on the levator muscle. The authors occasionally resurface the orbital roof with resorbable 0.25-mm polydioxanone (PDS) foil to avoid soft tissue catching on the overlying bone, particularly if there is a large defect into the floor of the frontal sinus (**Fig. 18**). The wound is then closed in 2 layers, with 6-0 resorbable sutures to reapproximate the orbicularis muscle and then the skin. If a CSF leak was repaired, the authors use a water-tight closure with running permanent suture.[28]

Medial Wall Fractures

Fractures of the medial wall are approached through a precaruncular incision[29] (**Fig. 19**). A precaruncular incision is preferred over a transcaruncular incision for improved healing and an optimal dissection plane on the deep surface of the posterior limb of the medial canthal tendon. Until the surgeon is experienced with the approach, lacrimal probes are placed into the canaliculi for protection and a corneal protector is placed on the lubricated cornea. The caruncle is grasped with forceps and gently lateralized, and a Westcott scissor is used to make an incision through the conjunctiva at the medial aspect of the caruncle. The scissor is then spread, entering the plane on the deep surface of the posterior limb of the medial canthal tendon. The incision is lengthened inferiorly into the inferior fornix (see the discussion on orbital floor approach later) to increase the surgical access. The incision can be extended superiorly for only a few millimeters because of the risk of damage to the superior fornix. Following this blunt dissection, the lamina papyracea is reached where a subperiosteal plane is entered under endoscopic visualization. The periosteum is then elevated from the medial wall, and the ethmoid arteries are cauterized with bipolar forceps and divided as needed. After visualization of the entire wall and optic nerve as indicated, the orbital contents are reduced out of the ethmoid sinuses, the fractured bone is repositioned or removed in order to prevent delayed sinus complications (**Figs. 20** and **21**), and an implant is placed. For very small

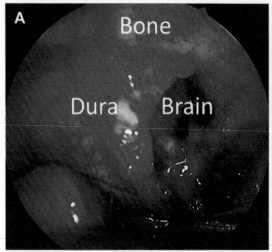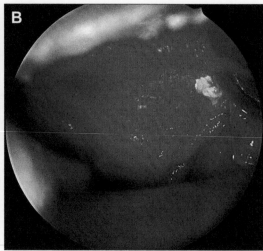

Fig. 17. Fracture of orbital roof. (*A*) Malleable retractor displacing orbital contents inferiorly; bone fragments have been removed revealing dura and defect in frontal lobe. (*B*) Dural matrix placed over bone defect.

fractures, the authors use a resorbable PDS foil, in 0.25-mm thickness. For larger defects, they use a thin titanium orbital implant mesh. This mesh is implanted and positioned and navigated with MIO to confirm that the position and shape are anatomic. The implant is then surfaced on its orbital side with 0.25-mm PDS sheet to prevent herniation of orbital fat through the titanium and provide a glide surface in case of contact with the orbital musculature. All aspects of the implant are inspected to confirm that the optic nerve is not compressed and there is no entrapment of orbital contents deep to the implant. Forced ductions are performed to confirm normal muscle

Fig. 18. Orbital roof reconstruction. Appearance looking from above downward through frontal sinus on PDS foil placed transorbital in the left orbital roof. View through endoscope placed into left frontal sinus through contralateral (*right*) orbital approach.

excursion and meticulous hemostasis is assured. The incision does not need to be closed. If the caruncle does not sit in the correct position, a single 6-0 fast-absorbing suture can be placed between the caruncle and medial skin to maintain it until the edema resolves.

Orbital Floor Fractures

Fractures of the orbital floor are approached through a transconjunctival inferior fornix incision. Although there are several alternative approaches, we prefer this approach as it protects the orbital septum and avoids postoperative lid retraction[30] (**Fig. 22**). This incision can be connected with the medial and lateral approaches as needed.

The cornea is protected with a lubricated clear corneal protector, and the lower lid is retracted anteriorly with Ragnell retractors. The incision is made at least 3 mm inferior to the tarsus, through orbital fat directly to the inferior orbital rim. Medially, the incision can be carried into a precaruncular incision as described earlier. Laterally, it can be connected with a lateral retro-canthal approach (see later discussion) or canthotomy/cantholysis incision. The periosteum of the orbital rim is incised, the periorbita is raised, and the dissection continues over the orbital floor with endoscopic visualization. Care is made to protect the infraorbital nerve may run inferior, within or above the orbital floor and is often involved with the fracture. If the fracture is large, the ligamentous attachments of the lateral portion of the inferior orbital fissure can be divided. Similarly, dissection can continue up the medial wall depending on the site and extent of the fracture. Dissection is performed circumferentially around the fracture before dissecting the

A

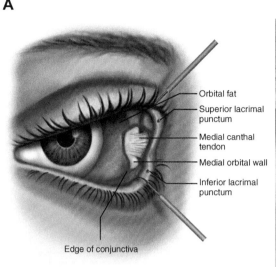

Orbital fat

Superior lacrimal punctum

Medial canthal tendon

Medial orbital wall

Inferior lacrimal punctum

Edge of conjunctiva

B

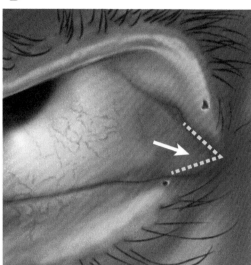

Fig. 19. (*A*) Anatomy of right precaruncular approach demonstrating posterior limb of medial canthal tendon, which is followed to the bone of the medial orbital wall. (*B*) Right precaruncular approach. Arrow indicates caruncle; dotted lines demonstrate incision.

orbital contents out of the maxillary sinus. Similar to medial wall fractures, the position of the bone fragments should be considered with regard to risk of future sinus complications and removed or repositioned as indicated. The orbital contents can be temporarily held in position using a variety of materials, including malleable retractors, PDS foil, Silastic sheeting, or saline-soaked cotton pledgets. The implant is then placed (thin titanium mesh),

positioned, and shaped. Once the implant is placed as desired, navigation is performed against the MIO template. The position and shape are then adjusted in situ until the implant is correct, matching the anatomy of the contralateral orbit. The implant is then lined with PDS foil as described earlier. For most fractures, when the implant is contoured to

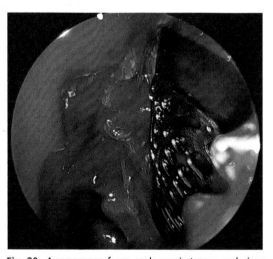

Fig. 20. Appearance from endoscopic transnasal view of left medial wall fracture after placement of implant through precaruncular approach. PDS foil (*blue*) is placed between the orbital contents and the implant. The PDS can bridge small gaps between the adjacent bone and the implant.

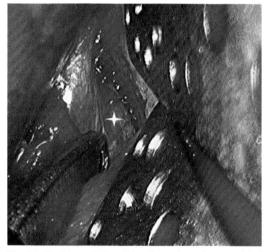

Fig. 21. Right medial wall implant viewed transorbital before placement of PDS foil. Note the proximity of the optic nerve (*star*) entering the optic canal at the tip of the suction Freer, just beyond the implant. It is essential to visualize all regions of the implant to be certain that it is not contacting critical structures or entrapping orbital contents before completing the procedure.

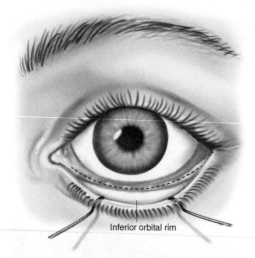

Fig. 22. Inferior deep fornix approach. The lid is retracted anteriorly, and the incision is made through orbital fat directly onto the inferior orbital rim.

fit the premorbid shape, it will sit within the orbit well supported by the adjacent bone. For large fractures, however, when significant bone gaps are spanned by the implant, it will require fixation to stable bone with 1 or 2 screws. The authors prefer self-drilling 3- or 4-mm screws for this, placed in the inferior orbital rim if possible. Endoscopy is used to examine the entire construct to eliminate the possibility of entrapment of the orbital contents under the implant. It is worth noting that anterior fixation of the orbital reconstruction plate can often cantilever the posterior aspect if it is not conformed exactly to the small inferior ledge on the back of the rim. This inadvertently elevates the back of the plate directly towards the optic nerve, and may not be well appreciated on direct visual examination.

The orbital floor is the region of the orbit with the highest anatomic variability. Although many patients have a spoon-shaped floor with a rise posteriorly in the apex, others are flatter in this region. It is critical to examine the contralateral (atraumatic) orbit to ascertain patients' individual contouring and match that on the reconstructed side. MIO is extremely helpful in this region and can provide individualized, highly accurate reconstruction.

The authors do not typically close the conjunctival incision after repair of orbital floor fractures. They do place gentle superior traction on the lower eyelid to prevent vertical overlap of the lamellae and check forced ductions to ensure normal muscular function. As described earlier, the authors complete the case by checking the globe position with exophthalmometry, expecting 2 to 3 mm of proptosis relative to the opposite globe. This typically resolves gradually over several weeks, depending on the size of the fracture (**Fig. 23**).

Lateral Wall Fractures

Fractures of the lateral orbital wall are very common as a component of zygomaticomaxillary complex fractures. In this case, the fracture proceeds from the frontozygomatic suture inferiorly to join

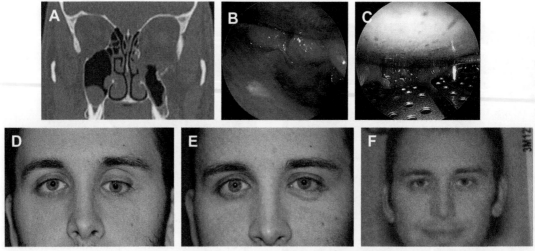

Fig. 23. A 28-year-old man presented with diplopia, enophthalmos, and hypoglobus after 2 repairs of extensive left orbital floor and medial wall fracture. Top row: (*A*) Coronal CT demonstrating appearance before correction, with Silastic implant in place. (*B*) Medial aspect of orbital floor fracture, Silastic removed, viewing into maxillary sinus. (*C*) Titanium mesh implant in place, in situ adjustment being performed with right angle hook to match with MIO virtual template. Bottom row: (*D*) Prerevision view. (*E*) Postoperative view: diplopia, enophthalmos, and hypoglobus resolved. Note the mild relative ptosis of the left upper eyelid creating visible asymmetry. (*F*) Preinjury driver's license photograph demonstrating that the ptosis in postoperative photograph existed before the original injury.

the orbital floor fracture (**Fig. 24**). In these cases, the lateral orbit is repositioned en bloc with the zygoma. They typically perform a lateral orbitotomy to check the alignment of these bones, but an implant is rarely needed in this region. Occasionally, with high-impact trauma, a fracture of the greater wing of the sphenoid bone may occur with compression of the orbital contents or impaction of bone fragments into the lateral rectus muscle. In these cases, decompression with removal of bone may be required. When bone is removed in this region, the authors place a layer of thin PDS foil across the bone defect to prevent adhesion between the orbital contents and the temporalis muscle in the infratemporal fossa.

There are 2 types of incisions to access the lateral orbital wall: a canthotomy with cantholysis or a canthal-sparing lateral retro-canthal approach.[31] Although a canthotomy and cantholysis approach provides excellent access, careful canthal reconstruction is required to prevent postoperative dehiscence and eyelid malposition or lateral canthal blunting as seen in **Fig. 25**. The lateral retro-canthal approach places the incision behind (or internal) to the lateral canthus and avoids this complication by preserving the lateral retinaculum, but exposure to the orbital floor is somewhat more limited (**Fig. 26**).

As described earlier, the authors use an endoscopic technique to lift the periorbita off the lateral orbital wall. The wall is exposed from the orbital roof to the inferior orbital fissure. For fractures extending to the orbital floor, the contents of the lateral aspect of the inferior fissure are ligated with bipolar forceps and divided, allowing extended exposure onto the orbital floor. Dissecting deeper toward the orbital apex, the superior fissure will be

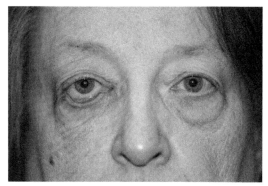

Fig. 25. Postoperative dehiscence of the lateral cantholysis leading to rounding of the canthus, canthal dystopia, and ectropion.

encountered at its confluence with the inferior fissure. The contents of the superior fissure, as noted earlier, include cranial nerves and should not be disturbed. After adequate exposure, the fracture fragments are then repositioned or removed, and the defect resurfaced with PDS foil as needed. The incision does not require closure unless a canthotomy and cantholysis were performed, in which case the authors reapproximate the inferior limb of the lateral canthal tendon to the superior limb using 5-0 monofilament resorbable suture.

Choice of Reconstruction Material

The authors choice of reconstructive materials varies based on the location and severity of fracture. There are several different types of materials suitable for reconstruction, including absorbable, nonabsorbable, porous and nonporous, bare titanium, and coated titanium. In general, they prefer thin titanium 3D orbital implants

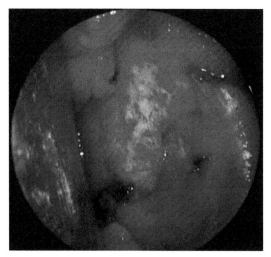

Fig. 24. Endoscopic view of left lateral orbital wall fracture after repositioning of bone fragments.

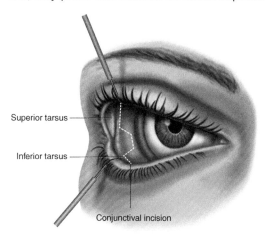

Superior tarsus

Inferior tarsus

Conjunctival incision

Fig. 26. The lateral retro-canthal approach in a right orbit. This conjunctival incision provides access to the lateral orbit without damage to lateral canthal tendon or lower eyelid support.

lined by PDS foil to provide a glide surface. A nonadherent surface is important in case of muscle contact, and use of a layer superficial to the titanium prevents herniation of fat through the mesh (which may also be a cause of muscle dysfunction) (**Fig. 27**). When the PDS resorbs, a thin nonadherent layer is left behind. Titanium implants have been particularly effective in reconstruction of more than 1 orbital surface (eg, orbital floor and medial wall or 3 wall fractures) to preserve orbital contour shape the orbital volume long-term. The authors avoid the use of porous polyethylene (PPE) implants when the implant is exposed to sinus cavity because of a lifelong risk of infection.

POSTOPERATIVE CARE

Patients are asked to use iced saline sponges or covered ice packs 20 minutes per hour for 48 hours after surgery. For patients with significant proptosis, the authors often prescribe a short course of oral steroids. If there is significant risk for significant postoperative chemosis, such as after repair of the orbital floor and both walls, the authors often place a temporary tarsorrhaphy suture at the lateral limbus until most of the chemosis resolves. The pupil can still be examined with this suture in place. Patients are seen in the clinic 7 and 14 days after surgery, then 6 weeks, 3 months, and 6 months after surgery.

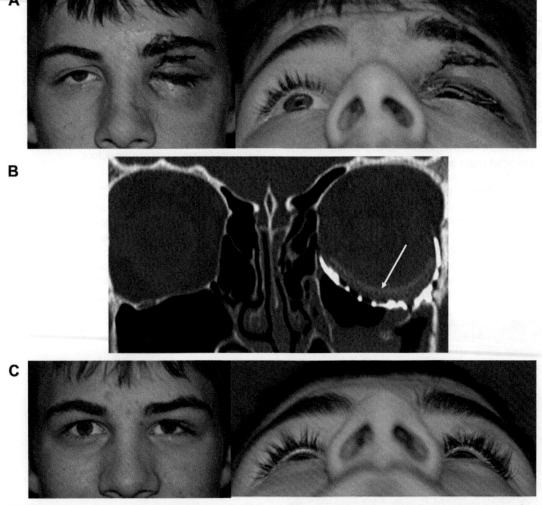

Fig. 27. A 14-year-old bull rider: left orbit impaled through the upper eyelid by a bull's horn causing severe fractures of the medial wall, floor, and lateral wall. (*A*) Preoperative appearance, 9 days after injury after significant resolution of edema. Note severe enophthalmos and levator injury preventing raising of the upper eyelid. Surgery was 17 days after injury, requiring double orbital implants to span the defect, using MIO guidance. (*B*) CT appearance 2 weeks after surgery. Arrow demonstrates PDS foil lining the implant before resorption. (*C*) appearance 1 year later, ptosis nearly resolved, Hertel exophthalmometry demonstrating symmetric globe position, diplopia resolved within 45° of central gaze.

Postoperative CT scans are not obtained unless there is concern of a possible complication. Hertel exophthalmometry is obtained at every clinic visit and compared with the measurements taken at the beginning and conclusion of surgery unless there are adjacent bone abnormalities that prevent accurate measurement.

When most of the surgical edema has resolved, patients are asked to begin mild physical therapy. This therapy includes gentle massage of the lower eyelid and exaggerated tight eye closure and opening (to keep the orbicularis oculi from retracting and/or tethering). If range-of-motion exercises are indicated, the authors ask patients to perform a full range of extraocular motions tracking their index finger (arm fully extended, head still) both vertically and horizontally to the extremes of gaze. This exercise should be done several times daily.

SURGICAL OUTCOMES

Outcome analysis in orbital reconstruction is challenging to perform and interpret because of the number of structures involved in the injury and disparity in reporting. The structures that may be involved in the injury include the eyelids and their support structures, the lacrimal system, the globe, the extraocular muscles and their corresponding motor nerves, the optic nerve, the orbital bones, and potentially the brain. Injury to most of these structures can have significant impact on postoperative outcomes. Yet the surgery that the authors perform in the initial setting (aside from repair of globe injuries by the ophthalmologist) is largely limited to the closure of lacerations and repair of fractures. Thus, a significant orbit fracture may result in damage to the adjacent fat, muscle, and nerves; but the surgery will restore only the bone alignment and orbital volume. Therefore, when evaluating postoperative results, it can be difficult to determine whether, and to what extent, a deficit is due to the initial injury versus suboptimal surgical technique.

In the postoperative setting, globe position, visual acuity, and degree of diplopia should be measured. Analysis of globe position and visual acuity are relatively straightforward; but diplopia, for the reasons discussed earlier, can be challenging to measure. Ophthalmologists often quantify diplopia with the use of prisms, but this is complex and less practical for other specialists. The authors' practice is to examine muscle function to rule out entrapment and note the degree at which diplopia occurs in each direction (15°, 30°, or 45° off neutral gaze). Some degree of binocular diplopia may be normal in the uninjured state, particularly at extremes of gaze, and is to be expected after fracture repair. There is disagreement on the amount, however; patients are seldom aware of their premorbid status. Various reporting methods have evaluated outcomes based on the presence of diplopia in primary gaze, 30° or 45°, or whether prism correction was required. The authors evaluate their outcomes based on the presence of diplopia within 45°. When patients complain of diplopia within this range 6 or more months after surgery, the authors obtain a CT scan to confirm proper implant position and contour and consider referral to a neuro-ophthalmologist for further evaluation. Monocular diplopia suggests injury to the globe and is an indication for referral to an ophthalmologist whenever it is discovered.

Although postoperative globe position is influenced primarily by bone and implant position, fat atrophy may occur after the injury and may also contribute to asymmetry. The degree of fat atrophy probably increases with the severity of injury, but this is challenging to quantify on imaging. The question may arise regarding intentional overcorrection of bone defect repair at the time of surgery, and some degree of this occurs when thicker PPE-coated implants are used. Given that the degree of fat atrophy cannot be measured or anticipated, the authors strive for exact restoration of premorbid bone anatomy and do not overcorrect. For patients with apparent postoperative orbital volume asymmetry despite appropriate anatomic correction, eyelid position should be carefully checked as ptosis or lid retraction can create an illusion of abnormal globe position. Patients should also be asked for a preoperative photograph (a driver's license may be sufficient) to evaluate for preexisting asymmetry unnoticed by patients, as seen in **Fig. 23**.

In the authors' experience, the surgical outcomes depend on the mechanism, severity, and extent of injury, as expected.[25] It is not reasonable to expect that all patients will be corrected to their premorbid state with normal vision and no diplopia because of the frequent presence of at least minimal neuromuscular damage. A reasonable goal, however, should be restoration of symmetric orbital contours and volume, using an implant that allows normal extraocular muscle function and has the lowest possible chance of future infection.

In a study of 113 consecutive patients with severe orbital fractures, the authors found that by using the techniques presented in this article (including orbital endoscopy, MIO, and intraoperative navigation), they achieved a statistically significant reduction in postoperative diplopia and a 4-fold reduction in their revision rate relative to historical controls. The outcomes in globe position were also markedly improved.[25]

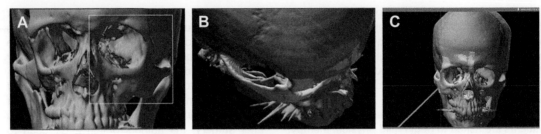

Fig. 28. Navigation-guided surgery and MIO in zygomatic and maxillary fractures. (*A*) right zygomaticomaxillary complex fracture, yellow square outlining normal anatomy for templating. (*B*) Oblique view, MIO in yellow. Note the deviation of the zygomatic arch. (*C*) after closed repositioning of the bone fragments, navigation is performed along the reconstruction to confirm accurate anatomic reduction. (*Blue line* represents navigation instrument on bone.)

COMPLICATIONS

The most common complications after orbital fracture repair are persistent globe malposition, diplopia, and sensory disturbance of the infraorbital nerve (numbness or worsening pain). Other complications include upper eyelid ptosis, lower eyelid malposition (entropion, ectropion, or cicatricial retraction), implant infection requiring removal and replacement, sinusitis, orbital

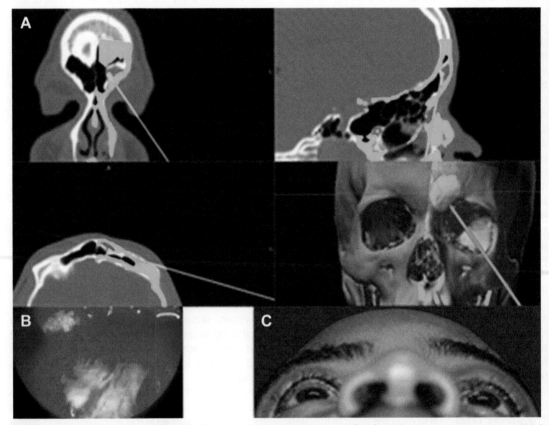

Fig. 29. (*A*) Fracture anterior table left frontal sinus, endoscopic transorbital repair. Green areas represent MIO plan over area of fracture. Blue line represents navigation instrument demonstrating surgical approach. The fracture is repaired endoscopically through a blepharoplasty approach through the floor of the frontal sinus. The fracture is reduced, and the bone is then navigated to confirm accurate reduction. (*B*) Endoscopic view using trans-orbital approach into the frontal sinus showing dissolvable packing supporting the reduced anterior table fragment. (*C*) Inferior view showing total resolution of bony indentation with a small amount of residual postoperative edema (7 days after injury).

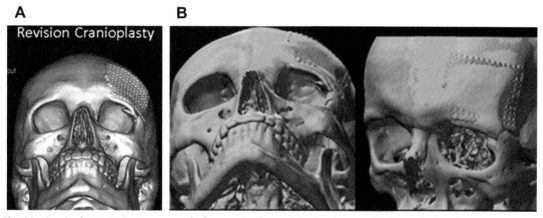

Fig. 30. Cranioplasty. Patient presented after cranioplasty with titanium mesh, dissatisfied with appearance. (A) Preoperative 3D CT scan. (B) Preoperative MIO surgical analysis; green areas represent overlay of contralateral normal structures. Note the areas of asymmetry, with overcorrection of the temporal region and undercorrection of the frontal bone. Patient underwent correction according to the plan, augmenting the construct with hydroxy-apatite cement.

cellulitis or abscess, CSF leak, diminished visual acuity, retrobulbar hemorrhage, and blindness. All of these issues, with the exception of implant infection, may be caused by the original injury as well.

Retrobulbar hemorrhage, in which patients present with worsening pain, proptosis, and decreasing visual acuity, is a surgical emergency. In this setting, lateral canthotomy and cantholysis should be performed immediately to relieve the intraocular pressure, while obtaining an ophthalmology consultation. Postoperative blindness is an extremely rare complication and demands an emergent ophthalmology evaluation with orbital exploration or radiographic imaging as indicated.

APPLICATION OF ENDOSCOPY, MIRROR-IMAGE OVERLAY, AND NAVIGATION TO OTHER TYPES OF CRANIOFACIAL RECONSTRUCTION

The techniques of endoscopic visualization, MIO planning, and navigation-guided reconstruction are applicable to related deformities that often occur in conjunction with orbital fractures. These applications include repair of zygomaticomaxillary fractures (**Fig. 28**), correction of frontal sinus and frontal bone fractures (**Fig. 29**), cranioplasty (**Fig. 30**), and navigation-guided rhinoplasty (**Fig. 31**). The authors have found that the use of these minimally disruptive techniques has decreased the extent and number of

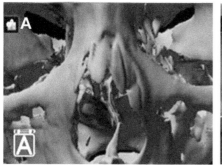
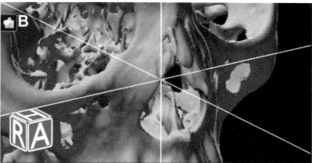

Fig. 31. Navigation-guide rhinoplasty: complex nasal fracture with esthetic and functional deformity. (A) 3D CT scan. (B) Navigation-guided osteotomies to mobilize fracture bone, allowing anatomic reconstruction of nasal bones. Navigation is used to mark the course of the osteotomies on the skin; the osteotomy is then created with a navigated osteotome with real-time monitoring similar to a global positioning system. Blue crosshairs indicate position of the tip of the osteotome as the right lateral osteotomy is begun.

incisions and amount of dissection that are needed and increased the accuracy of their reconstruction. This combination of techniques has provided a significant decrease in postoperative morbidity and a more rapid return of normal function.

REFERENCES

1. Yadav K, Cowan E, Wall S, et al. Orbital fracture clinical decision rule development: burden of disease and use of a mandatory electronic survey instrument. Acad Emerg Med 2011;18(3): 313–6.
2. Martinez AY, Como JJ, Vacca M, et al. Trends in maxillofacial trauma: a comparison of two cohorts of patients at a single institution 20 years apart. J Oral Maxillofac Surg 2014;72(4):750–4.
3. Kühnel TS, Reichert TE. Trauma of the midface. GMS Curr Top Otorhinolaryngol Head Neck Surg 2015;14:Doc06.
4. Puljula J, Cygnel H, Mäkinen E, et al. Mild traumatic brain injury diagnosis frequently remains unrecorded in subjects with craniofacial fractures. Injury 2012;43(12):2100–4.
5. Jelks GW, La Trentra G. Orbital fractures. In: Foster CA, Sherman JE, editors. Surgery of facial bone fractures. 17th edition. New York: Churchill Livingston; 1987. p. 67–91.
6. Ko MJ, Morris CK, Kim JW, et al. Orbital fractures: national inpatient trends and complications. Ophthal Plast Reconstr Surg 2013;29(4):298–303.
7. Joshi R, Johnson M, Willmore K, et al. Does sinus surgery increase the risk of orbital fractures in patients? Faseb J 2016;30(1 Supplement 1040.5).
8. Nagasao T, Miyamoto J, Nagasao M, et al. The effect of striking angle on the buckling mechanism in blowout fracture. Plast Reconstr Surg 2006;117(7): 2373–80.
9. Ahmad F, Kirkpatrick NA, Lyne J, et al. Buckling and hydraulic mechanisms in orbital blowout fractures: fact or fiction? J Craniofac Surg 2006;17(3): 438–41.
10. Rhee JS, Kilde J, Yoganadan N, et al. Orbital blowout fractures: experimental evidence for the pure hydraulic theory. Arch Facial Plast Surg 2002; 4(2):98–101.
11. Berens AM, Davis GE, Moe KS. Transorbital endoscopic identification of supernumerary ethmoid arteries. Allergy Rhinol (Providence) 2016;7(3):144–6.
12. Joseph JM, Glavas IP. Orbital fractures: a review. Clin Ophthalmol 2011;5:95–100.
13. Kikkawa DO, Lemke BN. Orbital and eyelid anatomy. In: Dortzback RK, editor. Ophthalmic plastic surgery: prevention and management of complications. New York: Raven Press; 1994. p. 1–29.
14. Doerr TD. Evidence based facial fracture management. Facial Plast Surg Clin North Am 2015;23: 335–45.
15. Wang JJ, Koterwas JM, Bedrossian EH, et al. Practice patterns in the use of prophylactic antibiotics following nonoperative orbital fractures. Clin Ophthalmol 2016;10:2129–33.
16. Hawes MJ, Dortzbach RK. Surgery on orbital floor fractures. Influence of time of repair and fracture size. Ophthalmology 1983;90:1066–70.
17. Harris GJ, Garcia GH, Logani SC, et al. Orbital blowout fractures: correlation of preoperative computed tomography and postoperative ocular motility. Trans Am Ophthalmol Soc 1998;96:347–53.
18. Higashino T, Hirabayashi S, Eguchi T, et al. Straightforward factors for predicting the prognosis of blow-out fractures. J Craniofac Surg 2001;22: 1210–4.
19. Schouman T, Courvoisier DS, Van Issum C, et al. Can systemic computed tomographic scan assessment predict treatment decision in pure orbital floor blowout fractures? J Oral Maxillofac Surg 2012;70: 1627–32.
20. Fan X, Li J, Zhu J, et al. Computer-assisted orbital volume measurement in the surgical correction of late enophthalmos caused by blowout fractures. Ophthal Plast Reconstr Surg 2003;19:207–11.
21. Whitehouse RW, Batterbury M, Jackson A, et al. Prediction of enophthalmos by computed tomography after 'blow out' orbital fracture. Br J Ophthalmol 1994;78(8):618–20.
22. Raskin EM, Millman AL, Lubkin V, et al. Prediction of late enophthalmos by volumetric analysis of orbital fractures. Ophthal Plast Reconstr Surg 1998;14: 19–26.
23. Choi SH, Kang DH, Gu JH. The correlation between the orbital volume ratio and enophthalmos in unoperated blowout fractures. Arch Plast Surg 2016;43(6): 518–22.
24. Balakrishnan K, Moe KS. Applications and outcomes of orbital and transorbital endoscopic surgery. Otolaryngol Head Neck Surg 2011;144(5): 815–20.
25. Bly RA, Chang SH, Cudejkova M, et al. Computer-guided orbital reconstruction to improve outcomes. Facial Plast Surg 2013;15(2):113–20.
26. Moe KS, Bergeron CM, Ellenbogen RG. Transorbital neuroendoscopic surgery. Neurosurgery 2010; 67(3):ons16–28.
27. Ellenbogen RG, Moe KS. Transorbital neuroendoscopic approaches to the anterior cranial fossa. In: Snyderman C, editor. Skull base surgery. Philadelphia: Walters Kluwer; 2015. p. 151–64.
28. Moe KS, Kim LJ, Bergeron CM. Transorbital endoscopic repair of complex cerebrospinal fluid leaks. Laryngoscope 2011;121:13–30.

29. Moe KS. The precaruncular approach to the medial orbit. Arch Facial Plast Surg 2003;5: 483–7.

30. Moe KS, Ellenbogen RG. Transorbital neuroendoscopic approaches to the middle cranial fossa. In: Snyderman C, editor. Skull base surgery. Philadelphia: Walters Kluwer; 2015. p. 343–56.

31. Moe KS, Jothi S, Stern R, et al. Lateral retrocanthal orbitotomy; a minimally invasive canthus-sparing approach. Arch Facial Plast Surg 2007;9(6):419–26.

Correction of Nasal Fractures

G. Nina Lu, MD[a], Clinton D. Humphrey, MD[a], J. David Kriet, MD[b],*

KEYWORDS

- Nasal fracture management • Open reduction internal fixation nasal fracture
- Nasomaxillary fracture • Facial trauma • Nasal bone

KEY POINTS

- Nasal fracture is the most common bony injury resulting from blunt facial trauma.
- Optimal management of nasal trauma in the acute setting is critical to restoring pretraumatic form and function and minimizing secondary nasal deformities.
- Evaluation of nasal fractures should include careful examination of the nasal septum because unsuccessful fracture management is often due to inadequate treatment of concurrent septal fracture.
- Complex traumatic nasal deformities, especially with significant septal involvement, may require more aggressive acute surgical management and an initial open surgical approach.
- The open treatment of isolated nasal fractures is a controversial subject without widely accepted indications for timing, patient selection, and surgical technique.

INTRODUCTION

Nasal fractures most commonly result from blunt facial trauma in events, such as motor vehicle accidents, sports-related injuries, assaults, and falls.[1] The nasal bones are the most frequently fractured facial bone, with a peak incidence during the second and third decades of life with boys and men more commonly affected than girls and women.[1–4] Isolated nasal fractures are defined as fractures involving the nasal bones with or without concomitant involvement of the nasal cartilages and nasal septum. Nasal septal fractures are associated with 39% to 96% of nasal fracture cases, with increasing severity associated with more frequent septal fractures.[5–7] In more severe cases, they can coincide with fractures of the nasomaxillary buttress, naso-orbitoethmoid (NOE) complex, and frontal sinus. For the purposes of this article, discussion is focused on the treatment of isolated nasal fractures.

ANATOMIC CONSIDERATIONS

The structural framework of the nose includes the nasal bones, the nasal septum, the nasal process of the frontal bone, the frontal process of the maxilla, the ethmoid bone, the vomer, and cartilaginous structures. The nasal bones are thicker above the intercanthal line as they meet the nasofrontal suture. Inferiorly, the thinner nasal bone serves as a cantilever point for the attached upper lateral cartilages (ULCs) and corresponds externally to the rhinion. The transition between the thicker and thinner nasal bone is a common fracture site.[8] Within the nasal cavity, the perpendicular plate of the ethmoid fuses with the nasal bones along the dorsum. External impact to the

Disclosure Statement: The authors have nothing to disclose.
a Department of Otolaryngology–Head and Neck Surgery, University of Kansas Medical Center, 3901 Rainbow Boulevard, MS 3010, Kansas City, KS 66160, USA; b Division of Facial Plastic and Reconstructive Surgery, Department of Otolaryngology–Head and Neck Surgery, University of Kansas Medical Center, 3901 Rainbow Boulevard, MS 3010, Kansas City, KS 66160, USA
* Corresponding author.
E-mail address: dkriet@kumc.edu

Facial Plast Surg Clin N Am 25 (2017) 537–546
http://dx.doi.org/10.1016/j.fsc.2017.06.005

nasal bones is transmitted to the septum through this connection leading to concomitant septal injury during nasal trauma.

The paired ULCs attach to the caudal aspect of the nasal bone and dorsal aspect of the quadrangular (septal) cartilage. Cephalically, the ULCs attach via fibrous union to the nasal bones and can overlap the undersurface of the nasal bones by as much as 11 mm.[9] Laterally, the ULCs are only loosely attached to the maxilla by a fibrous aponeurosis. Thus, the nasal bone and septal attachments of the ULCs are the main contributions to their stability and support of the middle vault. Internally, the ULCs help form the internal nasal valve and contribute to the midline support of the cartilaginous septum. The paired lower lateral cartilages (LLCs) provide little septal support but are essential in the aesthetics and contour of the nasal tip. In general, significant force is required to cause cartilaginous injury due to the soft and malleable quality of cartilage that allows the dissipation of force.

The nasal septum plays a crucial role in the nasal structure and understanding its anatomy is paramount in the management of nasal fractures. The quadrangular cartilage comprises the majority of the septum with bony contributions from the vomer inferiorly and perpendicular plate of the ethmoid posteriorly and superiorly. Inferiorly, the quadrangular cartilage thickens and lies within the bony groove of the maxillary nasal crest. The dorsal and posterior septal cartilage provides the primary support for the nasal dorsum and the caudal septum provides the primary support for the nasal tip. Correction of septal deformities secondary to trauma is crucial in re-establishing premorbid form and function. In children the septum remains as a major growth center for the face until approximately 12 to 13 years of age. Significant septal trauma can adversely affect midface development.[10]

The external and internal carotid arteries supply a rich vascular network in the nasal region. Branches of the maxillary artery (sphenopalatine, greater palatine, and infraorbital arteries), facial artery (superior labial and angular arteries), and ethmoid arteries (anterior and posterior) anastomose in a redundant fashion, predisposing nasal fracture patients to epistaxis. Anterior or posterior epistaxis may arise depending on the location of vessel injury, with anterior bleeds more commonly seen than posterior. In most cases, nasal hemorrhage is either self-limited or readily controlled with direct manual pressure, blood pressure management, and/or topical medications. Rare persistent cases can require nasal packing, operative intervention, or angiography with embolization.

FRACTURE PATTERNS

No universally accepted classification of nasal fracture pattern exists although many clinical, anatomic, and radiographic classifications have been proposed.[5,7,8,11,12] Nasal fractures can be classified in 2 broad categories based on impact force: lateral-type versus frontal-type injuries. Lateral-type injuries tend to be more common, have fewer residual anatomic and functional defects compared with frontal injuries, and are more amenable to closed reduction.[12,13] Frontal injuries classically produce a posteriorly depressed fracture where the nasal septum is always involved. They are more severe, have a higher risk of residual deformity postsurgery, and are often associated with NOE fractures.

Stranc and Robertson[12] proposed a classification of lateral and frontal injuries based on anterior-posterior depth of injury in relation to the nasal tip and concluded that deeper levels of injury portended worse prognosis. In 1989, Murray and colleagues[8] proposed a pathologic classification system with 7 types of nasal fractures based on a cadaver study. They illustrated that septal fractures occur if the nose is deviated more than one-half a nose breadth from its original position and emphasized the importance of septal management for successful reduction. The variety of injury patterns and complexity of classification have precluded universal practical clinical application of any of these schemes.

Most isolated nasal fractures can be evaluated with several major characteristics in mind:

1. Unilateral versus bilateral involvement and degree of comminution
2. Lateral-type versus frontal-type injury
   - Degree of bony deviation relative to nasal width
   - Degree of depression of nasal dorsum
3. Status of nasal septum
4. Presence of middle vault/cartilaginous dislocations

Nasal fractures vary along a continuum between a unilateral, nondisplaced, greenstick fracture to bilateral, severely comminuted, and depressed nasal bone fractures with significant septal involvement and concomitant adjacent fractures. More aggressive surgical management is necessary with increased severity. Closed and open treatments may have similar outcomes with appropriate patient selection for each operative treatment.[14] In general, closed fracture reduction techniques are still considered first line for mild nasal fractures.[15] Treatment outcomes from closed reduction, however, are often disappointing and secondary surgical corrections are necessary in a sizable subset of patients. Open structure stabilization and classic rhinoplasty techniques are advocated for initial management of severe fractures by some investigators.[16]

INITIAL EVALUATION

All patients evaluated for facial trauma should first be evaluated in the framework of airway, breathing, circulation, and disability of cervical spine and brain (ABCDs) as well as hemodynamic stability.[17] Once a patient is stabilized, a complete history and physical and review of systems should be performed. Any neurologic or ophthalmologic symptoms should result in prompt consultation and communication with the appropriate specialties. Regarding the nasal fracture, history should elicit the method of injury, pretrauma and posttrauma status of nasal airflow, history of sinus disease or allergies, and prior nasal injury or surgery. Brisk epistaxis, septal hematoma, and watery drainage indicative of possible cerebrospinal fluid (CSF) leak must be identified and treated appropriately.

Physical examination of the nose should be approached in a stepwise, routine fashion. The nose can be classified into thirds and should be examined from the frontal, lateral, oblique, and base views. In the upper third, examination should identify deviation of the nasal pyramid, collapse of the nasal bones, and broadening of the rhinion. Telecanthus, or widening of the intercanthal distance, should be noted as well. In the cartilaginous middle third, the ULCs may be collapsed medially or disarticulated from the nasal bones. The middle vault may also be deviated relative to the upper bony vault and nasal tip. In the lower third, the nasal tip and base view should identify nostril asymmetry, caudal septal deviation, tip deviation, and nostril collapse. Lateral inspection may reveal dorsal irregularities or telescoping of the nasal bones as manifested by a saddled dorsum, increased nasolabial angle, and nasal foreshortening. Bimanual palpation of the bony, middle, and lower vault for step-offs, crepitus, and mobility can localize fractures and elucidate structural instability or collapse.[18] Internally, the nasal septum should be examined for hematoma, fracture, and dislocation. Nasal endoscopy may be helpful for posterior septal abnormalities and for control of epistaxis.

It is imperative to evaluate concomitant paranasal fractures of the orbit, NOE complex, and skull base because these can dramatically change patient management and surgical approach.

Nasomaxillary fractures may be missed during the evaluation of obvious nasal fractures and isolated central facial injuries.[19,20] The fracture line does not extend to the medial canthal tendon or lacrimal bone as in the classic NOE fracture and exists in a more inferior location. Nasomaxillary fractures will cause tenderness along infraorbital rim and intraorally along piriform aperture and may be lead to deformities of the nose and orbit. Additionally, unrepaired nasomaxillary fractures are a common cause of persistent nasal obstruction despite nasal fracture treatment.

RADIOLOGY

Nasal fractures may be diagnosed with history and physical examination alone. Plain films have no role in the management of nasal fractures with high false-positive reading as well as the inability to distinguish old fractures.[21,22] With increasing severity of trauma and concern for multiple injuries, high-resolution CT (HRCT) is the most appropriate imaging modality in the management of nasal fractures. HRCT allows a physician to evaluate concomitant injuries, define the spatial alignment of displaced fragments, evaluate the bony septum, and aid in surgical planning. Additionally, 3-D reconstruction can be generated from HRCTs and provides helpful information in the anatomy of the fracture. In situations where CT is undesirable or unavailable, high-resolution ultrasound (HRUS) is an alternative with comparable sensitivity and specificity to CT.[23–25] HRUS use is limited by operator experience, study interpretation, and the fact that little information is provided other than nasal bone position.

MANAGEMENT RATIONALE

Treatment of nasal fractures, as with any facial fractures, is predicated on the severity of the fracture, with the primary objective of restoring premorbid form and function with the least invasive method available. Management options fall into 4 major categories from least to most invasive:

1. Observation
2. Closed reduction
3. Closed reduction with septoplasty
4. Open reduction with or without internal stabilization

The optimal timing for surgical treatment is within the first few hours after injury (often elapsed by time of patient presentation) or 7 days to 10 days after injury when acute edema has begun to resolve. Unlike in other maxillofacial fractures where the bony alignment is directly visualized, nasal fractures require palpation and inspection of dorsal alignment to assess the adequacy of reduction. The surgeon must balance the severity of soft tissue edema and the choice of treatment. Closed reduction is best performed before fibrosis of fracture lines, typically within 2 weeks after injury but up to 3 weeks after is described.[26] A delay of 6 weeks or more when planning first-line open septorhinoplasty has been advocated to ensure complete resolution of acute inflammation.[16]

OBSERVATION

Patients presenting with nondisplaced fractures of the nasal bone, nasal septum, and/or anterior nasal spine without clinically relevant nasal deformities or airway obstruction are managed with close observation. As in all nasal fractures, patients should be counseled to apply ice packs and elevate the head of their bed to improve edema. All patients should be followed until swelling is resolved to confirm that a deformity has not been missed. Patients are typically seen for follow-up 7 days to 10 days after their injury when edema is resolved but closed reduction is not precluded.

CLOSED REDUCTION

Closed reduction is effective for noncomminuted and mild nasal fractures with or without dorsal septal disruption. In the typical case, one side is laterally displaced, the opposite side is medially depressed, and free-floating segments may be centrally depressed. Some investigators still advocate local and topical anesthesia for closed reduction with unilateral or minimally displaced fractures.[27] If local anesthesia is desired, the nasal cavity is prepared with cotton pledgets soaked in a topical anesthetic and vasoconstrictor, an infraorbital nerve block injection is performed, and intravenous sedation can be administered if available for comfort. General anesthesia is commonly preferred over local anesthesia for management of nasal fractures with evidence supporting significant improvement in appearance and function of nose, decreased subsequent corrective surgeries, and patient satisfaction with anesthesia.[28] The authors have found that the time required for closed reduction with a short general anesthetic is significantly less than the time required to adequately locally anesthetize a patient in the office setting. Additionally, the comfort of both patient and surgeon is improved.

A Boies elevator is placed against the external nose to measure the distance from the medial canthus to the nostril rim. This prevents the surgeon from inserting the elevator too far superiorly and injuring the skull base. The elevator is inserted between the depressed nasal bone and the nasal septum, parallel to the nasal dorsum. The depressed bone is pulled laterally and guided into a neutral position. Centrally depressed fragments require an anterior lifting motion with the elevator. A palpable click may sometimes be appreciated after successful reduction. Asch or Walsham reduction forceps are helpful for reducing the nasal septum and elevating a centrally depressed fragment. Each arm of the forceps is inserted on either side of the septum parallel to the nasal dorsum. Using an upward and outward force perpendicular to the dorsum, the septum is guided back into a neutral positon. A judicious amount of force and placement of forceps anterior to the fracture line must be considered to avoid torque on the skull base and potential CSF leak. An external splint is fashioned over the nasal dorsum. Comminuted or loose nasal bones can be supported with intranasal packing between the nasal bones and septum. The authors typically prefer absorbable packing, such as a Nasopore (Stryker, Kalamazoo, MI, USA), cut to the desired size to avoid the need for packing removal. If nonabsorbable packing is used, antibiotics should be administered for toxic shock syndrome prophylaxis.

Early studies on patient outcomes with closed reduction found high rates of patient satisfaction, with only 3% to 9% of patients pursuing secondary septorhinoplasty after initial reduction.[29,30] Comparatively, surgeons were satisfied with their results on average 37% of the time compared with patient satisfaction 79% of the time in a summary of 13 early publications.[31] More recent studies have noted a persistent deformity and need for subsequent septorhinoplasty after closed reduction in 11% to 50% of patients.[32-35] The accurate measurement of true patient satisfaction has also come into question when considering the discrepancy between patient and surgeon satisfaction.[36]

CLOSED REDUCTION WITH SEPTOPLASTY

An unreduced septal fracture is widely accepted as the most common cause of residual deformity. Cadaver studies by Murray and colleagues[37] and Harrison[38] have illustrated a consistent C-shaped septal fracture accompanying nasal fractures deviated by at least half the nasal bridge width. Studies of prospectively analyzed patients reveal closed reduction with acute septoplasty yields significant improvement in nasal breathing quality of life as compared with closed reduction alone.[39]

Thus, deviation of the nasal bridge greater than 50% and/or septal injury causing nasal obstruction are indications for concurrent septoplasty. The authors typically use Doyle splints after septal work for additional support.

With the rise of endoscopic surgery, endoscopic submucosal septoplasty techniques have been applied to this paradigm as well. In a retrospective review of 90 patients undergoing closed reduction combined with endoscopic septoplasty, persistent nasal deformity requiring subsequent surgery was reduced to 3.3% and investigators noted improved visualization of posterior septum.[40] Radiologic aids, such as use of C-arm, fluoroscopy, and intraoperative ultrasound-guided reduction, have been studied, with some evidence supporting reduced complications and need for reoperation.[41–43]

In a retrospective review of 49 patients, the surgical revision rate was lower in patients with septal deformity treated with an open approach to the nasal pyramid compared with those treated with closed reduction and conventional septoplasty (75% vs 6.5%). The investigators hypothesize that patients requiring septoplasty have more severe nasal fractures, and subsequent revision can be decreased with an open approach to these patients. One crucial area to consider when evaluating a posttraumatic nasal septum is the L-strut. The L-strut refers to 1-cm strips along the caudal and dorsal aspects of the quadrangular cartilage that is critical to nasal tip and dorsum support as well as external nasal appearance. Septal deformities not involving the L-strut often cause airway obstruction but seldom affect nasal appearance.[16] Conventional septoplasty avoids manipulation or disruption of the nasal L-strut due to its critical role in nasal airway and framework. Accordingly, septal deviation due to L-strut deformity is often inadequately treated with conventional septoplasty alone. Open septorhinoplasty techniques, such as septal batten grafting and columellar strut manipulation, may be necessary in these cases. In nasal trauma patients, a higher degree of L-strut involvement should prompt the surgeon to consider an open approach to the nasal pyramid. The authors avoid conventional septoplasty on these patients to preserve tissue for future grafting.

OPEN TREATMENT PRINCIPLES

Historically, open treatment of traumatic nasal deformities was reserved for treatment failure after closed reduction. Surgery was typically delayed by at least 6 months after injury. Evolving rhinoplasty techniques and failures of closed reduction have resulted in support for the open treatment of nasal fractures as an initial management strategy. Consensus exists regarding the need for open treatment with increasingly complex nasal fractures. For example, in nasal fractures associated with an NOE or Le Fort II/III fracture, the use of open fixation techniques is well established. Controversy abounds, however, regarding indications, timing, and surgical techniques for the initial open treatment of isolated nasal fractures. Research is focused on accurately identifying patients who will inevitably fail closed reduction and would benefit from incurring the risks and costs of initial open treatment. Some investigators advocate a trial of closed reduction in the operating room followed by immediate conversion to open treatment if a deformity persists.[16,31]

Severe septal fractures, comminuted fractures, cartilaginous fractures, and a destabilized nasal framework are proposed indications for open reduction or open septorhinoplasty.[26,44] As with any patient, surgeons must integrate treatment goals, unique anatomic factors, concomitant injuries, and social circumstances with clinical judgment in formulating their management plan. Advantages of open treatment include direct visualization of tissues for diagnostic accuracy and surgical access for rigid stabilization. Early skeletal stabilization may also prevent further anatomic distortion from osseous malunion and soft tissue contracture that can complicate secondary surgical intervention. Conversely, delaying open treatment allows the septal fractures to heal and may increase the amount and quality of septal grafting material available. Concerns exist regarding stripping periosteum from severely comminuted nasal bone fractures that may cause devitalization and necrosis of the bone. The high initial cost of treatment and the higher risk of complication with more aggressive treatment must also be considered.

In contrast to traditional open reduction and internal fixation in other areas of maxillofacial trauma, plate or wire fixation is described but not preferentially used for isolated nasal fractures.[45,46] Implant complications include bone erosion, skin breakdown, hardware infection, migration, and localized pain. The need for hardware removal may further complicate future rhinoplasty procedures. The term, internal stabilization, as applied to acute treatment of nasal fractures, may include rhinoplasty techniques, such as grafting and suture fixation, to restore structural integrity. Intranasal splinting, such as Doyle splints, may be used on a case-by-case basis for additional support, especially if septal mucosal flaps are raised.

General anesthesia is recommended and timing for surgery can range from 1 week to more than 6 weeks after injury. Traumatic nasal deformities may be corrected using traditional septorhinoplasty techniques many months or years after injury as a secondary procedure. This article focuses on open reduction for nasal fractures in the acute setting.

OPEN SURGICAL APPROACHES

Several approaches may be considered for open repair, depending on the location of injury and type of reconstruction anticipated. Common approaches include

1. Coronal
2. Endonasal rhinoplasty
3. External rhinoplasty
4. Use of existing lacerations

The use of medial canthal and subciliary incisions have been reported but are less cosmetically favored and should be avoided.[47,48]

The coronal approach provides excellent exposure of the superior nasal complex as well as other upper facial skeletal injuries if concomitant zygomatic arch, NOE, and frontal sinus fractures exist. It also allows for calvarial bone harvest and reconstructions. The cartilaginous middle vault and tip of the nose are not well exposed or treated with this approach. The incision is well hidden in the hairline but may be complicated by alopecia or temporal wasting, and there is a small risk of frontal nerve injury.

The endonasal intercartilaginous approach allows for good dorsal nasal exposure but does not give the opportunity to address the nasal tip cartilages. Intercartilaginous incisions between upper and lower lateral cartilages meets a transfixion incision at the caudal end of septal cartilage. Subperiosteal dissection through the intercartilaginous incision allows for exposure of the nasal dorsum and root. Subperichondrial dissection along the septum allows for treatment of septal fractures. This approach avoids external incisions and addresses the septum as well as the middle vault. The exposure of the nasal bones and dorsum may be inadequate, however, for true fixation of these structures. An endonasal delivery approach provides similar dorsal exposure but also gives the surgeon control of the nasal tip. This approach combines intercartilaginous and marginal incisions, allowing the LLCs to be delivered as bipedicle chondromucosal flaps.

The external rhinoplasty approach involves bilateral marginal incisions along the caudal border of the LLC and a transcolumellar incision at the narrowest portion of the midcolumella. This approach provides excellent exposure and control of the nasal tip and cartilaginous middle vault in severe fractures. Septal fractures are readily addressed through this approach and the disrupted L-strut can be readily treated with cartilage grafting as needed. Similar to the endonasal approach, exposure of nasal bone fractures may be inadequate if reduction and fixation is required. In certain cases, extensive dorsal and alar lacerations may disrupt blood supply to columellar flap and preclude the use of this approach.

OPEN TREATMENT WITHOUT INTERNAL STABILIZATION

Open treatment without internal stabilization refers to fracture reduction with the creation of medial and/or lateral osteotomies. If a septal injury exists, septoplasty and septal reduction are performed first. Closed nasal bone reduction is then used. If persistent bony asymmetry exists, osteotomies are created for further reduction. The fracture line often presents an existing osteotomy. Depending on fracture location, medial/lateral osteotomies are created on the contralateral side. Dorsal hump reductions and rasping techniques can further smooth out the bony contour. Considering the destabilized nasal pyramid, rasping should be used gently. The osteotomies increase the surgeon's ability to manipulate the nasal bone position. Although effective at reduction, some surgeons argue that without internal stabilization, this technique further destabilizes the nasal skeleton and creates more variability in healing. In nontraumatic rhinoplasty patients, osteotomies are rarely performed in conjunction with a fixation technique due to continued periosteal and septal support. For trauma patients, varying disruption of periosteal and septal support may influence the success of osteotomies without fixation. Fibrin glue has been proposed as a method of potential stabilization for more comminuted fractures in some patients.[49,50]

OPEN TREATMENT WITH INTERNAL STABILIZATION
Grafting

Severe structural instability or significant loss of dorsal bone or cartilage requires additional cartilage or bone grafting (split calvarium). Bone or cartilage may be used to suspend the collapsed septum to the graft, resuspend LCLs, and reestablish the nasofrontal angle (105°–120°). Small bone fragments that no longer contribute to the structure of the nasal complex should be removed to avoid serving as further nidus for infection. A cantilever technique for a graft that extends from above the nasion to just beneath the cephalic border of the alar cartilages is frequently used (**Fig. 1**). Fixation to the stable nasal root is completed. Further plate fixation may be performed from distal undersurface of the graft to the anterior nasal spine.

Cartilage grafting from the posterior septum, ear, or rib may be used to correct asymmetry using traditional rhinoplasty techniques. Spreader grafts can be placed to lateralize depressed ULCs and support dorsal L-strut fractures (**Fig. 2**). Caudal septal battens or extension grafts may be used to support the deviated caudal L-strut and to control the projection and rotation of the LLCs and nasal tip. Cartilaginous lacerations or transection of the LLC may be supported with crural strut grafts.

Suture Fixation

With caudal septal dislocation along the maxillary crest, reduction of the septal cartilage and suture fixation to maxillary bone periosteum can be used for further fixation. When disarticulation of ULC occurs, the main aim is to suture the cartilages back to the nasal bone. Small-gauge drills may be used to fashion fixation holes within the nasal bones. Internal nasal packing should be used to further support the ULC and re-establish premorbid position.

POSTOPERATIVE MANAGEMENT

In the first postoperative week, patients are instructed to elevate the head during sleep, abstain from nose blowing, and avoid use of aspirin or blood thinners. Ice packs are used to minimize edema. If nonresorbable intranasal packing was used, antibiotics are given for toxic shock prophylaxis until removal. Nonresorbable sutures and the external nasal splint are removed 5 days to 7 days postoperatively. Patients may return to sports and normal activities 4 weeks after treatment. The future risk of nasal fracture is discussed and protective facial masks are suggested

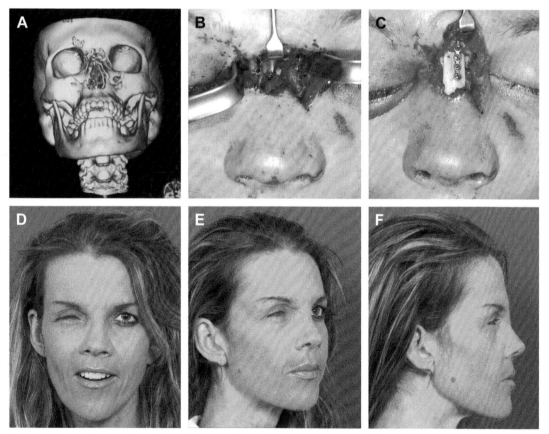

Fig. 1. (*A*) Severely comminuted nasal fractures in addition to type 2 NOE. (*B*) Plating of central bony segments with attached medial canthal tendons to frontal process. (*C*) Cantilever technique using split calvarial bone graft to replace severely comminuted nasal bones. (*D–F*) Frontal, oblique, and lateral views of patient 6 months post-surgery. On lateral view, the nasal radix is still slightly low but the patient declined revision.

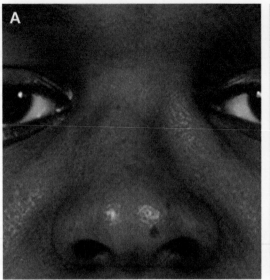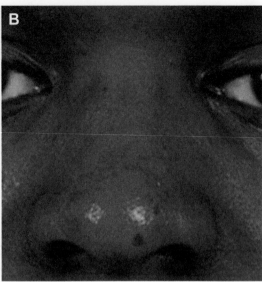

Fig. 2. (A) Nasal bony pyramid with deviation to the right and depression of left ULC. (B) Patient after closed reduction of nasal bones with endonasal spreader graft to ULC on the left.

to patients involved in sporting activities for 6 weeks to 8 weeks to prevent nasal reinjury.

POSTOPERATIVE IMAGING

Postoperative imaging is not typically performed except in severely comminuted fractures. Intraoperative cone beam CT imaging is helpful in assessing complex fracture reductions and allows for remanipulation of displaced fragments while still in the operating room. In centers where intraoperative imaging is not available, postoperative CT imaging can be performed.

SUMMARY

Isolated nasal fractures are the most common bony injury resulting from blunt facial trauma, resulting in a significant number of patients seeking treatment both in the acute and delayed settings. Neglect of septal deformities at the time of closed reduction often results in residual post-treatment deformities. Complex nasal fractures, especially associated with other maxillofacial injuries, may require more aggressive surgical treatment. Proper management in the acute setting can minimize secondary surgeries, lower overall health care costs, and increase patient satisfaction. The definition, however, of proper management for nasal fractures varies widely between surgeons. The open treatment of isolated nasal fractures is a particularly controversial subject with regard to timing, patient selection, and

surgical technique. More research is necessary to establish practice standards. Treating surgeon must integrate the utility of each technique with their surgical experience, the anatomic factors present, and patient goals in choosing the appropriate management plan.

REFERENCES

1. VandeGriend ZP, Hashemi A, Shkoukani M. Changing trends in adult facial trauma epidemiology. J Craniofac Surg 2015;26(1):108–12.
2. Hyman DA, Saha S, Nayar HS, et al. Patterns of facial fractures and protective device use in motor vehicle collisions from 2007 to 2012. JAMA Facial Plast Surg 2016;18(6):455–61.
3. Atisha DM, Burr T, Allori AC, et al. Facial fractures in the aging population. Plast Reconstr Surg 2016; 137(2):587–93.
4. Allareddy V, Itty A, Maiorini E, et al. Emergency department visits with facial fractures among children and adolescents: an analysis of profile and predictors of causes of injuries. J Oral Maxillofac Surg 2014;72(9):1756–65.
5. Hwang K, You SH, Kim SG, et al. Analysis of nasal bone fractures; a six-year study of 503 patients. J Craniofac Surg 2006;17(2):261–4.
6. Rhee SC, Kim YK, Cha JH, et al. Septal fracture in simple nasal bone fracture. Plast Reconstr Surg 2004;113(1):45–52.
7. Zhao Y, Zhu L, Ma F. CT analysis of classification of external nasal fracture and the influence of fractured position to nasal septum. Lin Chung Er Bi Yan Hou

Tou Jing Wai Ke Za Zhi 2014;28(8):527–30 [in Chinese].

8. Murray JA, Maran AG, Busuttil A, et al. A pathological classification of nasal fractures. Injury 1986;17(5): 338–44.

9. Parkes ML, Kanodia R. Avulsion of the upper lateral cartilage: etiology, diagnosis, surgical anatomy and management. Laryngoscope 1981;91(5):758–64.

10. Hall BK, Precious DS. Cleft lip, nose, and palate: the nasal septum as the pacemaker for midfacial growth. Oral Surg Oral Med Oral Pathol Oral Radiol 2013;115(4):442–7.

11. Won Kim S, Pio Hong J, Kee Min W, et al. Accurate, firm stabilization using external pins: a proposal for closed reduction of unfavorable nasal bone fractures and their simple classification. Plast Reconstr Surg 2002;110(5):1240–6 [discussion: 1247–8].

12. Stranc MF, Robertson GA. A classification of injuries of the nasal skeleton. Ann Plast Surg 1979;2(6): 468–74.

13. Daw JL, Lewis VL. Lateral force compared with frontal impact nasal fractures: need for reoperation. J Craniomaxillofac Trauma 1995;1(4):50–5.

14. Ondik MP, Lipinski L, Dezfoli S, et al. The treatment of nasal fractures: a changing paradigm. Arch Facial Plast Surg 2009;11(5):296–302.

15. Yilmaz MS, Guven M, Varli AF. Nasal fractures: is closed reduction satisfying? J Craniofac Surg 2013;24(1):e36–8.

16. Davis RE, Chu E. Complex nasal fractures in the Adult-A changing management philosophy. Facial Plast Surg 2015;31(3):201–15.

17. ATLS Subcommittee, American College of Surgeons' Committee on Trauma, International ATLS Working Group. Advanced trauma life support (ATLS(R)): the ninth edition. J Trauma Acute Care Surg 2013;74(5):1363–6.

18. Pollock RA. Nasal trauma. Pathomechanics and surgical management of acute injuries. Clin Plast Surg 1992;19(1):133–47.

19. Frodel JL. Avoiding and correcting complications in perinasal trauma. Facial Plast Surg 2012;28(03): 323–32.

20. Morgenstein KM, Bloom BS. Naso-maxillary fracture. Eye Ear Nose Throat Mon 1971;50(9):331–3.

21. Logan M, O'Driscoll K, Masterson J. The utility of nasal bone radiographs in nasal trauma. Clin Radiol 1994;49(3):192–4.

22. de Lacey GJ, Wignall BK, Hussain S, et al. The radiology of nasal injuries: problems of interpretation and clinical relevance. Br J Radiol 1977;50(594): 412–4.

23. Mohammadi A, Ghasemi-Rad M. Nasal bone fracture–ultrasonography or computed tomography? Med Ultrason 2011;13(4):292–5.

24. Atighechi S, Baradaranfar MH, Karimi G, et al. Diagnostic value of ultrasonography in the diagnosis of nasal fractures. J Craniofac Surg 2014;25(1):e51–3.

25. Lee IS, Lee JH, Woo CK, et al. Ultrasonography in the diagnosis of nasal bone fractures: a comparison with conventional radiography and computed tomography. Eur Arch Otorhinolaryngol 2016;273(2): 413–8.

26. Verwoerd CD. Present day treatment of nasal fractures: closed versus open reduction. Facial Plast Surg 1992;8(4):220–3.

27. Atighechi S, Baradaranfar MH, Akbari SA. Reduction of nasal bone fractures: a comparative study of general, local, and topical anesthesia techniques. J Craniofac Surg 2009;20(2):382–4.

28. Al-Moraissi EA, Ellis E 3rd. Local versus general anesthesia for the management of nasal bone fractures: a systematic review and meta-analysis. J Oral Maxillofac Surg 2015;73(4):606–15.

29. Crowther JA, O'Donoghue GM. The broken nose: does familiarity breed neglect? Ann R Coll Surg Engl 1987;69(6):259–60.

30. Illum P. Long-term results after treatment of nasal fractures. J Laryngol Otol 1986;100(3):273–7.

31. Staffel JG. Optimizing treatment of nasal fractures. Laryngoscope 2002;112(10):1709–19.

32. Basheeth N, Donnelly M, David S, et al. Acute nasal fracture management: a prospective study and literature review. Laryngoscope 2015;125(12):2677–84.

33. Higuera S, Lee EI, Cole P, et al. Nasal trauma and the deviated nose. Plast Reconstr Surg 2007;120(7 Suppl 2):64s–75s.

34. Rohrich RJ, Adams WP Jr. Nasal fracture management: minimizing secondary nasal deformities. Plast Reconstr Surg 2000;106(2):266–73.

35. Murray JA, Maran AG. The treatment of nasal injuries by manipulation. J Laryngol Otol 1980; 94(12):1405–10.

36. Fernandes SV. Nasal fractures: the taming of the shrewd. Laryngoscope 2004;114(3):587–92.

37. Murray JA, Maran AG, Mackenzie IJ, et al. Open v closed reduction of the fractured nose. Arch Otolaryngol 1984;110(12):797–802.

38. Harrison DH. Nasal injuries: their pathogenesis and treatment. Br J Plast Surg 1979;32(1):57–64.

39. Younes A, Elzayat S. The role of septoplasty in the management of nasal septum fracture: a randomized quality of life study. Int J Oral Maxillofac Surg 2016;45(11):1430–4.

40. Andrades P, Pereira N, Borel C, et al. A new approach to nasoseptal fractures: submucosal endoscopically assisted septoplasty and closed nasal reduction. J Craniomaxillofac Surg 2016; 44(10):1635–40.

41. Han DS, Han YS, Park JH. A new approach to the treatment of nasal bone fracture: the clinical

usefulness of closed reduction using a C-arm. J Plast Reconstr Aesthet Surg 2011;64(7):937–43.

42. Abu-Samra M, Selmi G, Mansy H, et al. Role of intraoperative ultrasound-guided reduction of nasal bone fracture in patient satisfaction and patient nasal profile (a randomized clinical trial). Eur Arch Otorhinolaryngol 2011;268(4):541–6.

43. Chen RF, Chen CT, Hao Chen C, et al. Optimizing closed reduction of nasal and zygomatic arch fractures with a mobile fluoroscan. Plast Reconstr Surg 2010;126(2):554–63.

44. Reilly MJ, Davison SP. Open vs closed approach to the nasal pyramid for fracture reduction. Arch Facial Plast Surg 2007;9(2):82–6.

45. Park HK, Lee JY, Song JM, et al. The retrospective study of closed reduction of nasal bone fracture. Maxillofac Plast Reconstr Surg 2014;36(6):266–72.

46. Kurihara K, Kim K. Open reduction and interfragment wire fixation of comminuted nasal fractures. Ann Plast Surg 1990;24(2):179–85.

47. Burm JS, Oh SJ. Indirect open reduction through intercartilaginous incision and intranasal Kirschner wire splinting of comminuted nasal fractures. Plast Reconstr Surg 1998;102(2):342–9.

48. Nunery WR, Tao JP. Medial canthal open nasal fracture repair. Ophthal Plast Reconstr Surg 2008;24(4):276–9.

49. Choi MS, Kim W, Youn S, et al. Concomitant open reduction of a nasal bone fracture combined with a zygomatic fracture through a subciliary incision. J Craniofac Surg 2012;23(1):e25–7.

50. Jeong HS, Moon MS, Lee HK, et al. Use of fibrin glue for open comminuted nasal bone fractures. J Craniofac Surg 2010;21(1):75–8.

Management of Zygomaticomaxillary Complex Fractures

E. Bradley Strong, MD[a],*, Celeste Gary, MD[b]

KEYWORDS

- Maxillofacial trauma • Zygoma • Fracture • Zygomaticomaxillary • Intra-operative imaging
- Navigation • Pre-surgical planning

KEY POINTS

- Zygomaticomaxillary complex fractures are one of the most common facial fractures.
- Thin-cut axial CT with sagittal, coronal, and 3-D reconstructions are recommended for accurate radiologic diagnosis.
- A thorough understanding of the bony tetrapod structure and fracture dynamics is critical for an accurate clinic diagnosis.
- Treatment options include closed and open reduction.
- Computer-aided applications can reduce operative morbidity and improve the accuracy of the bony reduction.

INTRODUCTION

Zygomaticomaxillary complex (ZMC) fractures account for approximately 25% of all facial fractures and are commonly the result of industrial accidents, sports injuries, and interpersonal altercations.[1–4] These injuries can result in both functional (trismus, diplopia, and paresthesias) and aesthetic deformities (malar flattening, midfacial widening, and globe malposition).[5,6] Although there is a significant body of literature studying ZMC fractures, there remains no clear consensus on surgical approaches or the type and location of hardware application. This article reviews pertinent anatomy, diagnostic modalities, principles of surgical repair (including indications, surgical approaches, fixation techniques, and computer-aided applications to optimize surgical management) and presents a treatment algorithm for surgical decision making.

ANATOMY

The ZMC occupies a prominent position in the facial skeleton. It provides height, width, and projection to the lateral face (**Fig. 1**). The ZMC has 4 attachments to the skull base: zygomaticofrontal, zygomaticosphenoidal, zygomaticomaxillary, and zygomaticotemporal (**Fig. 2**). For the purposes of discussion, the zygomaticomaxillary buttress is divided into 2 subregions: the inferior maxillary buttress and the superior orbital rim.

FRACTURE PATTERNS

ZMC fractures typically involve all 4 buttresses; passing through the suture lines and the infraorbital foramen (**Fig. 3**). Multiple fracture classification schemes have been developed.[7–9] One of the more commonly used systems was described by

Disclosure Statement: The authors have nothing to disclose.
[a] Department of Otolaryngology, University of California Davis School of Medicine, 2521 Stockton Boulevard, Suite 5200, Sacramento, CA 95817, USA; [b] Department of Otolaryngology, LSU Health New Orleans, 533 Bolivar Street, Suite 566, New Orleans, LA 70112, USA
* Corresponding author.
E-mail address: ebstrong@ucdavis.edu

Facial Plast Surg Clin N Am 25 (2017) 547–562
http://dx.doi.org/10.1016/j.fsc.2017.06.006

facialplastic.theclinics.com

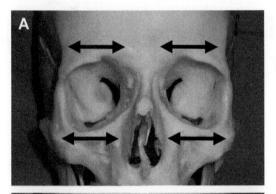

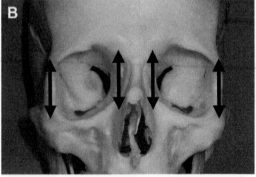

Fig. 1. (*A*) Horizontal buttresses of the facial skeleton; (*B*) vertical buttresses of the facial skeleton.

Zingg and colleagues[7] in 1992 (**Fig. 4**). Injuries were divided into 3 groups: type A — isolated injuries, type B — single-segment fractures, and type C — comminuted fractures. Unfortunately, classification systems are rarely applied in the clinical setting, because a physical description of the fracture is often more accurate and clinically

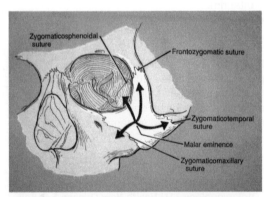

Fig. 2. Tetrapod structure of the ZMC. Buttresses include Frontozygomatic, zygomaticotemporal, zygomaticomaxillary, and zygomaticosphenoidal. (*From* Strong EB, Sykes JM. Zygoma complex fractures. Facial Plast Surg 1998;14(1);107; with permission.)

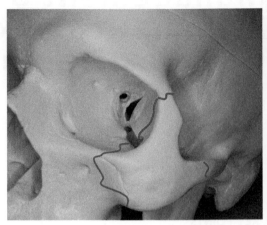

Fig. 3. Typical fracture patterns of the ZMC.

relevant. They can, however, be useful for education and research applications.

DIAGNOSIS

The initial assessment of facial trauma patients should include evaluation of critical structures: airway, hemodynamic stability, and cervical spine. Patients should receive a thorough history and physical examination.

History

The history should include documentation of

- Level of consciousness: can the patient give an accurate account of the traumatic event?
- Injury type (high velocity vs low velocity): high-velocity injuries are much more likely to result in complex fracture patterns involving multiple areas of the facial skeleton.
- Mechanism of injury (blunt or penetrating): blunt injuries are often localized, whereas penetrating trauma is more likely to involve deeper neurovascular structures. These can be less apparent on physical examination.
- Past medical history: this includes previous facial injuries.

Physical Examination

A complete head and neck examination should be performed with special attention given to

- Ophthalmologic examination: injury to the globe can result in profound long term morbidity.[6] The eye examination should include visual acuity, pupillary response, extraocular muscle function, gross examination of

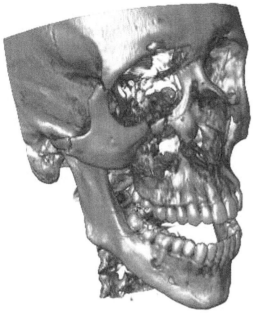

Fig. 8. 3-D reconstruction of right ZMC fracture. Note that the location of individual fractures and an intervening comminuted segment of the orbital rim are well visualized.

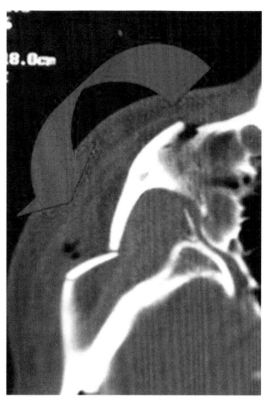

Fig. 10. Counterclockwise rotation of a low-velocity ZMC fracture.

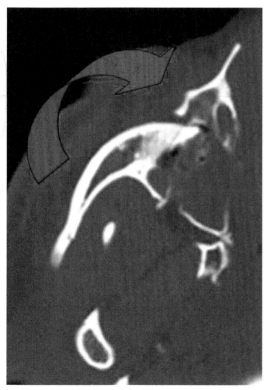

Fig. 9. Clockwise rotation of a low-velocity ZMC fracture.

whereas an elderly patient, in poor health, with thick skin, may decide against any intervention for even a moderately displaced injury. The decision for surgery must be made on an individual basis, combining the surgeon's assessment of risk for deformity and the patient's level of concern about the risk of long-term facial asymmetry.

Functional impairment

Depression of the zygomatic arch can result in impingement on the coronoid process and trismus. Orbital involvement can result in diplopia and globe malposition. Management of orbital injuries is addressed in Scott E Bevans and Kris. S. Moe's article, "Advances in the Reconstruction of Orbital Fractures," in this issue.

Computer-Aided Applications

Presurgical planning

Despite advances in surgical technique, surgeons still struggle with accurate fracture reduction, particularly in complex ZMC injuries. Computer-aided design and manufacturing

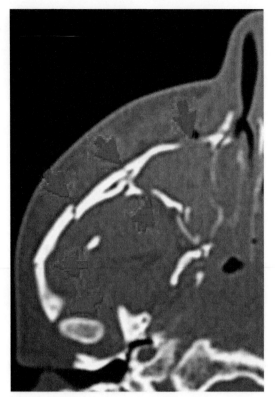

Fig. 11. Comminuted high-velocity ZMC fracture. Note the multiple bony segments with fractures (*arrows*) through the central body of the zygoma.

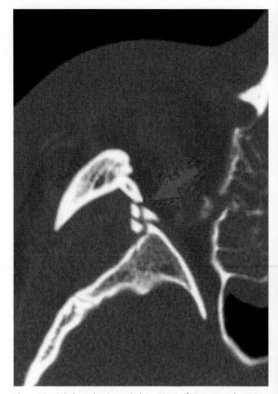

Fig. 12. High-velocity right ZMC fracture showing comminution and depression of the zygomaticosphenoidal buttress (*arrow*).

software can assist surgeons with virtual presurgical planning and visualization. Common planning techniques include segmentation of bone from soft tissue, isolation of specific bone segments from the facial skeleton, mirroring of uninjured skeletal segments to the contralateral side of injury for virtual surgical repair, and insertion of normative CT data to assist with a virtual repair of bilateral injuries.[13,14]

Intraoperative navigation

Facial incisions used in maxillofacial reconstruction are often far from the site of injury, limiting the surgeon's 3-D perspective on the anatomy. Although surgical navigation systems were developed to assist with delineation of anatomic landmarks during neurosurgical and rhinologic procedures, the technique is equally effective for use in maxillofacial reconstruction. Navigation allows the surgeon to confirm pertinent anatomic landmarks without clear visualization, improving the accuracy of reduction.[13–15]

Intraoperative imaging

Visualization of the entire ZMC is not possible using a single surgical approach. Consequently,

ZMC fracture reduction must be inferred from looking at individual buttresses, without complete visualization. Although intraoperative imaging is used primarily in orthopedic surgery, it is equally effective in maxillofacial reconstruction. It provides a real-time assessment of fracture reduction that is not possible with direct visualization, thus allowing for intraoperative correction of bony malreduction or implant malpositioning.[16–20] Average intraoperative revision rates for maxillofacial reconstructive procedures with the use of intraoperative imaging is approximately 22% (range 14%–28%).[18–21] Disadvantages of intraoperative imaging include cost, radiation exposure, and increased operative times. Although technical advances continue to minimize these issues, they still limit access and utility in maxillofacial reconstruction.

- Cost: at the time of publication, intraoperative imaging devices range from approximately $250,000 to $900,000.
- Operative time: historically intraoperative CT scanners were cumbersome and time consuming to use. Current portable imaging devices are much more efficient, with 1-minute to 2-minute scan times and rapid

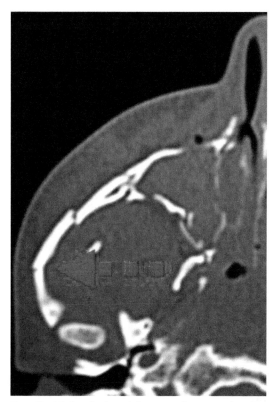

Fig. 13. High-velocity right ZMC fracture showing comminution and lateral displacement (*arrow*) of the zygomatic arch.

processing algorithms. Intraoperative imaging has been shown to add approximately 15 minutes per case.[19] In the authors' experience, factors that have the greatest influence on operative time include surgeon planning (bed, room, instrumentation set-up, and so forth) and support staff experience (ie, expertise using the imaging device).

• Radiation: there is a growing body of literature evaluating the potential risk of medical radiation exposure.[22] Although the literature is not clear on increase in lifetime risk for adults, a more conservative approach is likely indicated in children.[23,24] Current portable imaging devices offer a significant reduction in radiation exposure, while continuing to provide good image quality (**Fig. 14**). These devices can be divided into 2 different modalities: traditional axial CT (fan beam CT) and digital volume tomography (cone beam CT).[16]

○ Axial CT (fan beam CT): these devices use a collimator to generate a fan-shaped beam, passing through the patient, and recorded as axial slices on image detectors (ie, 32-slice, 64-slice, and 128-slice scanners) (**Fig. 15**). These 2-D slices can be viewed individually or reformatted to generate sagittal, coronal, and 3-D reconstructions.

Modality	Dosage (μSv – microseiverts)
Background Radiation (24 h)	8
Panorex	19
Cone Beam CT - Pediatric	27
Cone Beam CT - Adult	87
Dental Series	171
New York – Tokyo Flight	150
Fan Beam CT – Adult	860

Fig. 14. Radiation dosages from multiple modalities.

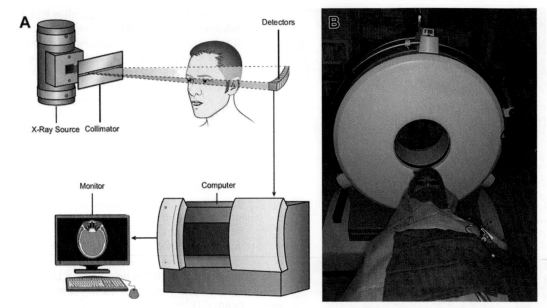

Fig. 15. Axial CT. (*A*) Illustration of fan beam CT. (*B*) Photograph of intraoperative fan beam CT scanner. (*From* Strong EB, Tollefson TT. Intraoperative use of CT imaging. Otolaryngol Clin N Am 2013;46:720; with permission.)

○ Digital volume tomography (cone beam CT): these devices emit a cone-shaped x-ray beam that is recorded as a 3-D volume on an image intensifier (**Fig. 16**). This volume can then be sliced into 2-D images in virtually any plane.

A comparison of the 2 modalities reveals that fan beam CT provides the greatest image resolution (ie, good visualization of both soft tissue and bone), whereas cone beam CT offers a significant reduction in radiation exposure but has poor soft tissue resolution. In summary, presurgical planning software, intraoperative navigation, and intraoperative imaging are powerful resources for maxillofacial reconstruction. Presurgical planning allows surgeons to plan the procedure in a virtual environment, intraoperative navigation confirms execution of the plan, and intraoperative imaging verifies that the plan has been achieved (**Fig. 17**).

Closed Versus Open Reduction

Fracture reduction can be achieved through both closed and open surgical approaches.

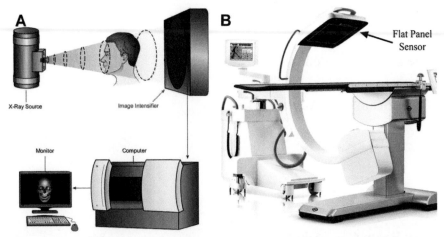

Fig. 16. Digital volume tomography. (*A*) Illustration of a cone beam CT. (*B*) Photograph of intraoperative cone beam CT scanner. (*From* Strong EB, Tollefson TT. Intraoperative use of CT imaging. Otolaryngol Clin N Am 2013;46:721; with permission.)

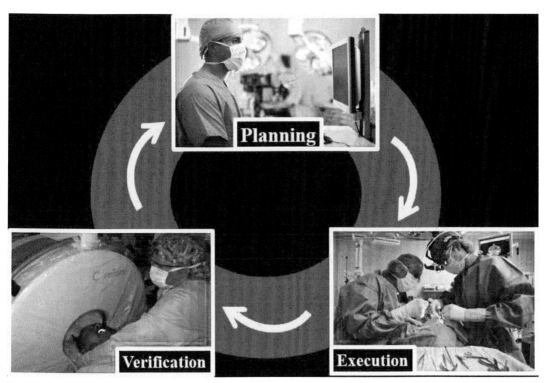

Fig. 17. Illustration of computer-aided surgery workflow. Presurgical planning allows the surgeon to plan the procedure in a virtual environment, intraoperative navigation confirms execution of the plan, and intraoperative imaging verifies that the plan has been achieved.

Lower-velocity injures may be amenable to closed reduction (without fixation) via limited incisions. Intraoperative imaging has expanded the indications for closed repair by confirming the accuracy of reduction without the need for direct visualization. In this scenario, there is an initial attempt at closed reduction followed by confirmation with intraoperative imaging. Open reduction is only required when a closed reduction cannot be achieved or is unstable. Higher-velocity injuries are more likely to require open reduction and internal fixation. Computer-aided applications, including presurgical planning, intraoperative navigation, and intraoperative imaging, can be helpful to optimize the surgical repair.

Buttress-Based Approach

Historically, surgeons have focused the number and location of buttresses that should be repaired for optimal ZMC fracture stability.[25–31] Although hardware can be applied to the zygomaticosphenoidal suture line, the remaining 3 ZMC buttresses are most commonly used for fracture stabilization (**Fig. 18**). The need for 1-point, 2-point, 3-point, or 4-point fixation should be

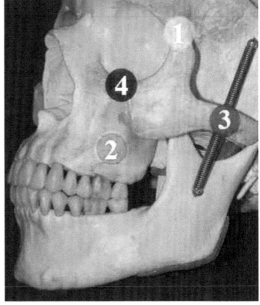

Fig. 18. Illustration of the most stable bony buttresses used for plating of ZMC fractures. (1) Zygomaticofrontal, (2) zygomaticomaxillary, (3) zygomaticotemporal, and (4) orbital rim.

based on fracture stability; applying the minimum amount of hardware to maintain fracture reduction throughout the process of healing. This approach has been termed, *functionally stable fixation*.

Incision-Based Approach

More recent thinking emphasizes an incision based approach for management of ZMC fractures.[32] The surgeon selects the minimum number incisions with the least iatrogenic morbidity, while still offering adequate access for optimal reduction and fixation. Of the 4 facial incisions commonly used for treatment of ZMC fractures, the least morbid is the sublabial, followed by the lateral blepharoplasty, lower eyelid, and finally the coronal incision (**Fig. 19**). With this approach, the surgeon often starts with the sublabial incision and adds additional incisions only when required for fracture reduction or stabilization.

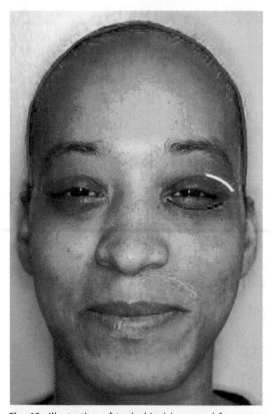

Fig. 19. Illustration of typical incisions used for access to ZMC fractures. An incision based approach uses the least morbid incision first; moving up to more invasive approaches as necessary. Incision morbidity: sublabial (*green*) < lateral blepharoplasty (*yellow*) < lower eyelid (*blue*) < coronal (*red*).

Closed Repair

Patients with simple, low-velocity injuries are good candidates for closed reduction. Fracture types include zygomatic arch and single-piece ZMC fractures (see **Fig. 4**, type A1 and type B). After closed reduction, intraoperative imaging can be used to confirm the accuracy of repair. Surgical approaches to these injuries include

- Temporal: a 2-cm incision is placed in the scalp of the temporal region approximately 4 cm above the zygomatic arch. The temporalis muscle fascia is exposed (**Fig. 20**). A Boise or Rowe elevator is used to dissect in a subfascial plane beneath the arch (**Fig. 21**). Lateral force is applied to and reduce the fracture. No pressure should be applied to the skull.
- Sublabial: a 2-cm sublabial incision is placed just above the mucogingival junction, eliminating the risk of alopecia, which can occur with the temporal approach. A subperiosteal dissection is performed, elevating deep to the zygomatic arch. A Boise or Rowe elevator is inserted under the arch to reduce the fracture, as described previously (see temporal approach) (**Fig. 22**).
- Percutaneous: a stab incision is placed in the cheek skin. A bone hook can be placed beneath the malar prominence,[33–35] or Carroll-Girard screw (**Fig. 23**) inserted directly into the zygoma.[3,36] The mobile bone segment is then reduced

Open Repair

Common approaches to the ZMC are listed in **Table 1**.

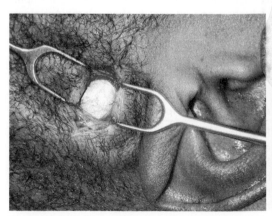

Fig. 20. Photograph of a 2-cm temporal incision with exposure of the temporalis muscle fascia.

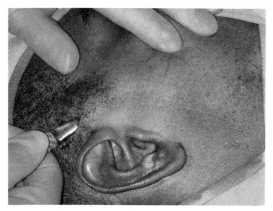

Fig. 21. Photograph of a Boise elevator placed through a temporal incision and under the zygomatic arch. Lateral force is applied to reduce the fracture. No pressure should be applied to the skull.

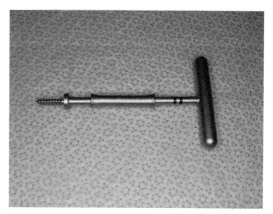

Fig. 23. Photograph of a Carroll-Girard screw. It is placed directly into the zygoma and provides control of the mobile ZMC.

Zygomaticomaxillary buttress

- Sublabial incision (inferior maxillary buttress): a 4-cm to 5-cm incision is placed just above the mucogingival junction, extending from approximately the lateral incisor to first molar, avoiding injury to the parotid duct (see **Figs. 2** and **19**). The dissection continues in a subperiosteal plane exposing the face of the maxilla. Superior dissection delineates the infraorbital nerve and often provides visualization of the inferior orbital rim. This incision is well hidden, provides excellent visualization, has minimal

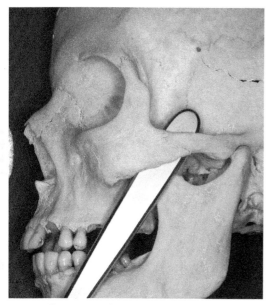

Fig. 22. Illustration of an elevator being placed sublabially below the zygomatic arch to reduce a ZMC fracture.

morbidity, and provides access the buttress with the greatest biomechanical advantage for maintenance of reduction.[3,25,27,37] Therefore, the sublabial incision is often the first choice for surgical exposure. Although comminution can occur at this buttress, accurate alignment can generally be achieved with a single miniplate (**Fig. 24**). Microplate application along the inferior orbital rim is possible in some patients depending on individual anatomy.

- Eyelid incision: there are 4 common surgical approaches to the inferior orbital rim: (1) transcutaneous subciliary, (2) transcutaneous subtarsal, (3) transconjunctival preseptal, and (4) transconjunctival postseptal. These approaches are described in greater detail in Scott E Bevans and Kris. S. Moe's article, "Advances in the Reconstruction of Orbital Fractures," in this issue. Fractures of the orbital rim are often comminuted. Careful reduction and application of a microplate will restore facial width and help with orbital floor alignment (**Fig. 25**). The orbital rim, however, provides only mild structural integrity.

Zygomaticofrontal buttress

- Lateral upper-lid blepharoplasty incision: the lateral upper-lid blepharoplasty incision is the best choice for access to the zygomaticofrontal buttress (see **Figs. 2** and **19**). Unlike the eyebrow incision, which can result in alopecia and a prominent scar, this incision provides good exposure with minimal scarring risk. An approximately 2-cm skin incision is placed along a natural skin crease on the outer third of the upper eyelid, at least 10 mm to 12 mm above the lid margin. The incision is carried

Table 1
Surgical approaches to the zygomaticomaxillary buttresses

Buttress	Surgical Approach
Zygomaticomaxillary (inferior maxillary buttress)	Intraoral sublabial
Zygomaticomaxillary (orbital rim)	Eyelid incision (transconjunctival/transcutaneous)
Zygomaticofrontal	Lateral upper-lid blepharoplasty or coronal
Zygomaticosphenoidal	Lateral upper-lid blepharoplasty or coronal
Zygomaticotemporal	Coronal

through the skin and orbicularis muscle. Traction on the forehead skin then elevates the upper lid until the skin incision lies over the zygomaticofrontal buttress. A needle-point electrocautery on a low setting is then used to dissect through the underlying soft tissue and periosteum. For more complex injuries where a coronal incision is required, this buttress can be accessed via the coronal approach (see coronal incision, discussed later). The zygomaticofrontal buttress is a primary landmark for ZMC reduction. Comminution rarely occurs at this location. Because this is a narrow buttress, fracture reduction restores ZMC width and height but gives little information about fracture rotation. The overlying skin is relatively thick and a 4-hole to 5-hole miniplate can be used for fracture fixation. The initial screw is partially inserted into the frontal process of the zygoma (inferior to the fracture on the mobile bone segment). Upward force is then applied to reduce the fracture while the superior screw is inserted on stable bone at the skull base (**Fig. 26**). The initial screw insertion is then completed. This

2-screw configuration allows for some mobility while reducing and fixating the other buttresses. After the other buttresses have been plated, the final 2 screws are placed at the periphery of the frontozygomatic buttress plate.

Zygomaticosphenoidal buttress

- Lateral upper-lid blepharoplasty incision: The primary access to the zygomaticosphenoidal buttress is via the lateral upper-lid blepharoplasty incision (see zygomaticofrontal buttress discussed previously) (see **Figs. 2 and 19**). Once the lateral orbital rim is exposed, a periosteal elevator can be used to expose lateral orbital wall and zygomaticosphenoidal buttress. The zygomaticosphenoidal buttress is extremely stable; however, comminution can occur with high-velocity injuries. Reduction at this site restores ZMC projection, width, and rotation, making it one of the most reliable indicators of accurate fracture reduction (**Figs. 27** and **28**).[31,38,39] Internal fixation is challenging; however, placement of a 3-hole miniplate is possible with more aggressive surgical exposure. Plate

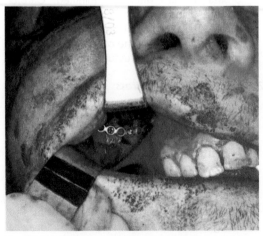

Fig. 24. Photograph of a maxillary buttress miniplate placed through a sublabial incision.

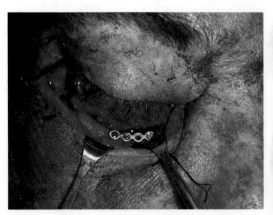

Fig. 25. Photograph of an inferior orbital rim microplate.

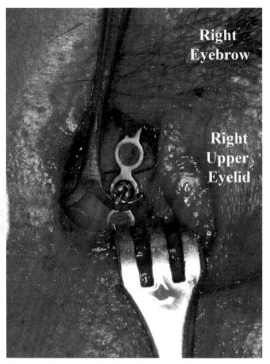

Fig. 26. Photograph of hardware application to zygomaticofrontal buttress. The first screw is partially inserted on the mobile ZMC. Upward force is then applied to reduce the fracture while the superior screw is inserted on stable bone at the skull base.

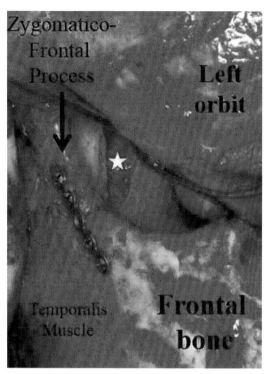

Fig. 27. Superior view of an unreduced zygomaticosphenoidal buttress fracture. Note the white star in the soft tissue where the fracture is distracted laterally.

application at this site is more easily achieved through a coronal incision (see coronal incision, discussed later).

Zygomaticotemporal buttress

- Coronal incision: The primary access for the zygomaticotemporal buttress is through coronal incision (see **Figs. 2** and **19**). It does, however, carry a greater risk of iatrogenic sequelae, such as alopecia, paresthesias, and facial nerve injury. Therefore, this approach is usually reserved for complex fractures requiring 4-point fixation. A coronal incision is marked out at least 4 cm to 6 cm behind the hairline. The hair can be banded and need not be shaved. The incision may be straight line or zig-zag. The zig-zag incision can assist with scar camouflage, taking advantage of inferior hair follicle alignment to cover the transverse arms of the scar. An intimate knowledge of the temporal anatomy is required to preserve the temporal branch of the facial nerve, minimize alopecia, and reduce the risk of temporal hollowing (**Fig. 29**). The lateral dissection continues

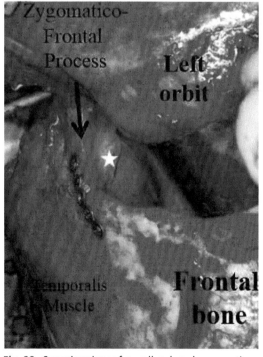

Fig. 28. Superior view of a well reduced zygomaticosphenoidal buttress fracture. The white star sits just lateral to the reduced fracture prior to hardware application across the fracture line.

A

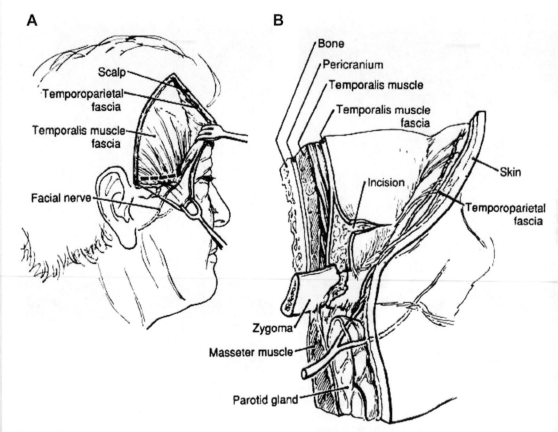

B

Fig. 29. Illustration of a coronal incision. (*A*) The incision should be 6 cm behind the hairline and expose the temporalis muscle facia, protecting the temporal branch of the facial nerve. (*B*) A transverse incision is placed through the temporalis muscle fascia, 2 cm above the arch and the dissection is continued in a plane superficial to the temporal fat pad.

below the temporal line, leaving the temporalis muscle fascia intact to a level approximately 2 cm above the zygomatic arch. The fascia is then incised and the dissection continues toward the arch, just superficial to the temporal fat pad. This is a dense dissection plane that does not elevate easily. Once the zygomatic arch is exposed, the periosteum is incised on the superior border to protect the temporal branch of the facial nerve. The periosteum is carefully elevated to expose the zygomaticotemporal buttress. The buttress is thin and comminution is relatively common. Fracture reduction with a miniplate restores malar projection but gives little information about width or rotation. Miniplates can be used along the arch, and a single fixation screw can be placed to stabilize buttress fractures at the skull base (**Fig. 30**). After fracture repair, the closure is performed in layers, resuspending the temporal scalp to prevent long-term ptosis.

Timing of Repair

Early repair of ZMC fractures offers the greatest opportunity for an accurate reduction. Scar tissue has not formed and bony fracture contours

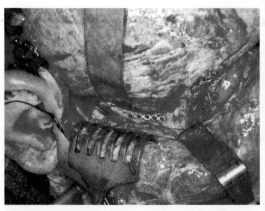

Fig. 30. Photograph of a miniplate placed along the zygomaticotemporal buttress. Note the position screw fixating the zygomatic root at the skull base.

are readily visible. Unfortunately, facial edema often makes surgical visualization extremely difficult. In such cases, repair should be performed at 7–10 days after much of the edema has resolved but before significant bone healing has occurred. Fractures reduction in the subacute timeframe (2–6 weeks) can still be achieved, but anatomic landmarks are significantly less clear. Secondary fracture repair (>6 weeks) can be extremely challenging with marked distortion of normal anatomic landmarks. The use of presurgical planning, intraoperative navigation, and intraoperative imaging is highly recommended.

REFERENCES

1. Kostakis G, Stathopoulos P, Dais P, et al. An epidemiologic analysis of 1,142 maxillofacial fractures and concomitant injuries. Oral Surg Oral Med Oral Pathol Oral Radiol 2012;114(5 Suppl):S69–73.

2. Ellis E, El-Attar A, Moos KF. An analysis of 2,067 cases of zygomatico-orbital fracture. J Oral Maxillofac Surg 1985;43(6):417–28.

3. Ellis E 3rd, Kittidumkerng W. Analysis of treatment for isolated zygomaticomaxillary complex fractures. J Oral Maxillofac Surg 1996;54(4):386–400 [discussion: 400–1].

4. Marinho RO, Freire-Maia B. Management of fractures of the zygomaticomaxillary complex. Oral Maxillofacial Surg Clin N Am 2013;25(4):617–36.

5. Timashpolsky A, Dagum AB, Sayeed SM, et al. A prospective analysis of physical examination findings in the diagnosis of facial fractures: determining predictive value. Plast Surg (Oakv) 2016;24(2):73–9.

6. Jamal BT, Pfahler SM, Lane KA, et al. Ophthalmic injuries in patients with zygomaticomaxillary complex fractures requiring surgical repair. J Oral Maxillofac Surg 2009;67(5):986–9.

7. Zingg M, Laedrach K, Chen J, et al. Classification and treatment of zygomatic fractures: a review of 1,025 cases. J Oral Maxillofac Surg 1992;50(8):778–90.

8. Knight JS, North JF. The classification of malar fractures: an analysis of displacement as a guide to treatment. Br J Plast Surg 1960;13:325–39.

9. Fujii N, Yamashiro M. Classification of malar complex fractures using computed tomography. J Oral Maxillofac Surg 1983;41(9):562–7.

10. Tanrikulu R, Erol B. Comparison of computed tomography with conventional radiography for midfacial fractures. Dentomaxillofac Radiol 2001;30(3):141–6.

11. Laine FJ, Conway WF, Laskin DM. Radiology of maxillofacial trauma. Curr Probl Diagn Radiol 1993; 22(4):145–88.

12. Roth FS, Kokoska MS, Awwad EE, et al. The identification of mandible fractures by helical computed tomography and panorex tomography. J Craniofac Surg 2005;16(3):394–9.

13. Pham AM, Rafii AA, Metzger MC, et al. Computer modeling and intraoperative navigation in maxillofacial surgery. Otolaryngol Head Neck Surg 2007; 137(4):624–31.

14. Fuller SC, Strong EB. Computer applications in facial plastic and reconstructive surgery. Curr Opin Otolaryngol Head Neck Surg 2007;15(4): 233–7.

15. Strong EB, Rafii A, Holhweg-Majert B, et al. Comparison of 3 optical navigation systems for computer-aided maxillofacial surgery. Arch Otolaryngol Head Neck Surg 2008;134(10):1080–4.

16. Strong EB, Tollefson TT. Intraoperative use of CT imaging. Otolaryngol Clin North Am 2013;46(5):719–32.

17. Strong EB. Intraoperative computed tomography for repair of facial fractures. Arch Facial Plast Surg 2012;14(3):159–61.

18. Stanley RB Jr. Use of intraoperative computed tomography during repair of orbitozygomatic fractures. Arch Facial Plast Surg 1999;1(1):19–24.

19. Shaye DA, Tollefson TT, Strong EB. Use of intraoperative computed tomography for maxillofacial reconstructive surgery. JAMA Facial Plast Surg 2015; 17(2):113–9.

20. Wilde F, Lorenz K, Ebner AK, et al. Intraoperative imaging with a 3D C-arm system after zygomatico-orbital complex fracture reduction. J Oral Maxillofac Surg 2013;71(5):894–910.

21. Hoelzle F, Klein M, Schwerdtner O, et al. Intraoperative computed tomography with the mobile CT Tomoscan M during surgical treatment of orbital fractures. Int J Oral Maxillofac Surg 2001;30(1): 26–31.

22. Shuryak I, Lubin JH, Brenner DJ. Potential for adult-based epidemiological studies to characterize overall cancer risks associated with a lifetime of CT scans. Radiat Res 2014;181(6):584–91.

23. Brenner DJ. Estimating cancer risks from pediatric CT: going from the qualitative to the quantitative. Pediatr Radiol 2002;32(4):228–31 [discussion: 242–4].

24. Brenner D, Elliston C, Hall E, et al. Estimated risks of radiation-induced fatal cancer from pediatric CT. AJR Am J Roentgenol 2001;176(2):289–96.

25. Fujioka M, Yamanoto T, Miyazato O, et al. Stability of one-plate fixation for zygomatic bone fracture. Plast Reconstr Surg 2002;109(2):817–8.

26. Czerwinski M, Martin M, Lee C. Quantitative topographical evaluation of the orbitozygomatic complex. Plast Reconstr Surg 2005;115(7):1858–62.

27. Yonehara Y, Hirabayashi S, Tachi M, et al. Treatment of zygomatic fractures without inferior orbital rim fixation. J Craniofac Surg 2005;16(3):481–5.

28. Hwang K. One-point fixation of tripod fractures of zygoma through a lateral brow incision. J Craniofac Surg 2010;21(4):1042–4.

29. Kim ST, Go DH, Jung JH, et al. Comparison of 1-point fixation with 2-point fixation in treating tripod fractures of the zygoma. J Oral Maxillofac Surg 2011;69(11):2848–52.

30. Kim JH, Lee JH, Hong SM, et al. The effectiveness of 1-point fixation for zygomaticomaxillary complex fractures. Arch Otolaryngol Head Neck Surg 2012; 138(9):828–32.

31. Rana M, Warraich R, Tahir S, et al. Surgical treatment of zygomatic bone fracture using two points fixation versus three point fixation–a randomised prospective clinical trial. Trials 2012;13:36.

32. Ellis E 3rd, Perez D. An algorithm for the treatment of isolated zygomatico-orbital fractures. J Oral Maxillofac Surg 2014;72(10):1975–83.

33. Kovacs AF, Ghahremani M. Minimization of zygomatic complex fracture treatment. Int J Oral Maxillofac Surg 2001;30(5):380–3.

34. Zingg M, Chowdhury K, Lädrach K, et al. Treatment of 813 zygoma-lateral orbital complex fractures: new aspects. Arch Otolaryngol Head Neck Surg 1991; 117(6):611–20.

35. O'Sullivan ST, Panchal J, O'Donoghue JM, et al. Is there still a role for traditional methods in the management of fractures of the zygomatic complex? Injury 1998;29(6):413–5.

36. Evans GR, Daniels M, Hewell L. An evidence-based approach to zygomatic fractures. Plast Reconstr Surg 2011;127(2):891–7.

37. Shumrick KA, Kersten RC, Kulwin DR, et al. Criteria for selective management of the orbital rim and floor in zygomatic complex and midface fractures. Arch Otolaryngol Head Neck Surg 1997;123(4): 378–84.

38. Hollier LH, Thornton J, Pazmino P, et al. The management of orbitozygomatic fractures. Plast Reconstr Surg 2003;111(7):2386–92 [quiz: 2393].

39. Kelley P, Hopper R, Gruss J. Evaluation and treatment of zygomatic fractures. Plast Reconstr Surg 2007;120(7 Suppl 2):5S–15S.

Updates in Management of Craniomaxillofacial Gunshot Wounds and Reconstruction of the Mandible

 CrossMark

Baber Khatib, MD, DDS[a,b,c,]*, Savannah Gelesko, MD, DDS[c],
Melissa Amundson, DDS[c,d], Allen Cheng, MD, DMD[c,d,e],
Ashish Patel, MD, DDS[c,d,f], Tuan Bui, MD, DDS[g],
Eric J. Dierks, MD, DMD[c,d], R. Bryan Bell, MD, DDS[c,d,f,h]

KEYWORDS

- Gunshot wounds - Mandible reconstruction - Facial trauma - Ballistic trauma
- Virtual surgical planning - Computer-aided surgery

KEY POINTS

- Mandibular injuries have been treated effectively for generations using closed reduction and open reduction with internal fixation.
- With advances in computer-aided surgery, complex and difficult surgeries are now possible with the precision and accuracy once achieved by only a select few seasoned surgeons.
- The increasing research and applications of custom hardware, patient-specific planning, and virtual surgery has led to, and will continue to lead to, improved patient function, improved esthetics, decreased operative times, decreased costs, and most importantly beneficial patient outcomes.

INTRODUCTION

Mandibular injuries have been treated effectively for generations using closed reduction and open reduction with internal fixation. Recently, there have been several notable advances in surgical management that have added substantially to a facial surgeon's ability to tackle simple as well as complex mandibular injuries more effectively.

Recent hardware advances in closed reduction include maxillomandibular fixation (MMF) screws in lieu of arch bars and hybrid systems that combine traditional arch bars with screw fixation. Open reduction and fixation has seen some very

Disclosure statement: The authors have nothing to disclose.
[a] Advanced Craniomaxillofacial and Trauma Surgery/Head and Neck Oncologic and Microvascular Reconstructive Surgery, Department of Surgery, Legacy Emanuel Medical Center, 2801 N Gantentenbein Avenue, Portland, OR 97227, USA; [b] Providence Portland Hospital, 4805 NE Glisan Street, Portland, OR 97213, USA; [c] Head & Neck Surgical Associates, 1849 NW Kearney Street #302, Portland, OR 97209, USA; [d] Department of Surgery, Trauma Service, Legacy Emanuel Medical Center, 2801 N Gantentenbein Avenue, Portland, OR 97227, USA; [e] Head and Neck Cancer Program, Legacy Good Samaritan Medical Center, 1015 NW 22nd Avenue, Portland, OR 97210, USA; [f] Providence Oral, Head and Neck Cancer Program and Clinic, Providence Cancer Center, 4805 NE Glisan Street, Portland, OR 97213, USA; [g] Oral and Maxillofacial Pathology, Sanford Health, E - 1717 S University Drive Fargo, ND 58103, USA; [h] Robert W. Franz Cancer Research Center, Earle A. Chiles Research Institute at Providence Cancer Center, 4805 NE Glisan Street, Portland, OR 97213, USA
* Corresponding author. 1849 Northwest Kearney Street, #300, Portland, OR 97209.
E-mail address: baber.khatib@gmail.com

exciting applications of technology that include prebent and custom patient plates.

As a result of their complexity, treatment planning for facial ballistic injuries has seen an increase in the use of virtual surgery, patient-specific surgical guides, and intraoperative navigation and/or imaging to yield predictable and consistently repeatable results, once only achievable by seasoned surgeons.

The authors briefly review updates in management of mandibular trauma and reconstruction as they relate to MMF screws, custom hardware, virtual surgical planning (VSP), and protocols for use of computer-aided surgery and navigation when managing composite defects from gunshot injuries to the face.

Advances in Closed Reduction

MMF has a long history in the treatment of facial fractures dating back to 460 BC when Hippocrates used gold wire to fixate teeth for a mandible fracture.[1] Over the years there have been many modifications, including Barton bandage, suspension wires, Ivy loops, arch bars, MMF screws, and embrasure loops.[1–3] Erich arch bars (Karl Leibinger Co, Mulheim, Germany) continue to be the most commonly used technique. MMF screw fixation has the benefit of speedy application, decreased risk of puncture injury to the surgeon, less damage to the periodontium, and simple application and removal.[2,4–6] Their use is not without complications. The most commonly reported complications include screw loosening, iatrogenic damage to tooth roots, screw fracture, and ingestion.[7] A combination between MMF screws and arch bars known as *hybrid systems* are the newest advances to closed reduction. Commonly used systems include the SmartLock System Hybrid MMF (Stryker, Kalamazoo, MI), the MatrixWave (DePuy Synthes West Chester, PA), and the OmniMax MMF System (Zimmer Biomet, Jacksonville, FL). These systems are approved by the Food and Drug Administration for use in adults and children with fully erupted permanent dentition as a temporary means of fixation.[8–10] These systems allow expeditious placement associated with MMF screws while maintaining lugs at crown level, allowing traction vectors closer to the occlusal table. Potential complications are similar to those of MMF screws. Although the hybrid systems are much costlier than Erich arch bars, Kendrick and colleagues'[11] cost analysis of the Stryker SmartLock system versus traditional arch bars found no difference when accounting for operating room time, cost, and time saved.

Advances in Open Reduction

Virtual surgical planning/Stereolithography

Among the greatest technological advances in craniomaxillofacial (CMF) surgery is computer-aided CMF surgery. Bell[12] divides computer-aided CMF surgery into 3 main categories: (1) computer-aided presurgical planning, (2) intraoperative navigation, and (3) intraoperative computed tomography (CT)/MRI imaging. Computer-aided presurgical planning in mandibular trauma and reconstruction involves computer-aided design and computer-aided manufacturing (CAD/CAM) technology and VSP, which can then be applied to the fabrication of stereo-lithographic models and custom plates.[12–15]

Even in basic mandible fractures, intraoperative bending and contouring of reconstruction plates can be time consuming and inaccurate. Complex, multi-segment, and/or avulsed mandibular defects make this task much more difficult and potentially frustrating.

Although originally developed for industry, initial medical applications of CAD/CAM included neurosurgery and radiation therapy. CAD/CAM has since proven indispensable in the reconstruction of complex mandibular trauma and other CMF surgery.[16] CAD/CAM software enables the clinician to import 2-dimensional CT data in Digital Imaging and Communications in Medicine (DICOM) format to a computer workstation and to generate an accurate 3-dimensional (3D) representation of the skeletal and soft tissue anatomy. These digital models can be manipulated by virtual surgery allowing restoration of bony segments to their pretraumatic positions. Stereo-lithographic models of the virtually reduced mandible are then fabricated and can be used to manufacture custom cutting guides, plates, and splints.[12] These models have been reported to be accurate within 1 mm and have shown to decrease operative time and wound exposure time when used in the planning stage.[17,18]

Despite this degree of precision, there are a few areas where significant inaccuracies can be introduced. One critical area of inaccuracy is in the dental occlusion. CT scans, whether medical grade or cone beam, are unable to accurately capture occlusal anatomy. If accurate occlusal relationships are critical for surgical planning, then separate impressions must be taken from patients. These impressions can be done using traditional analog techniques with alginate/polyvinyl siloxane and stone or using newer digital impression techniques. Analog models are scanned into digital information. The dental and occlusal data can then be fused with the maxillofacial CT. Fusion can be done manually by a computer surgical planning engineer. However, if more precision is necessary, an occlusal fiduciary marker (a marker embedded in a bite registration or a bite registration mounted with a registration device) should be used when obtaining the maxillofacial CT and scanning the models. The fiduciary helps in accurately registering the models to the maxillofacial CT.

A second area of inaccuracy is in plate bending. The inherent rigidity of reconstruction plates makes them difficult to bend accurately, particularly when attempting to match the irregular contours of a mandible. Although smoothing osteoplasty can be performed on a model and subsequently transferred to patients, performing the same osteoplasty on patients potentially introduces another source of error. Repeated plate bending decreases fatigue resistance and increases the risk of plate fracture.[19,20] By combining the use of VSP, various CAD/CAM techniques, and novel surgical hardware manufacturing, it is now possible to implant custom plates that require little to no bending.

Custom plates
There are 3 main processes of manufacturing custom plates applicable to CMF surgery and mandible reconstruction: prebent plates, milled (subtractive manufacturing) plates, and additive layer manufacturing (ALM).

Prebent plates
In the infancy of stereo lithography (SLA), a well-documented technique involved printing a corrected stereo-lithographic model to which a reconstruction plate would be hand bent. Prebending decreases operative time and improves accuracy yet still introduces areas of fatigue more prone to failure with cyclic loading. Although the cause of plate fracture is multifactorial, limiting the number of bends to the plate should help maintain the original plate strength. The use of custom milled or printed plates substantially reduces the need for bending, often completely.

Subtractive and additive manufactured plates
The creation of milled plates is a subtractive technique that uses high-precision drills to cut a solid titanium/titanium alloy billet into the desired shape. Computer numerical control (CNC) machining dates back to the early 1940s when Parsons first created numerical control for the aerospace industry. CNC is the computer automation of machining tools, which eliminates the need for manual instrumentation. The 1940 CNC prototype engineered by Parsons at the Massachusetts Institute of Technology is the forbearer of this technology today.[21]

ALM, commonly known as 3D printing, is the newest technique used in plate fabrication. There are 2 main divisions within ALM: sintering and melting. Sintering involves heating metal powder to a temperature just before liquefaction, which allows cohesion to occur at the molecular level. This process allows control of porosity, which may later result in bone growth into the final structure. Melting involves the complete liquefaction of the metal within an accurately shaped container that results in a homogenous structure. These fabrication techniques are further divided into SLA, selective laser melting, selective laser sintering, and electron beam melting/direct metal printing. Current materials used in fracture and reconstruction plates include pure titanium and titanium, aluminum vanadium alloy (Ti6Al4V). Stainless steel 316L and cobalt chrome alloys have also been used in other applications.

Regardless of the additive method used, the basic steps are similar. A CT scan is taken after which the DICOM files are imported into a surgical planning software program. After the mandible is virtually reduced or reconstructed, the surgeon and the engineer collaborate, usually in the form of an online meeting, to design the plate. Once the final design is established, a software program slices the plate digitally into multiple horizontal layers. These data are then entered into a production machine that contains metal powder. A computer-guided laser runs over the powder and solidifies it layer by layer, from the bottom up. Any leftover powder can be reused, which is one major difference between ALM and milling. With milling, the shavings can be reused only after specialized processing, which is costly.

In both the subtractive and additive techniques, the plate is fully customizable and is designed over a digital workflow with an engineer and surgeon. Options for customization in both techniques include plate thickness, shape, screw hole position, number of screw holes, and varied thickness within the same reconstruction plate.

Navigation/intraoperative computed tomography
The digital workflow makes it possible to visualize the entire mandibular and facial skeleton, which is somewhat unrealistic. Unfortunately, these conditions do not translate directly to the operating room. Blood, edema, and avulsive soft and hard tissue defects can make it difficult to see appropriate landmarks for repair. A custom-fabricated plate that looks perfect during VSP can result in malocclusion, facial asymmetry, and poor bony adaptation if the implant does not seat in its exact planned position. The use of navigation systems

has helped bridge the gap between virtual planning and reality.

As described by Bell,[12] navigation is analogous to global positioning systems (GPSs) in a car. The localizer represents a satellite in space; the instrument/probe represents track waves emitted by the GPS unit in the car; the preloaded CT scan represents the map.[12] Intraoperative navigation systems were initially developed for use in neurosurgery as a rigid system known as framed stereotaxy. Since its development, newer technology allows for navigation without rigid head frames, making the tool more accessible to other applications. Frameless stereotaxy is now used commonly in endoscopic surgery and in CMF surgery.[22–26] In CMF surgery, navigation is most commonly used in orbital reconstruction and has been reported to be accurate to within 1 to 2 mm.[27–29] By manipulating the surgical instrument affixed to a probe, one can precisely correlate a position on a computer surgically planned CT scan with patients in coronal, axial, and sagittal views. This ability allows for an intraoperative verification (evaluative phase) after the initial 3 phases of computer-aided CMF surgery have been completed (planning, modeling, surgery). The surgeon has the ability to adjust and verify in real time the positioning of bone and fixation, potentially avoiding an unnecessary return to the operating room if inconsistencies are seen on postoperative imaging.

Complex mandible reconstruction related to ballistic trauma

Gunshot wounds (GSWs) to the craniofacial region result in devastating functional disabilities and esthetic deformities, which are further magnified by the associated psychological trauma. Because most of these patients return to work, return to their preinjury lifestyle, and have a low rate of suicide recidivism, adequate reconstruction is essential to their comprehensive rehabilitation.[30,31]

Although most GSWs involve injuries to extremities, most self-inflicted GSWs are to the head and neck.[32] The infrequency of these injuries, combined with their enormous complexity, makes their reconstruction a daunting task. The complexity of these injuries prompted Rene Le Fort to exclude them in his classic article, reporting GSWs as "veritable explosions in the face" and "without surgical interest."[33] The reported mortality is 15%, with complications in those who survive as high as 30%.[34,35] Survivors have a long road to recovery that ideally involves a large multidisciplinary care team that includes surgeons, medicine, psychiatry, physical therapy, occupational therapy, speech/language pathology, case management, and social work.

In 2014, Shackford and colleagues[34] published an 11-year, 720-patient, multicenter retrospective review of GSW injuries to the face. Of the 720 patients, 20% died within 48 hours. Of those who survived the first 48 hours, 15% were ultimately discharged or transferred. The remaining 85% underwent surgical reconstruction. 41% of these injuries were the result of low-velocity handguns and 40% involved the mandible. Patients with mandibular trauma required an average of 1.7 operations. This finding was consistent with Taher's[36] review of 1135 facial gunshot injuries requiring an average of 1.5 operations.[34]

The tissue damage caused by high-velocity bullets (>1200 feet per second [fps], military/hunting weapons) results in tremendous soft and hard tissue defects both from immediate damage and progressive die-back phenomenon. Low-velocity bullets (<1200 fps) may not cause the same avulsive defects and rarely result in a significant die-back phenomenon but can result in comminution. Traditionally, external fixation was used in this setting to prevent further devascularization of bone secondary to periosteal stripping and to temporarily maintain large bony defects without soft tissue retraction until definitive repair. This procedure has been largely replaced with rigid internal fixation but is still a useful adjunct in the armamentarium for treatment of complex GSWs to the mandible. The significant defects caused by gunshot injuries to the mandible are not unlike those defects caused by ablative tumor surgery or necrotizing infection. Many of the techniques used in the reconstruction of ablative tumor defects can be applied to gunshot injuries to the mandible.

For those cases in which the soft tissue and hard tissue mandibular defects are amenable to primary repair, local flaps, and/or nonvascularized bone grafts, aided by VSP, can expedite the surgical process. In grossly comminuted fractures or continuity defects, the contralateral mandible can be mirrored to the injured side to approximate the mandible's pretraumatic form, which can then be used as described earlier to prebend plates or design custom plates.

The workflow starts with establishing stable reference points by placing patients in maxillomandibular fixation and taking a CT scan using the specific VSP protocol (typically 1-mm cuts) (www. medicalmodeling.com).[37] As mentioned earlier, stone models of the dentition can be sent to the surgical planning engineers and merged with the CT data for added accuracy. Next, a Web-based planning session is scheduled. The fractured and displaced bony segments are aligned virtually by an engineer guided by a surgeon. If any adjustments need to be made, they are done during the

Web meeting. Once the virtual reduction has been completed and confirmed by the surgeon, the placement of the plate is virtually planned. If a custom plate is to be used, the surgeon can decide the shape of the plate, thickness (which can be varied across the length of the plate), and number of holes. Stereo-lithographic models are made to aid in reduction in the operating room. In some instances, positioning guides with predictive holes for the reconstruction plate can help with reduction. In segmental defects, cutting guides are made to precisely freshen the edges of the defects to allow for easy buttressing with reconstructed tissue (**Fig. 1A–H**).

For complex composite mandibular defects, microvascular reconstruction has become a mainstay. Ever since Hidalgo[38] reported the use of the fibula free flap for mandibular reconstruction, it has become the workhorse for such defects. Other flaps used in mandibular reconstruction include the deep circumflex iliac artery (DCIA) flap, scapula, and osteo-cutaneous radial forearm. For many reasons outside the scope of this article, the fibula flap is the most versatile and frequently used. The DCIA flap, scapula flap, and osteo-cutaneous radial forearm flaps have their specific indications but are used much less frequently in the authors' practice.[39]

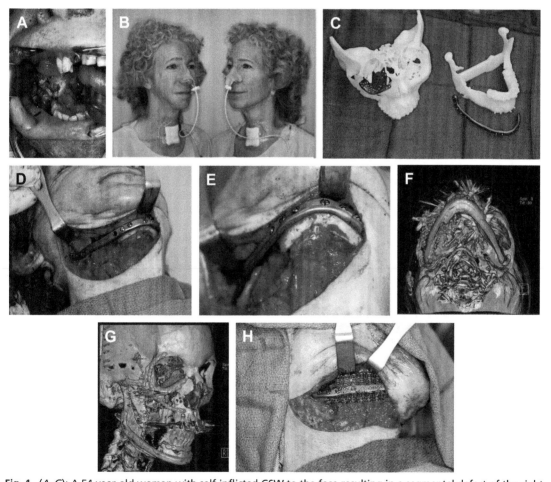

Fig. 1. (*A–G*): A 54-year-old woman with self-inflicted GSW to the face resulting in a segmental defect of the right mandibular body and orbital floor fracture reconstructed with custom orbital floor plate and mandibular reconstruction plate. Segmental defect grafted with autogenous iliac crest, platelet rich plasma (PRP), and bone morphogenetic protein (BMP). (*A*) Intraoral photograph showing comminution of right mandible. (*B*) One month after MMF, tracheostomy, debridement, wound closure, and feeding tube placement. (*C*) Custom printed mandibular reconstruction plate and orbital floor plate on stereo-lithographic models. (*D*) Custom mandibular reconstruction plate in situ. (*E*) Intimate adaptation of custom mandibular reconstruction plate. (*F*) Axial view of facial CT with plate in place. (*G*) The 3D reconstruction of CT with custom hardware in place. (*H*) Autogenous iliac bone graft/PRP/BMP in titanium mesh 3 months after initial injury.

There is some controversy over the method of fixation used for these reconstructions. Some investigators advocate fixation of the neo-mandible with mini-plates, whereas others prefer reconstruction plates.[38–41] Advocates of mini-plates argue that a stress-shielding phenomenon occurs with load-bearing reconstruction plates that impedes osseous healing. However, reconstruction plates have been shown to have less need for removal, lower infection rates, and greater ability to accurately shape the neo-mandible to mimic the native mandible.[41,42]

The mandible, when viewed from above, is shaped like an omega, with an irregular contour (**Fig. 2**). A common problem with adapting the fibula to the shape of the mandible is the discrepancy between the curved mandible and the straight fibula. Traditionally, multiple osteotomies were made to account for this discrepancy. However, recent cadaveric studies suggest that maintaining bone segments 2 cm or greater has a more reliable chance of containing a periosteal vessel then smaller segments (94% vs 65% in 1.0 cm).[43] One method to address the discrepancy, while also limiting the number of fibula osteotomies required, is to take a subunit approach to mandibular reconstruction. The mandibular defect is divided into subunits (body, symphysis, condyle, and ramus). Fibula osteotomies are performed allowing for a straight segment to replace each of these subunits, as necessary. Therefore, a hemi-mandibular defect would only require 2 closing osteotomies and 3 segments, each with sufficient length to maintain vascularity. In addition, this simplifies adaptation of the reconstructive plate to the neo-mandible.

Early on, a stereo-lithographic model could be made by mirroring the contralateral mandible and ground to a flat surface, simulating the fibula. Now, data from stock fibulas can be loaded into the surgical planning software, which can then be printed directly into the stereo-lithographic model for prebending. Alternatively, patient-specific fibula data taken from CT angiograms of the extremities can be loaded into the surgical planning software, for greater accuracy.

In addition, computer-aided surgical planning allows accurate reconstruction in 3 dimensions.[15] Establishing the correct transverse, anterior-posterior, and vertical dimension of the lower face, while simultaneously positioning the neo-mandible to the opposing dental arch at the correct vertical dimension of occlusion, used to be incredibly difficult with the limitations of our surgical approaches to the facial skeleton. Now, this accurate positioning in 3 dimensions is easily verified using virtual models and replicated intraoperatively using guides, navigation, and/or intraoperative CT. These techniques have proven to be accurate, cost saving, and efficient.[44–46] Furthermore, these techniques allow for more predictable implant supported prosthetic rehabilitation while preventing overprojection of the mandible.[12]

Much of the bench work has been moved to the virtual realm with advances in CAD/CAM software and additive manufacturing of surgical guides and custom plates. In 2009, Hirsch and colleagues[47] described the use of Surgi Case CMF software (Materialise, Leuven, Belgium) to virtually plan a mandibular resection and reconstruction with a free fibula flap. The virtually planned osteotomies were incorporated into a surgical guide designed using planning software, then manufactured using a 3D printer, thereby transferring the virtual plan into an intraoperative tool. These surgical guides were then used to create the virtually planned osteotomies in vivo (Medical Modeling, Inc, Golden, CO). This practice allowed the vascularized composite tissue to reconstruct the mandible with ideal anterior/posterior, vertical, and transverse positioning. Levine and colleagues[48] and Hirsch and colleagues[47] have taken this a step further, developing a protocol for Jaw in a Day. In this protocol, they are able to virtually plan a mandibular segmental resection, reconstruction with a fibula free flap, guided placement of dental implants into the fibula, and a fixed provisional hybrid prosthesis that is immediately placed and loaded, all in one surgery.[48] This procedure has been successfully replicated at several institutions, including the authors' own. It has allowed surgeons to take patients to premorbid form and function in 1 day, an end point that previously

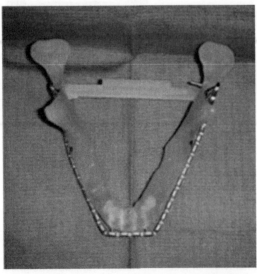

Fig. 2. Omega shape of mandible versus straight fibula.

would require 1 or more years.[49,50] This concept could be applied to mandibular traumatic defects.

Composite mandibular defects can also be managed with the use of distraction osteogenesis (DO). The technique was first described for mandibular reconstruction in 1920 by Rosenthal but did not become popularized until the Ilizarov protocols on limb DO in 1951.[51] It proved advantageous for reconstruction of the facial skeleton in its ability to address both hard and soft tissue deficiencies. A common difficulty associated with this technique is the unpredictable control of the regenerative chamber vector. With stock distraction prostheses, a set linear trajectory is built into the prosthesis dictated by the screw. Bidirectional screws, endless screws, and multi-planar 3D distraction have been described; however, their application to GSW injuries is limited by the inability to locate precise anatomic landmarks.[52,53]

With the advent of computer surgical planning, DO is once again a useful tool in the reconstructive armamentarium. Benateau and colleagues[54] described the use of computer-assisted custom distraction devices and cutting guides for reconstruction of the lower face after gunshot injury.[54] Similar to computer surgical planning discussed earlier, planning for DO facilitates management of the spatial position of the neo-mandible in reference to the dentition and occlusal plane of the maxilla. Akin to the authors' experience with self-inflicted mandible GSW injures, Benateau and colleagues[54] found the ramus/condyle unit tends to be spared. The segments were repositioned virtually; osteotomy lines were planned; and predictive markers were used on the cutting guides for placement of the distraction device. The 2 cases reported showed excellent symmetry and reconstruction of an 8.5-cm and 10.0-cm defect.

In comparison with fibula free flaps, Wojcik and colleagues[55] showed that there was less cost associated with standard DO because of the shorter hospitalization these procedures required. Even though the overall duration of treatment was longer, the duration of hospitalization was shorter on average by 10 days.[55] Another point to consider is the impact of failed therapy. The morbidity associated with failed distraction is significantly less than that of a failed fibula, with the added drawback of donor site morbidity. Nonetheless, case selection is important and the fibula free flap remains the workhorse for reconstruction of composite mandibular defects.

Protocol for Computer-Aided Surgical Reconstruction of Massive Craniomaxillofacial Gunshot Wounds: Focus on Composite Mandibular Defects

At the authors' institution, patients are initially evaluated and managed in accordance to the advance trauma life support system (**Fig. 3**). Particular importance is placed on the airway, as bleeding into the tight compartmentalized spaces of the neck, avulsion of the tongue's attachments, tongue edema, blood, bone, debris, and foreign objects can result in rapidly progressive airway compromise. Oral intubation is often successful with few patients requiring emergent cricothyrotomy or tracheostomy. This finding is consistent with Shackford and colleagues'[34] and Demetriades and colleagues'[35] studies, which reported 83% of patients with facial GSWs were successfully orally intubated and only 5% required a surgical airway.[34,35] Once patients are stabilized, an elective tracheostomy is performed for definitive airway management for the reconstruction phase. A thorough head and neck examination is performed in conjunction with the primary and secondary survey. In patients with penetrating neck injury, the authors follow a selective neck exploration protocol.[56] Those with hard signs of vascular injury, including expanding hematoma, massive

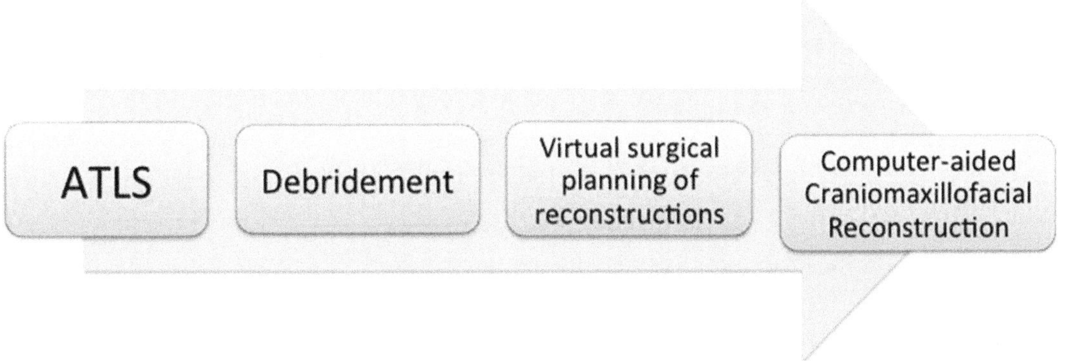

| ATLS | Debridement | Virtual surgical planning of reconstructions | Computer-aided Craniomaxillofacial Reconstruction |

Fig. 3. CMF GSW protocol. ATLS, advanced trauma life support.

subcutaneous emphysema, exsanguinating hemorrhage, shock, or airway compromise, and those with respiratory and hemodynamic stability with violation of the platysma and positive computer angiography tomography (CTA) findings warrant surgical exploration (**Fig. 5**A).

After patients are stabilized, they are taken for debridement, damage control surgery, elective tracheostomy, and feeding tube placement often the same day as arrival. This practice involves washout of the wound, examination under anesthesia (direct laryngoscopy, rigid esophagoscopy and/or esophagogastroduodenoscopy) surgical hemostasis, conservative debridement of frankly necrotic tissues, and wound closure and/or packing. Occasionally, some bony fixation may be applied, if it can be done easily and quickly. The primary objective is to achieve control of the wound and perform an initial assessment. During the time immediately after injury, while patients are marginally stable and in a profound inflammatory state, extended and lengthy procedures should be avoided. Damage control surgeries may require daily short trips to the operating room, particularly with evolving injuries, as is seen in ballistics or burn injuries (see **Fig. 5**B–D).

At this point, a maxillofacial CT scan with 1-mm fine cuts is taken. If a fibula flap is required, a CT angiogram of the lower extremities is also taken. The data are uploaded to the surgical planning software. The maxillofacial surgery team then schedules a Web meeting with an engineer to virtually plan the reconstructions.

The authors' goal is to complete as much of the skeletal and soft tissue reconstruction as possible during the initial hospitalization, with the understanding that revisions will certainly occur later. The authors prefer to stage the computer-aided CMF reconstruction in the following sequence (**Fig. 4**).

The authors begin with the midfacial and orbital reconstruction because of their importance in establishing proper facial width. A reciprocal relationship exists between anterior-posterior projection of the zygoma and facial width. By straightening the zygomatic arch, zygoma projection increases with a resultant decrease in facial width.[57] Stereo-lithographic models are created after virtually reducing midfacial fractures and plates are contoured to them intraoperatively. Intraoperative navigation facilitates accurate reduction and fixation (**Fig. 5**E–H).

Once the bizygomatic width is established, the authors focus on oromandibular reconstruction. The authors find that in self-inflicted GSWs, the condyle ramus unit tends to be spared. This preservation facilitates establishing the vertical dimension of the lower face against the already established transverse width by virtually seating the condyles in the fossa. Composite defects are then reconstructed with a fibula and custom reconstruction plate or custom plate alone in the case of adequate soft tissue and bone for a non-vascularized bone grafts (see **Fig. 1**D).

When planning for fibula reconstruction, the authors prefer butt joints between native mandible and reconstruction to facilitate flap inset. These butt joints are virtually created at the junction of reconstructive subunits (see **Fig. 5**I). Attention is then drawn to the 3D virtual fibula created from preloaded CTA data of the lower extremity.

Depending on the location of recipient vessels in the neck, location of the soft tissue defect and the need for anterior versus posterior positioning of the pedicle the ipsilateral or contralateral fibula is used. For body defects, body and symphysis defects, or angle to angle defects with ipsilateral recipient vessels available, the authors typically have the vessels run posterior. When the condylar ramus subunit needs to be reconstructed, the

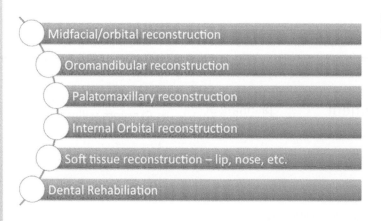

Fig. 4. CMF GSW reconstruction protocol.

Midfacial/orbital reconstruction

Oromandibular reconstruction

Palatomaxillary reconstruction

Internal Orbital reconstruction

Soft tissue reconstruction – lip, nose, etc.

Dental Rehabiliation

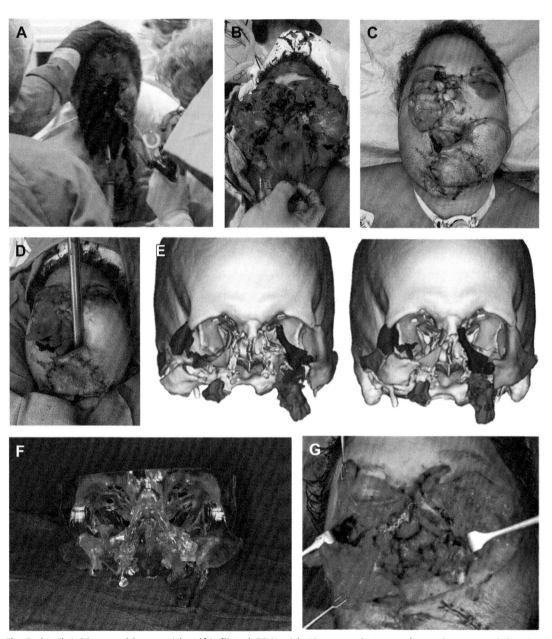

Fig. 5. (*A–P*) A 30-year-old man with self-inflicted GSW with 12-gauge shotgun who underwent stabilization and staged reconstruction following the authors' protocol. (*A*) Patient orally intubated and being stabilized by advanced trauma life support protocol. (*B*) Wound exploration, washout, conservative debridement, tracheostomy. (*C*) Wound closure, damage control. (*D*) Rigid esophagoscopy, direct laryngoscopy. (*E*) Virtual reduction of nasoorbitalethmoidal (NOE) and Le Fort III fractures. (*F*) Stereo-lithographic model with reduced NOE/Le Fort III fractures. (*G*) Open feeding gastrostomy tube placement, open reduction internal fixation Le Fort III fractures, NOE fractures, medial canthopexy. (*H*) Intraoperative navigation facilitates transfer of virtual plan to operating room. (*I*) Virtual surgical cutting guides to create butt joints at native mandible fibula junction. (*J*) Virtual planning of fibula osteotomies. (*K*) Fibula is placed intermediately between alveolus and inferior border at body region. (*L*) Left to right: mandible cutting guide, stereo-lithographic native mandible/maxilla (*pink*), neo-mandible model (*white*) with custom reconstruction plate. (*M*) Cutting guides on fibula (*top*) mandible (*bottom*). (*N*) Fibula inset with perfect adaptation of custom reconstruction plate. (*O*) Virtual planning for maxilla reconstruction with a fibula. (*P*) Use of intraoperative navigation during maxillary reconstruction.

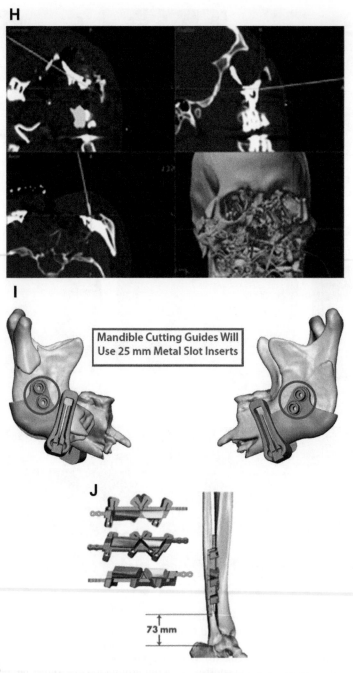

Fig. 5. (*continued*)

authors prefer vessels run anteriorly as this mitigates the need for hairpins in the vessels around the skull base. The engineer then virtually performs a distal osteotomy 6 to 7 cm from the malleolus and closing osteotomies to allow the defect to be filled from posterior to anterior restoring each missing subunit (see **Fig. 5J**). The remaining bone on the proximal fibula is removed and represents pedicle length. The authors choose to place the fibula at an intermediate point between the alveolus and inferior border of the mandible when reconstructing the body and at the inferior border and slightly lateral for reconstruction of the angle. This location allows for ideal placement of dental implants under the maxillary alveolus, providing adequate soft tissue for closure while still maintaining facial symmetry and facial contour (see **Fig. 5K**).

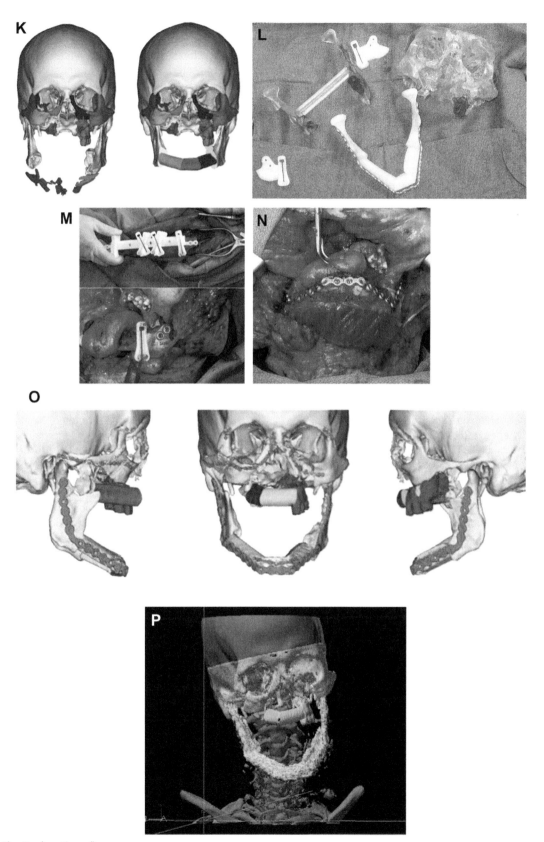

Fig. 5. (continued)

After this reconstructive planning phase, the engineer-surgeon team designs cutting guides and 3D prints them for use intraoperatively. The mandibular cutting guides are fixated on the lateral native mandible with mono-cortical screws and include a removable metal insert allowing for saw placement at the osteotomy site. Predictive holes are made that facilitate placement of the custom reconstruction plate. The fibula cutting guide is preferentially designed to rest on the lateral side of the fibula, which aids in protection of the pedicle during osteotomies and with a 0.5-mm relief to account for soft tissue. A mark is placed on the cutting guide to designate an arbitrarily selected distance from the lateral malleolus, to aid in fitting the fibula guide at the appropriate position along the proximal-distal axis. Finally, a custom 3D-printed reconstruction plate is engineered that matches predictive holes placed on the surgical guides. Templates are also fabricated of the bone graft and plate to assure the actual osteotomies match the computer-simulated plan. Lastly, the VSP data are merged with the original CT scan and overlaid for use with intraoperative navigation (see **Fig. 5**I, L).

Intraoperatively, a 2-team approach is used: one to perform the mandibular osteotomies, place the custom reconstruction plate, and locate recipient vessels while the second team harvests the fibula and shapes it to the computer-aided surgical plan (see **Fig. 5**M). The fibula is then inset, and the microvascular anastomosis is completed (see **Fig. 5**N). If the lip is being reconstructed with the soft tissue pedicle, a tensor fascia lata sling is suspended from the maxilla with Mitek mini anchors (Mitek Products Inc, Westwood, MA). The reconstruction is compared with planned reconstruction with bone graft templates and intraoperative navigation. At the completion of this phase, a postoperative CT scan is taken for the next phase of VSP.

Palatomaxillary reconstruction follows a subunit protocol similar to Brown and colleagues'[58] classification and Bell's[12] VSP approach. If composite reconstruction is planned, the digital workflow is similar to fibula reconstruction of the mandible. Reconstruction of maxilla in the correct 3D orientation is limited by accessibility and visibility in a confined space. An area of particular difficulty is abutting the fibula to the pterygoid plates, which can result in widening and a cant of the maxilla. Intraoperative navigation is an indispensable tool in this aspect. Other reconstructive options include the scapula tip or anterior lateral thigh/radial forearm for soft tissue only (see **Fig. 5**O, P).

Internal orbital reconstruction begins by comparing the internal orbital volume measured by the computer planning engineer. Virtual correction is then made using the uninjured or anatomically correct side by creating a mirror image that superimposes the traumatized side. In bilateral fractures, the least comminuted orbit is virtually corrected and then mirror imaged to the contralateral side. Custom orbital plates and/or stereo-lithographic models are then fabricated using the virtually corrected orbits. With stereo-lithographic models, a mesh plate is contoured preoperatively. Intraoperatively, the plates are positioned with the aid of navigation to locate the posterior orbital ledge. Navigation is then used to confirm its position in relation to the computer-simulated plan in the following sequential systematic protocol: malar eminence, infraorbital rim, lateral orbital rim, orbital floor, medial internal orbit/posteromedial orbital bulge, lateral internal orbit, posterior orbit/orbital apex, and finally globe projection. The authors find this technique reliably establishes orbital contour, volume, anterior bulge, and posterior medial bulge.[12,59–62]

Following a period of healing and establishment of a bony foundations, patients then undergo soft tissue reconstruction. Soft tissue procedures include rotational flaps, fat grafts, injectable fillers, and magnetic implant–supported prosthesis and are beyond the scope of this article.

Lastly, dental rehabilitation and reconstruction of a functional occlusion are performed. This process involves dental implants, hybrid prosthesis fabrication, and communication between the facial surgeon and the prosthodontist.

With this protocol, the authors find they get the best chance of establishing proper facial width, projection, and contour to produce a functional and reasonably esthetic facial reconstruction.

SUMMARY

With advances in computer-aided surgery, complex and difficult surgeries are now possible with the precision and accuracy once achieved by only a select few seasoned surgeons. The increasing research and applications of custom hardware, patient-specific planning, and virtual surgery has led to, and will continue to lead to, improved patient function, improved esthetics, decreased operative times, decreased costs, and most importantly beneficial patient outcomes.

REFERENCES

1. Mukerji R, Mukerji G, McGurk M. Mandibular fractures: historical perspective. Br J Oral Maxillofac Surg 2006;44(3):222–8.
2. Hollows P, Brennan J. Temporary intermaxillary fixation: a quick reliable method. Br J Oral Maxillofac Surg 1999;37(5):422–3.

3. Karlis V, Glickman R. An alternative to arch-bar maxillomandibular fixation. Plast Reconstr Surg 1997; 99(6):1758–9.

4. Arthur G, Berardo N. A simplified technique of maxillomandibular fixation. J Oral Maxillofac Surg 1989; 47(11):1234.

5. Onishi K, Maruyama Y. Simple intermaxillary fixation for maxillomandibular osteosynthesis. J Craniofac Surg 1996;7(2):170–2.

6. Schneider AM, David LR, DeFranzo AJ, et al. Use of specialized bone screws for intermaxillary fixation. Ann Plast Surg 2000;44(2):154–7.

7. Hashemi HM, Parhiz A. Complications using intermaxillary fixation screws. J Oral Maxillofac Surg 2011;69(5):1411–4.

8. DePuy synthes FDA approval. Available at: https://www.accessdata.fda.gov/cdrh_docs/pdf14/K141165.pdf. Accessed January 11, 2016.

9. Stryker Corp. Stryker craniomaxillofacial. Available at: http://www.accessdata.fda.gov/cdrh_docs/pdf12/K122313.pdf. Accessed January 11, 2016.

10. 510K Summary_Revised_12-10-2015-FDA. Available at: https://www.accessdata.fda.gov/cdrh_docs/pdf15/K152326.pdf. Accessed January 11, 2016.

11. Kendrick DE, Park CM, Fa JM, et al. Stryker SMART-Lock hybrid maxillomandibular fixation system: clinical application, complications, and radiographic findings. Plast Reconstr Surg 2016;137(1): 142e–50e.

12. Bell RB. Computer planning and intraoperative navigation in cranio-maxillofacial surgery. Oral Maxillofac Surg Clin North Am 2010;22(1):135–56.

13. Bell RB, Weimer KA, Dierks EJ, et al. Computer planning and intraoperative navigation for palatomaxillary and mandibular reconstruction with fibular free flaps. J Oral Maxillofac Surg 2011;69(3):724–32.

14. Bui TG, Bell RB, Dierks EJ. Technological advances in the treatment of facial trauma. Atlas Oral Maxillofac Surg Clin North Am 2012;20(1):81–94.

15. Markiewicz MR, Bell RB. The use of 3D imaging tools in facial plastic surgery. Facial Plast Surg Clin North Am 2011;19(4):655–82, ix.

16. Schramm A, Wilde F. Computer-assisted reconstruction of the facial skeleton. HNO 2011;59(8):800–6 [in German].

17. Barker TM, Earwaker WJ, Lisle DA. Accuracy of stereolithographic models of human anatomy. Australas Radiol 1994;38(2):106–11.

18. Mehra P, Miner J, D'Innocenzo R, et al. Use of 3-d stereolithographic models in oral and maxillofacial surgery. J Maxillofac Oral Surg 2011;10(1):6–13.

19. Martola M, Lindqvist C, Hänninen H, et al. Fracture of titanium plates used for mandibular reconstruction following ablative tumor surgery. J Biomed Mater Res B Appl Biomater 2007;80(2):345–52.

20. Alberts LR, Phillips KO, Tu HK, et al. A biologic model for assessment of osseous strain patterns and plating systems in the human maxilla. J Oral Maxillofac Surg 2003;61(1):79–88.

21. History of CNC milling and turning machines. Available at: http://www.cam-machine.com/history-of-cnc-milling-and-turning-machines/. Accessed June 11, 2016.

22. Hassfeld S, Muhling J. Computer assisted oral and maxillofacial surgery–a review and an assessment of technology. Int J Oral Maxillofac Surg 2001; 30(1):2–13.

23. Drake JM, Joy M, Goldenberg A, et al. Computer- and robot-assisted resection of thalamic astrocytomas in children. Neurosurgery 1991;29(1):27–33.

24. Mosges R, Klimek L. Computer-assisted surgery of the paranasal sinuses. J Otolaryngol 1993;22(2): 69–71.

25. Ossoff RH, Reinisch L. Computer-assisted surgical techniques: a vision for the future of otolaryngology-head and neck surgery. J Otolaryngol 1994;23(5): 354–9.

26. Barnett GH. Surgical management of convexity and falcine meningiomas using interactive image-guided surgery systems. Neurosurg Clin N Am 1996;7(2): 279–84.

27. Metzger MC, Rafii A, Holhweg-Majert B, et al. Comparison of 4 registration strategies for computer-aided maxillofacial surgery. Otolaryngol Head Neck Surg 2007;137(1):93–9.

28. Luebbers HT, Messmer P, Obwegeser JA, et al. Comparison of different registration methods for surgical navigation in cranio-maxillofacial surgery. J Craniomaxillofac Surg 2008;36(2):109–16.

29. Austin RE, Antonyshyn OM. Current applications of 3-d intraoperative navigation in craniomaxillofacial surgery: a retrospective clinical review. Ann Plast Surg 2012;69(3):271–8.

30. Ozturk S, Bozkurt A, Durmus M, et al. Psychiatric analysis of suicide attempt subjects due to maxillofacial gunshot. J Craniofac Surg 2006;17(6):1072–5.

31. Shuck LW, Orgel MG, Vogel AV. Self-inflicted gunshot wounds to the face: a review of 18 cases. J Trauma 1980;20(5):370–7.

32. Cunningham LL, Haug RH, Ford J. Firearm injuries to the maxillofacial region: an overview of current thoughts regarding demographics, pathophysiology, and management. J Oral Maxillofac Surg 2003;61(8):932–42.

33. Tessier P. The classic reprint. Experimental study of fractures of the upper jaw. I and II. Rene Le Fort, M.D. Plast Reconstr Surg 1972;50(5):497–506 contd.

34. Shackford SR, Kahl JE, Calvo RY, et al. Gunshot wounds and blast injuries to the face are associated with significant morbidity and mortality: results of an 11-year multi-institutional study of 720 patients. J Trauma Acute Care Surg 2014;76(2): 347–52.

35. Demetriades D, Chahwan S, Gomez H, et al. Initial evaluation and management of gunshot wounds to the face. J Trauma 1998;45(1):39–41.

36. Taher AA. Management of weapon injuries to the craniofacial skeleton. J Craniofac Surg 1998;9(4): 371–82.

37. 3D systems cranio-maxillofacial CT scanning protocol. Available at: http://www.medicalmodeling.com/downloads. Accessed November 6, 2016.

38. Hidalgo DA. Fibula free flap: a new method of mandible reconstruction. Plast Reconstr Surg 1989;84(1):71–9.

39. Disa JJ, Cordeiro PG. Mandible reconstruction with microvascular surgery. Semin Surg Oncol 2000; 19(3):226–34.

40. Hidalgo DA, Pusic AL. Free-flap mandibular reconstruction: a 10-year follow-up study. Plast Reconstr Surg 2002;110(2):438–49 [discussion: 450–1].

41. Bell RB, Dierks EJ, Potter JK, et al. A comparison of fixation techniques in oro-mandibular reconstruction utilizing fibular free flaps. J Oral Maxillofac Surg 2007;65(9):39.

42. Al-Bustani S, Austin GK, Ambrose EC, et al. Miniplates versus reconstruction bars for oncologic free fibula flap mandible reconstruction. Ann Plast Surg 2016;77(3):314–7.

43. Fry AM, Laugharne D, Jones K. Osteotomising the fibular free flap: an anatomical perspective. Br J Oral Maxillofac Surg 2016;54(6):692–3.

44. Toto JM, Chang EI, Agag R, et al. Improved operative efficiency of free fibula flap mandible reconstruction with patient-specific, computer-guided preoperative planning. Head Neck 2015;37(11): 1660–4.

45. Metzler P, Geiger EJ, Alcon A, et al. Three-dimensional virtual surgery accuracy for free fibula mandibular reconstruction: planned versus actual results. J Oral Maxillofac Surg 2014;72(12):2601–12.

46. Weijs WL, Coppen C, Schreurs R, et al. Accuracy of virtually 3D planned resection templates in mandibular reconstruction. J Craniomaxillofac Surg 2016; 44(11):1828–32.

47. Hirsch DL, Garfein ES, Christensen AM, et al. Use of computer-aided design and computer-aided manufacturing to produce orthognathically ideal surgical outcomes: a paradigm shift in head and neck reconstruction. J Oral Maxillofac Surg 2009;67(10): 2115–22.

48. Levine JP, Bae JS, Soares M, et al. Jaw in a day: total maxillofacial reconstruction using digital technology. Plast Reconstr Surg 2013;131(6):1386–91.

49. Qaisi M, Kolodney H, Swedenburg G, et al. Fibula jaw in a day: state of the art in maxillofacial reconstruction. J Oral Maxillofac Surg 2016;74(6):1284. e1–15.

50. Monaco C, Stranix JT, Avraham T, et al. Evolution of surgical techniques for mandibular reconstruction using free fibula flaps: the next generation. Head Neck 2016;38(Suppl 1):E2066–73.

51. Cope JB, Samchukov ML, Cherkashin AM. Mandibular distraction osteogenesis: a historic perspective and future directions. Am J Orthod Dentofacial Orthop 1999;115(4):448–60.

52. Labbe D, Nicolas J, Kaluzinski E, et al. Gunshot wounds: two cases of midface reconstruction by osteogenic distraction. J Plast Reconstr Aesthet Surg 2009;62(9):1174–80.

53. Gateno J, Teichgraeber JF, Aguilar E. Distraction osteogenesis: a new surgical technique for use with the multiplanar mandibular distractor. Plast Reconstr Surg 2000;105(3):883–8.

54. Benateau H, Chatellier A, Caillot A, et al. Computer-assisted planning of distraction osteogenesis for lower face reconstruction in gunshot traumas. J Craniomaxillofac Surg 2016;44(10): 1583–91.

55. Wojcik T, Ferri J, Touzet S, et al. Distraction osteogenesis versus fibula free flap for mandibular reconstruction after gunshot injury: socioeconomic and technical comparisons. J Craniofac Surg 2011; 22(3):876–82.

56. Bell RB, Osborn T, Dierks EJ, et al. Management of penetrating neck injuries: a new paradigm for civilian trauma. J Oral Maxillofac Surg 2007;65(4): 691–705.

57. Gruss JS, Van Wyck L, Phillips JH, et al. The importance of the zygomatic arch in complex midfacial fracture repair and correction of posttraumatic orbitozygomatic deformities. Plast Reconstr Surg 1990; 85(6):878–90.

58. Brown JS, Shaw RJ. Reconstruction of the maxilla and midface: introducing a new classification. Lancet Oncol 2010;11(10):1001–8.

59. Bell RB, Markiewicz MR. Computer-assisted planning, stereolithographic modeling, and intraoperative navigation for complex orbital reconstruction: a descriptive study in a preliminary cohort. J Oral Maxillofac Surg 2009;67(12): 2559–70.

60. Markiewicz MR, Dierks EJ, Bell RB. Does intraoperative navigation restore orbital dimensions in traumatic and post-ablative defects? J Craniomaxillofac Surg 2012;40(2):142–8.

61. Markiewicz MR, Dierks EJ, Potter BE, et al. Reliability of intraoperative navigation in restoring normal orbital dimensions. J Oral Maxillofac Surg 2011; 69(11):2833–40.

62. Markiewicz MR, Gelesko S, Bell RB. Zygoma reconstruction. Oral Maxillofac Surg Clin North Am 2013; 25(2):167–201.

Current Management of Subcondylar Fractures of the Mandible, Including Endoscopic Repair

Alexis M. Strohl, MD*, Robert M. Kellman, MD

KEYWORDS

• Subcondylar • Trauma • Fracture • Endoscopic • Mandible

KEY POINTS

- When patients can be placed into their normal occlusion, closed management with elastic maxillomandibular fixation and physical therapy is likely sufficient treatment.
- Several studies have shown better outcomes for subcondylar fractures treated with open reduction, internal fixation compared with closed management. When the occlusion cannot be reduced, open treatment is advised.
- Endoscopic-assisted open reduction with or without fixation achieves the benefits of open repair while minimizing risk.

GENERAL OVERVIEW

Proper management of subcondylar fractures has been a subject of debate for many years. Access to the condyle is technically challenging with risks of serious side effects. In the past, this has led to a trend of treating these patients via a closed approach.[1] However, there is no general consensus about what the best treatment is for various fracture patterns.[2] Recently, paradigms have begun to shift with several studies suggesting that open reduction leads to better outcomes[3–6] and advances in endoscopic technology are improving visualization and decreasing surgical risks.

Subcondylar fractures encompass 25% to 45% of all mandible fractures.[7] Traditional mechanisms of injury include bicycle accidents, motor vehicle accidents, fall from standing, and assault. It is common for other concomitant facial trauma to be present, including other mandible fractures. It is important to differentiate between condylar head, coronoid, condylar neck, subcondylar, and ramus fractures, as treatment options depend on fracture location. By definition, a subcondylar fracture extends from the mandibular notch to the posterior border of the ramus.[8]

IMAGING

Several imaging modalities can be used for adequate visualization of the mandible. The panorex is helpful to show fracture locations, as the entire mandible is imaged. Because of its 2 dimensions, it may be difficult to determine comminution and length of the proximal segment. Radiographic images have somewhat fallen out of favor. The Townes view (30° anteroposterior view) provides better visualization of the condyles and can show the mediolateral positioning of the condylar

Disclosure statement: The authors have nothing to disclose.
Department of Otolaryngology and Communication Sciences, State University of New York Upstate Medical University, 241 CWB, 750 East Adams Street, Syracuse, NY 13210, USA
* Corresponding author. 601 Elmwood Avenue, Box 629, Rochester, NY 14642.
E-mail address: alexis_strohl@urmc.rochester.edu

Facial Plast Surg Clin N Am 25 (2017) 577–580
http://dx.doi.org/10.1016/j.fsc.2017.06.008
1064-7406/17/Published by Elsevier Inc.

segments. Computed tomography (CT) scanning has become the new gold standard for imaging. With the advent of 3-dimensional (3D) reconstruction, CT images can be both informative and instructional for preoperative planning. Viewing the condyle can be challenging with radiograph or panorex because of the bony overlap. Three-view CT scans and 3D images provide the precise orientation and angle of the condyle, which is important to determine when deciphering what treatment is indicated.

METHODS OF TREATMENT

Treatment options for subcondylar fractures are generally divided into 2 groups: closed versus open management. Closed treatment involves some form of maxillomandibular fixation (MMF) with either rigid or elastic interdental fixation. There has been a trend toward using elastic fixation to encourage early temporomandibular joint mobilization and discourage long-term joint arthroses. Additionally, the use of elastics allows the occlusion to be retrained to a normal relationship. Typically, in closed management the fracture is not actually reduced; but it is possible to place patients in their normal occlusion without reduction. It is the authors' preference to use arch bars and elastic interdental fixation to retrain the musculature and guide normal occlusive relationships.

There are many different approaches that have been developed over the years for open treatment of subcondylar fractures. These approaches include retromandibular, submandibular, preauricular, and transoral incisions. With the advent of endoscopes, the transoral endoscopic approach to the condyle was developed. This method may be used with angled instruments or with transbuccal stab incisions to assist with rigid fixation.

In the past, most fractures were managed with closed treatment, which was mainly because of limitations in surgical access and risks associated with open procedures. It was thought that the risk of opening the area outweighed the benefits. Over time, paradigms began to shift with the idea that open management may achieve superior outcomes in some circumstances. Eckelt and colleagues[3] multi-institutional prospective randomized controlled trial challenged the idea that open and closed management achieved similar results by assigning patients to one of 2 treatment arms: closed treatment with MMF versus open surgical treatment. This study was stopped early because of the clear benefit being seen in open procedures over closed procedures, specifically in relation to mandibular shortening, angulation,

protrusion, and maximal interincisal distance. There were more reported occlusal disturbances from both the patients' perspective and physician evaluation in the closed treatment group. There was also more pain reported at 6 months in the closed group. The study concluded that all condylar fractures with angulation and mandibular shortening should be repaired with open reduction, internal fixation. One caveat to Eckelt and colleagues's[3] study is that experienced maxillofacial trauma surgeons were performing the procedures and complication rates in general were low. It is unclear if all cranio-maxillofacial trauma surgeons would achieve similar outcomes.

Zrounba and colleagues's[4] study looked retrospectively at 5 years of data treating condylar and subcondylar fractures via an open approach. From the results, they supported open repair stating there is a low complication rate while achieving better reduction and secure placement of plates. Furthermore, a meta-analysis by Kyzas and colleagues[5] showed that open reduction is as good as conservative management in all cases and may be the superior treatment option in select cases. This finding needs to be viewed in relation to a potential selection bias that would likely have shown an advantage for closed reduction.

There are no definitive recommendations for when endoscopic repair is indicated. In general, noncomminuted fractures with lateral override are considered easier to repair endoscopically than their counterparts. Bilateral fractures pose the additional challenge of reestablishing mandibular height. Edentulous patients also create the challenge of determining the height and position of the mandible without the guidance of the occlusion. High subcondylar or condylar head fractures are also challenging because of the difficulty plating these fractures.

Kokemueller and colleagues's[6] prospective study compared closed treatment twith endoscopic repair in patients with condylar neck fractures with or without dislocation. In the short-term, the patients treated with closed management reported less pain and dysfunction than the endoscopic group. However, at the 1-year follow-up, there were significantly fewer symptoms overall in the endoscopic group in regard to pain, occlusal disturbances, and articulation, suggesting that these patients benefit from endoscopic repair.

Endoscopic repair of subcondylar fractures has been described using both a transoral and a submandibular approach. Although the submandibular approach provides a more head-on view of the fracture, it the authors' preference to perform a transoral approach and, hence, avoid an external incision. Schön and colleagues[9] performed a series of open repairs on 17 patients, 8 of whom were treated with an endoscopic transoral approach. He showed that the transoral approach was a reliable form of treatment of subcondylar fractures and that, once trained in this technically challenging approach, it can be much faster than an open approach.

ENDOSCOPIC SURGICAL TECHNIQUE

The surgery begins by placing arch bars and putting patients in MMF. The mucosa overlying the ramus in infiltrated with lidocaine with epinephrine. An incision is made over the anterior border of the ramus and extended to the oblique line. The periosteum and masseter are then elevated over the lateral surface of the mandible from the angle to the condylar neck. Keeping the periosteum intact decreases bleeding and improves visualization. Once a pocket is created, the endoscope is introduced. A 4-mm, 30° rigid telescope is used through a brow lift sheath. Elevation is continued until the fracture site is encountered. Care is taken to elevate along the lateral border of the proximal segment.

Furthermore, to facilitate downward traction on the mandible, a stab incision parallel to the facial nerve is made and a trocar is placed at the angle. A self-tapping, self-drilling screw is placed in the bone and a wire is twisted around the screw to help manipulate the distal segment.[10] An alternative is creating a small submandibular incision and placing a drill hole. A 24-gauge wire may be threaded through the hole to use for manipulation when attempting reduction.[11]

Once there is adequate visualization, the fracture is ready to be reduced. Patients need to be released from MMF to accomplish this. Downward traction is applied to the distal segment by either pushing downward on the mandibular teeth or using one of the previously described methods. A bite block may be placed between the ipsilateral molar dentition while attempting to place the anterior dentition in occlusion. This placement will lengthen the ramus and aid in reduction. Medially displaced fractures can be more difficult to reduce, and it may be necessary to move the proximal segment laterally first. A transbuccal stab incision is placed, and a trocar is introduced. Once the fragment is lateralized, instruments introduced through the trocar may be used to help reduce the fracture. A second stab incision may be placed, and a threaded fragment manipulator may be secured to the proximal segment for better control of the fragment if necessary. However, if this is used, great

care must be taken not to fracture the screw portion of the device.

When possible, 2-plate fixation has been advised because of the risk of bony fracture displacement and/or plate fracture.[12] If only one plate is possible because of patient anatomy and fracture characteristics, elastic MMF may be required postoperatively to offset some of the dynamic force on the plate. Typically, 2-0 zygomatic plates are used with a goal of 2 holes placed on either side of the fracture (Fig. 1). Resorbable plates have been discussed; however, they have not proven to be strong enough to withstand the occlusal loading of the condyle and there is a risk of refracture.[4,12] There may be a role for their use in combination with elastic MMF, but data are limited.[4]

Postoperatively, patients may require elastic MMF until the natural occlusion is restored. Rigid fixation is typically not required. A soft diet is advised for 4 to 6 weeks. Physical therapy is often indicated, particularly when there is concern for temporomandibular joint arthroses or malocclusion. The need for postoperative imaging is not clearly defined. The authors prefer to obtain a coronal CT scan to ensure the condylar fragment is reduced into the glenoid fossa.

COMPLICATIONS

Facial nerve injury is possible with transoral endoscopic repair but, in theory, should be much less of a risk than with open repair. No facial nerve injury was reported in several studies.[2,3,10,12,13] Lee and colleagues[14] reported a single temporary facial nerve injury that fully recovered, and Kang and colleagues[12] reported 3 temporary facial palsies that improved over time. These findings

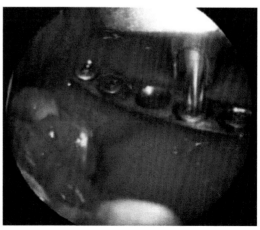

Fig. 1. Endoscopic placement of final screw in the distal segment of a subcondylar fracture.

are in comparison with the 12% to 48% risk of facial nerve injury in an open approach.[15] Scarring is also minimized by only using stab incisions on the external skin, which generally heal well.

SUMMARY

In the past, the treatment of subcondylar fractures was heavily biased toward closed management. This bias was likely due to the technical difficulty of open repairs with high risks of complications, including facial nerve injury. Recent literature suggests that open repair achieves better functional outcomes overall. The advent of endoscopic repair has provided a mechanism to perform open reduction while minimizing surgical risk. Overall, this will lead to better outcomes for patients.

REFERENCES

1. Zide MF, Kent JN. Indications for open reduction of mandibular condyle fractures. J Oral Maxillofac Surg 1983;41(2):89–98.
2. Schneider M, Erasmus F, Gerlach KL, et al. Open reduction and internal fixation versus closed treatment and mandibulomaxillary fixation of fractures of the mandibular condylar process: a randomized, prospective, multicenter study with special evaluation of fracture level. J Oral Maxillofac Surg 2008; 66(12):2537–44.
3. Eckelt U, Schneider M, Erasmus F, et al. Open versus closed treatment of fractures of the mandibular condylar process-a prospective randomized multi-centre study. J Craniomaxillofac Surg 2006; 34(5):306–14.
4. Zrounba H, Lutz JC, Zink S, et al. Epidemiology and treatment outcome of surgically treated mandibular condyle fractures. A five years retrospective study. J Craniomaxillofac Surg 2014;42(6):879–84.
5. Kyzas PA, Saeed A, Tabbenor O. The treatment of mandibular condyle fractures: a meta-analysis. J Craniomaxillofac Surg 2012;40(8):e438–52.
6. Kokemueller H, Konstantinovic VS, Barth EL, et al. Endoscope-assisted transoral reduction and internal fixation versus closed treatment of mandibular condylar process fractures–a prospective double-center study. J Oral Maxillofac Surg 2012;70(2): 384–95.
7. Dahlstrom L, Kahnberg KE, Lindahl L. 15 years follow-up on condylar fractures. Int J Oral Maxillofac Surg 1989;18(1):18–23.
8. Brandt MT, Haug RH. Open versus closed reduction of adult mandibular condyle fractures: a review of the literature regarding the evolution of current thoughts on management. J Oral Maxillofac Surg 2003;61(11):1324–32.
9. Schön R, Gutwald R, Schramm A, et al. Endoscopy-assisted open treatment of condylar fractures of the mandible: extraoral vs intraoral approach. Int J Oral Maxillofac Surg 2002;31(3):237–43.
10. You HJ, Moon KC, Yoon ES, et al. Clinical and radiological outcomes of transoral endoscope-assisted treatment of mandibular condylar fractures. Int J Oral Maxillofac Surg 2016;45(3):284–91.
11. Kellman RM. Endoscopically assisted repair of subcondylar fractures of the mandible: an evolving technique. Arch Facial Plast Surg 2003;5(3):244–50.
12. Kang SH, Choi EJ, Kim HW, et al. Complications in endoscopic-assisted open reduction and internal fixation of mandibular condyle fractures. Oral Surg Oral Med Oral Pathol Oral Radiol 2012; 113(2):201–6.
13. Gonzalez-Garcia R, Sanroman JF, Goizueta-Adame C, et al. Transoral endoscopic-assisted management of subcondylar fractures in 17 patients: an alternative to open reduction with rigid internal fixation and closed reduction with maxillomandibular fixation. Int J Oral Maxillofac Surg 2009;38(1):19–25.
14. Lee C, Stiebel M, Young DM. Cranial nerve VII region of the traumatized facial skeleton: optimizing fracture repair with the endoscope. J Trauma 2000; 48(3):423–31 [discussion: 431–2].
15. Shi D, Patil PM, Gupta R. Facial nerve injuries associated with the retromandibular transparotid approach for reduction and fixation of mandibular condyle fractures. J Craniomaxillofac Surg 2015; 43(3):402–7.

Issues in Pediatric Craniofacial Trauma

Srinivasa R. Chandra, MD, BDS, FDSRCS[a],*, Karen S. Zemplenyi, MD, DDS[b]

KEYWORDS

- Maxillofacial • Craniofacial • Craniomaxillofacial trauma • Pediatric trauma
- Pediatric craniofacial development

KEY POINTS

- The ratio of calvarium to facial skeleton affects incidence and location of craniomaxillofacial trauma in comparing patterns of trauma in children and adults.
- Fixation principles differ in pediatric cases as compared with adults to minimize potential growth restrictions and perturbations.
- The location of permanent tooth follicles must be considered in repair of Maxillomandibular injuries in individuals with primary or mixed dentition.
- Most common pediatric maxillofacial fractures for ages 0 to 18 are mandible (32.7%), nasal bone (30.2%), and maxilla and zygoma (28.6%).
- "Less-is-more" is often the best modus operandi in pediatric trauma treatment.

EPIDEMIOLOGY

In the setting of pediatric maxillofacial trauma, the age group of focus specifically includes children from birth to skeletal maturity (ages 16–18). Death is a common sequelae of trauma in children. However, the incidence of facial trauma is around 15%, far more uncommon than among adults. Pediatric facial fracture types are linked with age-related levels of activity—for example, learning to walk, ride a bike, and contact sports. Child abuse must be considered in cases of multiple facial fractures at various stages of healing with a pattern notable for dentoalveolar injuries and delayed presentation for treatment. With age, there is an overall increase in facial fracture incidence and a decrease in cranial fracture incidence.

The main insults resulting in maxillofacial injury are motor vehicle accidents and falls, making up 50% and 23% of mandibular injuries, respectively, in this age group.[1] The most common pediatric maxillofacial fractures for children ages 0 to 18 years old are mandible (32.7%), nasal bone (30.2%), and maxilla and zygoma (28.6%).[2] Some studies report orbital fractures to be the second most prevalent fracture type; however, nasal fractures are often underreported. Two-thirds of facial injuries occur in boys.[3]

GROWTH AND SURGICAL CONSIDERATIONS

At birth, the cranial vault consists of plates of intramembranous bone with interposed fibrous connective tissue. Embryologically, the midfacial skeleton and cranial vault are derived from intramembranous growth, whereas the skull base and mandibular growth centers derive from endochondral ossification. The intramembranously derived bones heal via fibrous union and subsequent ossification as compared with endochondrally derived

Disclosure Statement: The authors have nothing to disclose.
[a] Oral Maxillofacial–Head and Neck Oncologic Microvascular Reconstructive Surgery, University of Washington, Seattle, WA, USA; [b] Department of Oral Maxillofacial Surgery, University of Washington, Seattle, WA, USA
* Corresponding author. Harborview Medical Center, 325 9th Avenue, Box 359893, Seattle WA 98104.
E-mail addresses: chandra4@uw.edu; ramachandra.srini@gmail.com

Facial Plast Surg Clin N Am 25 (2017) 581–591
http://dx.doi.org/10.1016/j.fsc.2017.06.009

bones, which ossify through a cartilaginous intermediate. Any trauma or vascular changes to these zones of ossification have the potential to curtail growth. This potential starts as early as birth, at which time any insult or injury to the craniomaxillofacial skeleton might impede or interrupt the multifactorial complex facial bony development. The birthing process itself possesses inherent trauma because the cranial fontanelles must telescope over one another during fetal passage through the vaginal canal. Developmental anatomy in the pediatric patient impacts craniomaxillofacial injury patterns and, as such, the epidemiologic incidence and location of facial fractures varies with skeletal maturity.

Pediatric maxillofacial fractures themselves are relatively rare owing to anatomic differences between the juvenile and adult skulls. First, children's bone is less calcified than that of adults, making fracture less likely than "greenstick" flexing of the bone upon subjection to a force. Second, the facial sinuses are not well-developed until the teenage years (**Fig. 1, Table 1**).[3–5] These pneumatized barriers, which would otherwise cushion impact energy to brain, are less developed in children, leading to an increased number of cranial injuries as opposed to shattering of facial bones. Third, the overall ratio of cranial to facial volume decreases with age- 8:1 at birth, 4:1 at 5 years of age, and 2:1 for adults, which further explains why adults would exhibit proportionately more facial trauma as opposed to neurologic injury.[6] Fourth, children have more fat pads around the maxilla and mandible, allowing for increased

cushioning of forces leading to reduced fracture rate and enhancing the greenstick fracture effect.[7]

At birth, the mandible has relatively thin cortices with primary tooth buds comprising the majority of the mandibular volume (**Fig. 2**). Cortical bone thickens with growth and the tooth buds occupy relatively less volume with age. The mandibular vectors of growth are controlled by a constellation of interworking factors, including cartilaginous growth centers and soft tissue pull of the surrounding musculature—the "functional matrix."[8] The primary mandibular cartilaginous growth center is in the condyle, which grows in a superior and posterior direction, resulting in an anterior and inferior translation of the mandible with maturity. From birth to 3 years of age, elongation of the mandibular body occurs via labial bony deposition and lingual resorption. With eruption of the primary dentition from 6 months through 3 years of age, and the subsequent establishment of dental occlusion, comes increases in alveolar bone height and width. Notably, the location of the mental foramen in children younger than 3 years old is relatively anterior, presenting in the region between the primary canine and second deciduous molar. The last primary tooth root to form is that of the canine at an average age of 3.25 years (**Table 2**). On average, teeth take 2 to 3 years from crown formation to eruption and root completion.

By the age of 5 to 6 years old, the growth of the mandibular ramus has achieved its maximal rate, increasing the anterior–posterior projection of the mandible, paralleling the growth of the pharynx and maxilla.[9] This lengthening of the arch is

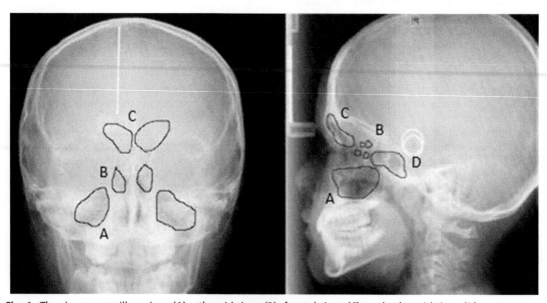

Fig. 1. The sinuses: maxillary sinus (A), ethmoid sinus (B), frontal sinus (C), and sphenoid sinus (D).

Table 1
Sinus development

Sinus	Status at Birth	Age at Which Adult Size Achieved
Maxillary sinus	Present	15 y
Ethmoid sinus	Present	12 y
Frontal sinus	Absent	Postpubertal
Sphenoid sinus	Absent	14 y

Data from Shah RK, Dhingra JK, Carter BL, et al. Paranasal sinus development: a radiographic study. Laryngoscope 2003;113(2):205–9.

necessary to accommodate the permanent molar, which erupts distally to the primary dentition around the age of 6. With the permanent dentition, the teeth per quadrant increases from 5 to 8. This lengthening results in a mental foramen near its adult position—inferior to the second premolar. By age 12, all permanent teeth have erupted with full root completion around age 15 (third molars, or "wisdom teeth," erupt from ages 17–21 years). Pubertal growth spurts result in increased condylar height and vertical orientation of the ramus.[9]

AIRWAY

The pediatric airway is significantly different compared with that of an adult. The mandible, in comparison, is not as prominent, but the tongue volume is larger with a more oblong and U-shaped epiglottis (**Fig. 3**). In addition, the tonsils and adenoids are more prominent in children as compared with adults. Other pediatric airway characteristics include a funnel-shaped larynx, which is narrow at the subglottic region, less compliant upper respiratory airway, higher respiratory rates, and the lesser total lung volume. Taken together, these qualities equate to less free air space and lower threshold for airway collapse.

SKELETAL INJURIES
Skull and Calvarial Injuries

Skull injuries in the pediatric population are a result of direct impact to the calvarium. The proportion of the skull to the face and mandible in the early years is close to 90% (**Fig. 4**). This is significant because of the associated intracranial injury, leading to traumatic death and disability in childhood.[10] The neurovisceral injuries are due to high force impact, such as those from motor vehicle collisions, and often present with associated midfacial and mandibular trauma.

Frontal Sinus Fractures

The frontal sinus is the last paranasal sinus to complete pneumatization at the end of the second decade of life, beginning between the ages of 5 and 8 years.[4,5,11] Isolated frontal bone injury is fairly common owing to its prominent overhang (**Fig. 5**). The management of pediatric frontal sinus injury is similar to that of adult fracture treatment. Neurosurgical needs are paramount as posterior wall fractures can be associated with cerebrospinal fluid leak. Close follow-up is necessary

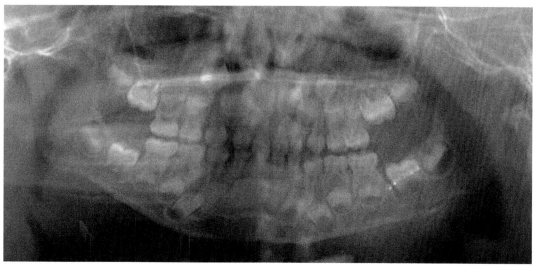

Fig. 2. Panoramic radiograph and permanent detention. This panoramic radiograph of a 5-year-old girl shows primary dentition with full complement of permanent dental follicles below. Note the proximity of the permanent follicles to the inferior border of the mandible.

Table 2
Developmental milestones of primary teeth (mean ages)

	Central Incisor	Lateral Incisor	Canine	First Molar	Second Molar
Maxillary					
Crown completed	1.5 mo	2.5 mo	9 mo	6 mo	11 mo
Eruption	10 mo	11 mo	19 mo	16 mo	29 mo
Root completed	1.5 y	2 y	3.25 y	2.5 y	3 y
Mandibular					
Crown completed	2.5 mo	3 mo	9 mo	5.5 mo	10 mo
Eruption	8 mo	13 mo	20 mo	16 mo	27 mo
Root completed	1.5 y	1.5 y	3.25 y	2.5 y	3 y

if no sinus obliteration is carried out to watch for mucocele development. It should be noted that complications such as mucocele development, osteomyelitis, or abscess formation after frontal sinus injuries are rare occurrences.[12]

MIDFACE INJURIES
Orbital Fractures

The pattern of orbital injuries is different in a child and growing teenager compared with an adult. In children younger than age 6 to 7 years, orbital floor and rim fractures are infrequent owing to a lack of maxillary and frontal sinus pneumatization (see **Fig. 5**). An increased incidence of orbital floor fractures coincides with maxillary sinus pneumatization.[6,10] However, owing to the propensity of children toward greenstick flexing of bone rather than fractures, orbital floor trauma may present with acute entrapment of the inferior muscular adipose tissue—a "trapdoor" effect (**Fig. 6**).[13] This pinching of tissue can lead to "white globe

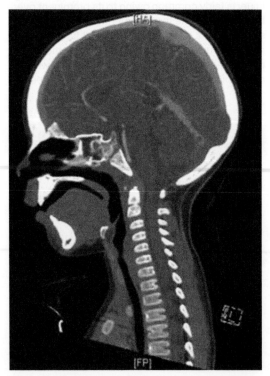

Fig. 3. Pediatric airway. Sagittal computed tomography scan of 3-year-old boy depicting large tongue volume and elongated soft palate and epiglottis.

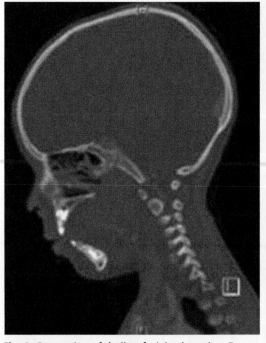

Fig. 4. Proportion of skull to facial volume in a 5-year-old child. Sagittal computed tomography scan of 5-year-old child notable for cranial volume in excess of the mid and lower facial volumes. Also note the lack of frontal sinus at this time.

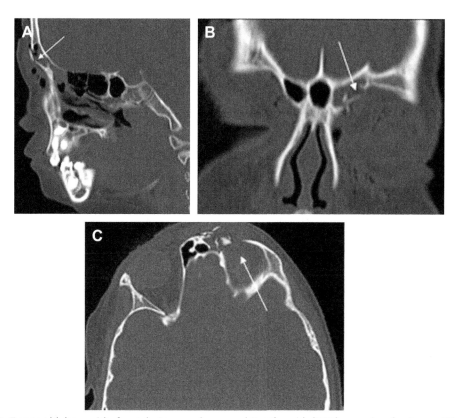

Fig. 5. A 7-year-old boy with frontal sinus and naso-orbitoethmoid (NOE) complex fractures. (*A*) Sagittal computed tomography (CT) scan indicating frontal sinus anterior table fracture (*arrow*). (*B*) Coronal CT scan indicating comminuted left orbital rim fracture (*arrow*). (*C*) Axial indicating left NOE and orbital rim fractures (*arrow*).

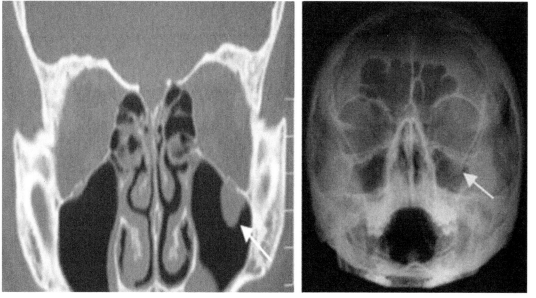

Fig. 6. Orbital floor fracture: "trapdoor" effect. Orbital contents noted herniating into maxillary sinus as would be seen in orbital floor fracture. *Arrows* pointing to the left orbital floor (right is the coronal CT scan and left a plain film sinus view) fracture with a tear drop herniation of soft tissue orbital contents. (*From* Cobb AR, Murthy R, Saiet J, et al. The tear-drop sign: a trap door for the unwary? Br J Oral Maxillofac Surg 2008;46(7):605–6; with permission.)

syndrome," an occulocardiac phenomena, in which every effort of superior gaze leads to bradycardia and associated nausea and syncope with extreme pain.[14] This injury often requires urgent management. Surgical release of the extraocular muscle fibers or the fibrous orbital connective tissue from the bony fragments is necessary. For bony defects that persist, resorbable orbital floor graft can be placed. An ophthalmology review is necessary preoperatively and postoperatively.

Nasal Injuries

Nasal fractures are often underreported in children. Closed management is common after a thorough speculum examination of the septum and soft tissues. Open fractures and high-velocity injuries involving the soft tissue are managed with esthetic guidance and subunit principles of reconstruction. Secondary corrections with rhinoplasty are undertaken after facial growth is complete. Full nasal projection is not usually achieved until ages 16 to 18 in females and 18 to 20 in males.[15]

Maxillary and Zygomatic Injuries

This subset of fractures is rare in children. High-velocity motor vehicle collisions as well as firearm-associated injuries are the leading causes of midface fractures. Sinus pneumatization, progress in teeth eruption, and vertical elongation by forward and downward projection of the face increases the incidence of zygomaticomaxillary fractures with facial maturity.

Mandible Fracture

With the incidence of facial fractures increasing with age, fracture patterns of 16- to 18-year-olds mirror the adult pattern, owing to achievement of skeletal maturity. For pediatric mandible fractures, the condylar region is most commonly affected.[1] Subtle condylar fractures can be easily missed, but will often be accompanied by laceration or contusion on the chin—a force exerted upward on the chin often causes bilateral condylar fractures (**Fig. 7**). The incidence of mandibular body and angle fractures increases with skeletal maturity.[16] When considering the techniques used for

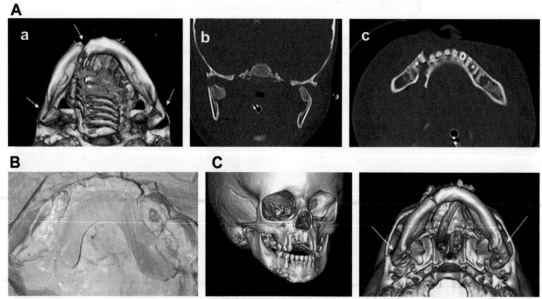

Fig. 7. (A) Mandibular fractures in 3-year-old boy. (a) Three-dimensional CT reconstruction, worm's eye view of displaced right mandibular and bilateral subcondylar fractures in 3-year-old boy (arrows). (b) Coronal computed tomography (CT) scan cut showing bilateral displaced subcondylar fractures. (c) Axial CT scan showing oblique displaced right mandibular fracture extending through buccal and lingual plates. (B) Lingual splint. Fabrication of a lingual splint used for mandibular body fracture reduction in this case. Holes can be drilled into the splint material through which wires are placed and secured to dentition and/or circummandibularly. (C) Mandibular fractures in 3-year-old boy: postoperative results. Postoperative 3-dimensional constructions of this 3-year-old boy after open reduction internal fixation of right mandibular body fracture and closed reduction of bilateral subcondylar fractures. (Right) Worm's eye view indicating anatomic reduction of mandibular body fracture and mandibular condyles. Note bony remodeling of condyles (arrows).

treatment of pediatric fractures, the great capacity for growth in children allows for judicious surgical intervention and greater efficacy of no intervention, compared with wide exposure and rigid internal fixation as the standard treatment for adults. Minimizing manipulation of periosteum and muscular attachments reduces scarring, thereby, diminishing constrictions to normal growth. Growth potential also affects the timing of fracture repair, requiring more expedient reduction in children. Whereas a 3-week window is accepted for repair in adults, manipulation of fractures becomes difficult beyond 1 week for children, after which bony callouses begin forming. The ideal window for repair is in the first 48 hours.[17]

Arch bars for intermaxillary fixation in children, although ubiquitous for adult fractures, are often untenable because the bulbous form of primary dentition and presence of partially erupted teeth in a mixed dentition make secure wire attachments difficult in stabilizing arch bars. Primary teeth can be extracted unintentionally by the pull of intermaxillary fixation. Retaining primary dentition, where possible, is important for future positioning of the adult dentition. Because primary teeth serve as place holders for adult teeth, premature loss of deciduous teeth often results in malocclusion and crowding later in the life. According to Smartt and colleagues,[16] the use of arch bars in children older than 11 years will minimize risk of tooth avulsion because sufficient root structure has formed in the permanent dentition by this age. The eyelet technique or Risdon wiring can be used for children less than 11 years old, using 24-gauge stainless steel wires. Splints may also be useful to aid with fracture reduction and stabilization on the lingual aspect of the mandible (see **Fig. 7**B). These splints are then secured to dentition or in a circummandibular fashion with wires. A downside to the fabrication of these appliances is the need for general anesthesia or sedation on 3 separate instances to make intraoral impressions, secure the splint after fabrication, and remove the splint after an appropriate healing window.

For fractures to be treated with closed reduction, the concern arises for intraarticular hemarthrosis and subsequent ankyloses in the temporomandibular joint with immobilization of the jaws. In children, 2 to 3 weeks may be sufficient for interdental wiring, as compared with the 4- to 6-week immobilization often used for adults. Ten-year follow-up studies for pediatric patients having undergone conservative treatment for mandibular condylar fractures showed no cases of ankyloses or serious asymmetry for closed reduction of 4 to 5 weeks. Reduced ramus height, deviation of the mandibular midline, and irregularly

shaped condyles were noted but did not correlate with severity of dysfunction (see **Fig. 7**C).[18] Behavior compliance is a definite obstacle for closed treatment of young children. Importantly, all cases of closed fracture immobilization must be followed with months of jaw physiotherapy after fixation is removed.

Open Reduction and Internal Fixation

Although many mandibular injuries in children are often greenstick (**Fig. 8**), those due to great forces may result in displaced or comminuted fractures (**Fig. 9**). Open reduction and internal fixation is useful for grossly displaced fractures, condylar neck fractures, fractures which impeded jaw movements, and fractures in non–tooth-bearing regions. As mentioned, the developing permanent tooth buds at the inferior border are of great concern when placing rigid fixation; therefore, only monocortical screws should be applied and directed posteromedially. Often, low-profile midfacial plates are used. Bicortical screws should not be placed until after 12 years of age, at which point there is space between the distal aspect of tooth roots and the inferior border.[16] Internal fixation, when applied judiciously, has the advantage of reducing immobilization time and faster progression to soft diet compared with closed reduction. The concern exists for rigid fixation constricting facial growth and the recommendation of hardware removal with a second surgery remains controversial.[19]

Biodegradable Plates

Controversy over rigid fixation in pediatric facial fractures arises owing to concerns for restricted growth when fixation plates are placed over bony suture lines. However, there has been recent

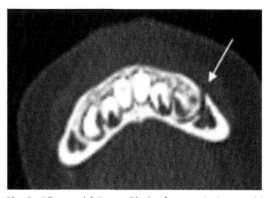

Fig. 8. "Greenstick" mandibular fracture in 3-year-old boy. Axial computed tomography scan showing "greenstick' left mandibular fracture. Nondisplaced fracture in vicinity of dental follicle (*arrow*).

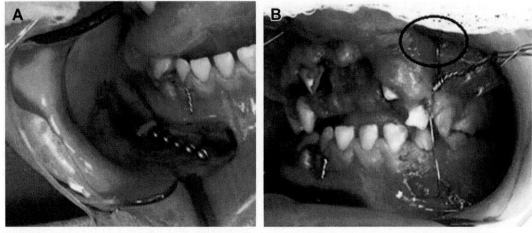

Fig. 9. Open reduction internal fixation of grossly displaced mandibular fractures. (*A*) Titanium plate fixation of right mandibular fracture with right mental nerve isolation and preservation. A midface low-profile plate was used and placed at inferior border to avoid permanent dental follicles. Bridle wire was used to reduce open fracture between right primary molar and incisor. (*B*) Intermaxillary fixation achieved with circummandibular wiring and piriform wiring (*circle*).

debate over the degree to which rigid fixation actually restricts growth. Work in rabbits showed no effect on vertical or sagittal mandibular growth when growth with rigid fixation for symphyseal fracture was compared with no fixation.[20] Only relatively recently has the use of biodegrable fixation in the form of polylacetate polymers been chronicled for maxillofacial surgery. These materials are unique in their ability to provide initial fracture stability and strength to the bony fragments, but dissolution with time and bony healing allows for physiologic force transference to bone without further dependence on a foreign material (**Fig. 10**).[21] A concern with biodegradable fixation is the inflammatory response created by the polymer itself. Localized inflammation is necessary for degradation of the plates, but must be controlled so as not to cause swelling, erythema, or fluid collection. A second concern is with the overall

strength of these biodegradable materials relative to that of standard titanium plates. For plating of zygomatic fractures, biodegradable plates have been shown to be both functional and esthetic.[22] A review of 745 patients over 10 years with biodegradable fixation for craniomaxillofacial surgery found a failure rate of 6%, which is comparable with titanium failure rates.[21] This study found that instances of failure were located exclusively in the mandible and resulted from breakage of screws. Inflammation requiring removal accounted for 4% of the 6%. A separate study using a tripolymer osteosynthesis system on 40 pediatric mandibular fractures confirmed that bioresorbable plates have satisfactory strength to withstand masticatory forces. Only 20% of patients exhibited mobility of fracture segments at the 1-month follow-up and no mobility was noted at 3 months.[23] In placing biodegradable plates, as with any plating system, patient compliance must be stressed—adherence to a soft diet and abstention from contact sports until clinical and radiographic confirmation of healing.

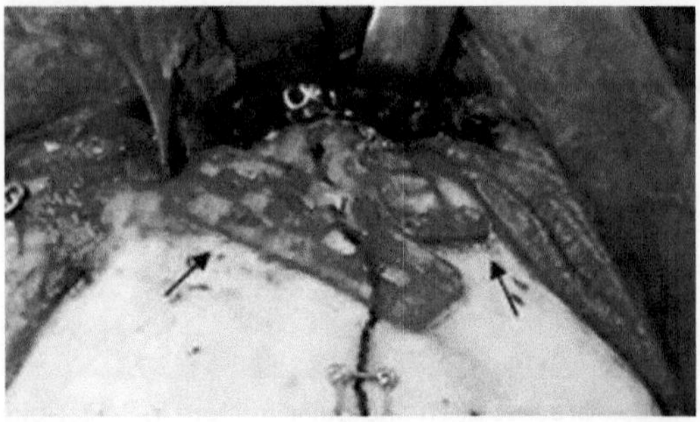

Dentoalveolar Fractures

Dentoalveolar fractures are common in the 0- to 18-year-old age group, with falls as the major cause of injury. Injuries include those to the teeth themselves and/or to the alveolar bone supporting the dentition. In the initial evaluation of a patient, all avulsed teeth should be accounted for so as to rule out potential for aspiration—a chest radiograph may be warranted. Avulsed primary teeth are not reimplanted for fear of damaging the

Fig. 10. Biodegradable plates. Cranial fractures fixed with biodegradable plates (*arrows*) in addition to titanium plates.

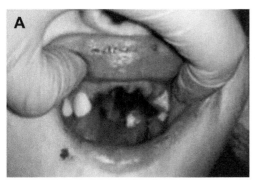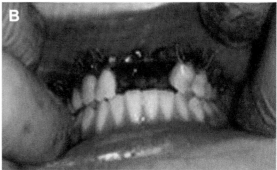

Fig. 11. Dentoalveolar trauma: composite splint and arch bar placement. (*A*) Dentoalveolar trauma in a 12-year-old girl. Maxillary central incisors and right later incisor were completely avulsed and unrestorable. Left maxillary canine and premolar were lingually intruded along with displaced palatal bone fragment. (*B*) Teeth and bone fragments were repositioned. The canine and premolar were splinted to the stable teeth behind the 24-guage wire and dental composite. The splint was then secured to an arch bar spanning from first molar to first molar with circumdental wiring engaging the palatal segments. Note proper dental occlusion is restored.

underlying permanent tooth bud. Avulsed permanent teeth should be stored in a physiologic storage media (saliva, saline, Hank's Balanced Salt Solution, whole milk) during transit to the nearest emergency department or dental office. Permanent teeth with an extraoral dry time of more than 60 minutes have poor long-term prognoses. Subluxed and luxated dentition should be repositioned and secured to surrounding stable dentition. This placement can be accomplished with nonrigid splints fabricated with orthodontic wire and dental cements or composites (**Fig. 11**). If alveolar bone mobility exists alongside dental mobility, an arch bar can be placed in addition to

dental splinting. Once mobile fragments are stabilized, the patient should be instructed to maintain a soft diet and follow-up with a dental professional for evaluation of tooth vitality and alignment.

SOFT TISSUE INJURIES

Minimizing scar tissue is of upmost importance, because extensive soft tissue injury may place constraints on the growing functional matrix of the facial skeleton. The majority of soft tissue injuries in children are circumoral and to the tongue, followed by injury to the chin then periorbital region and forehead.[24] In exposure of orbital or midfacial

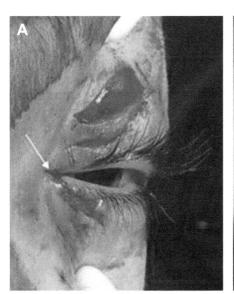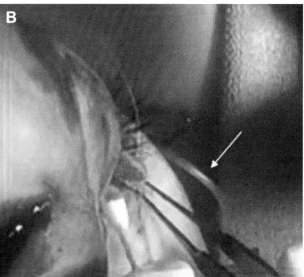

Fig. 12. Ocular soft tissue injuries. (*A*) Ocular examination exposes a canalicular detachment of the left eye after an avulsion injury. Canaliculus was reattached (*arrow*). (*B*) Repair of ocular injuries with monocanalicular stent (*arrow*).

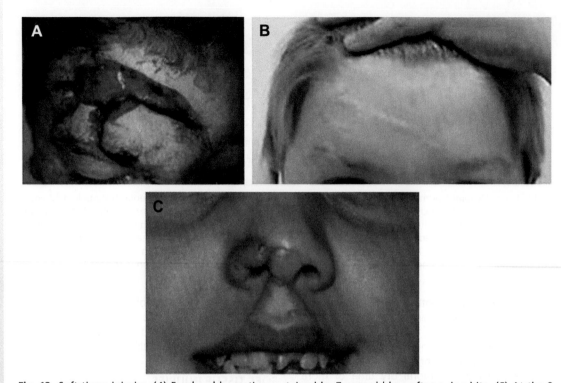

Fig. 13. Soft tissue injuries. (*A*) Forehead laceration sustained by 7-year-old boy after a dog bite. (*B*) At the 9-month follow-up, the patient has undergone primary repair. Follow-up shows appropriate healing with scar maturation. (*C*) Soft tissue crush injury to midface from automobile collision after primary repair. Follow-up for secondary revisions to lower nasal complex are advised at a later date, as would be recommended in an adult patient.

fractures, attention must be placed on avoiding injury to the orbital septum so as to prevent ectropion and entropion. All periocular injuries should undergo thorough examination under anesthesia to exclude any ocular trauma (**Fig. 12**). In general, soft tissue defects in children are best repaired primarily when possible without using rotational flaps at the initial encounter (**Fig. 13**). Defects should then be revisited secondarily to plan for flap or graft reconstructions. Considering pediatric healing capabilities, one should allow scars a full year of healing before consideration of scar revision procedures, because many skin defects improve considerably in this time.

SUMMARY

Pediatric craniofacial trauma differs from that of adults owing to differences in anatomy and the dynamism of the growing skull. Growth potential must always be considered when addressing pediatric trauma and often times a "less-is-more" approach is best. Regardless of the treatment modality, pediatric trauma cases must be followed through healing progress until skeletal maturity.

REFERENCES

1. Posnick JC, Wells M, Pron GE. Pediatric facial fractures: evolving patterns of treatment. J Oral Maxillofac Surg 1993;51:836–44.
2. Imahara SD, Hopper RA, Wang J, et al. Patterns and outcomes of pediatric facial fractures in the United States: a survey of the National Trauma Data Bank. J Am Coll Surg 2008;207(5):710–6.
3. Haug RH, Foss J. Maxillofacial injuries in the pediatric patient. Oral Surg Oral Med Oral Pathol Oral Radiol Endod 2000;90(2):126–34.
4. Shah RK, Dhingra JK, Carter BL, et al. Paranasal sinus development: a radiographic study. Laryngoscope 2003;113(2):205–9.
5. Scuderi AJ, Harnsberger HR, Boyer RS. Pneumatization of the paranasal sinuses: normal features of importance to the accurate interpretation of CT scans and MR images. AJR Am J Roentgenol 1993;160(5):1101–4.
6. Hatef DA, Cole PD, Hollier LH Jr. Contemporary management of pediatric facial trauma. Curr Opin Otolaryngol Head Neck Surg 2009;17(4):308–14.
7. Morris C, Kushner GM, Tiwana PS. Facial skeletal trauma in the growing patient. Oral Maxillofacial Surg Clin N Am 2012;24(3):351–64.

8. Moss ML. The functional matrix hypothesis revisited. 4. The epigenetic antithesis and the resolving synthesis. Am J Orthod Dentofacial Orthop 1997; 112(4):410–7.

9. Smartt J, Low D, Bartlett S. The pediatric mandible: I. A primer on growth and development. Plast Reconstr Surg 2005;116(1):14e–23e.

10. Totonchi A, Sweeney WM, Gosain AK. Distinguishing anatomic features of pediatric facial trauma. J Craniofac Surg 2012;23(3):793–8.

11. Hengerer AS. Embryologic development of the sinuses. Ear Nose Throat J 1984;63:134–6.

12. Freeman JL, Winston KR. Breach of posterior wall of frontal sinus: management with preservation of the sinus. World Neurosurg 2015;83(6):1080–9.

13. Cobb AR, Murthy R, Saiet J, et al. The tear-drop sign: a trap door for the unwary? Br J Oral Maxillofac Surg 2008;46(7):605–6.

14. Ethunandan M, Evans B. Linear trapdoor or "white-eye" blowout fracture of the orbit: not restricted to children. Br J Oral Maxillofac Surg 2011;49(2): 142–7.

15. Boyette JR. Facial fractures in children. Otolaryngol Clin North Am 2014;47(5):747–61.

16. Smartt J, Low D, Bartlett S. The pediatric mandible: II. Management of traumatic injury or fracture. Plast Reconstr Surg 2005;116(2):28e–41e.

17. Siy R, Brown R, Koshy J, et al. General management considerations in pediatric facial fractures. J Craniofac Surg 2011;22(4):1190–5.

18. Nørholt S, Krishnan V, Sindet-Pedersen S, et al. Pediatric condylar fractures: a long-term follow-up study of 55 patients. J Oral Maxillofac Surg 1993; 51(12):1302–10.

19. Fernandez H, Osorio J, Russi M, et al. Effects of internal rigid fixation on mandibular development in growing rabbits with mandibular fractures. J Oral Maxillofac Surg 2012;70(10):2368–74.

20. Bayram B, Yilmaz A, Ersoz E, et al. Does the titanium plate fixation of symphyseal fracture affect mandibular growth? J Craniofac Surg 2012;23(6):E601–3.

21. Turvey T, Proffit W, Phillips C. Biodegradable fixation for craniomaxillofacial surgery: a 10-year experience involving 761 operations and 745 patients. Int J Oral Maxillofac Surg 2011;40(3):244–9.

22. Mahmoud SM, Liao HT, Chen CT. Aesthetic and functional outcome of zygomatic fractures fixation comparison with resorbable versus titanium plates. Ann Plast Surg 2016;76(Suppl 1):S85–90.

23. Singh G, Mohammad S, Chak RK, et al. Bio-resorbable plates as effective implant in paediatric mandibular fracture. J Maxillofac Oral Surg 2011;11(4):400–6.

24. Bede S, Ismael W, Al-Assaf D. Patterns of pediatric maxillofacial injuries. J Craniofac Surg 2016;27(3): E271–5.

Emergent Soft Tissue Repair in Facial Trauma

 CrossMark

Melissa Marks, DO[a], Derek Polecritti, DO[a], Ronald Bergman, DO[b],
Cody A. Koch, MD, PhD[c],*

KEYWORDS

- Facial trauma • Reconstruction • Soft tissue

KEY POINTS

- Soft tissue injuries to the face are frequently encountered by the plastic surgeon and can have significant implications for patients both functionally and aesthetically.
- Management of soft tissue injuries to the face ranges from simple to very challenging based on the complexity of the injury and underlying structures that may be involved.
- A thorough evaluation and appropriate treatment plan are vital to ensuring the optimal aesthetic and functional outcome for each individual patient.

INTRODUCTION

Acute soft tissue injuries to the face are commonly encountered in the emergency setting as isolated injuries or with concomitant facial skeletal trauma. The most common etiology of facial soft tissue injuries varies based on the population studied; however, all facial soft tissue injuries can lead to poor cosmesis, loss of function, and/or social stigmata.[1] Facial soft tissue injuries require thorough evaluation, planning, and surgical treatment to achieve optimal functional and aesthetic outcomes while minimizing the risk of complications.

Facial soft tissue injuries are classified into multiple categories including closed versus open, facial subunit(s) involved, and the presence of additional injuries to related structures (eg, nerve, parotid duct). The classification of the wound guides appropriate treatment as well as helps predict postrepair form and function.

Soft tissue injuries can initially be classified as open or closed wounds. A closed wound is one that damages underlying tissue and/or structures without breaking the skin. Examples of closed wounds include hematomas, contusions, and crush injuries. In contrast, open wounds involve a break in the skin, which exposes the underlying structures to the external environment. Open wounds include simple and complex lacerations, avulsions, punctures, abrasions, accidental tattooing, and retained foreign body.

Injuries to the head and neck are also classified according to the subunit(s) involved. The major aesthetic subunits are the scalp, forehead, nose, periorbital, cheek, perioral, auricle, and neck.[1] Additionally, the major subunits are frequently divided into smaller subunits by location. The optimal aesthetic result is frequently achieved when individual subunits are reconstructed separately when possible and appropriate.

Due to the frequency, varying complexity, and impact on the patient of facial soft tissue injuries, knowledge of the appropriate evaluation and management of these injuries is vital for all health care personnel involved in their care. This review will discuss the evaluation, general principles of management, and specific treatment considerations and potential complications pertinent to individual

Disclosures: The authors have nothing to disclose.
[a] Department of Plastic and Reconstructive Surgery, Mercy Medical Center, 1111 6th Avenue, Des Moines, IA 50314, USA; [b] Department of Plastic and Reconstructive Surgery, Bergman Folkers Plastic Surgery, 2000 Grand Avenue, Des Moines, IA 50314, USA; [c] Department of Plastic and Reconstructive Surgery, Koch Facial Plastic Surgery, 4855 Mills Civic Parkway, West Des Moines, IA 50265, USA
* Corresponding author.
E-mail address: codykoch@kochmd.com

subunits. Additionally, evaluation and treatment considerations of injuries to underlying soft tissue structures, such as the facial nerve and parotid duct are discussed.

EVALUATION AND ASSESSMENT

All patients with trauma initially should be assessed and managed according to the principles of Advanced Trauma Life Support. Soft tissue injuries of the face and neck can be accompanied by significant soft tissue swelling as well as underlying injuries to the skeletal and laryngotracheal complex, leading to airway compromise. Emergency personnel should have a low threshold for securing the airway, which includes awake tracheotomy if necessary. The patient also should be assessed for associated ophthalmologic, intracranial, and cervical spine injuries, which might alter the management plan[2] (**Fig. 1**).

History

Once the patient has been evaluated for life-threatening injuries and stabilized as necessary,

a thorough yet focused history and physical examination of the face should be performed by the plastic surgeon. A systematic history elucidates the timeline and mechanism of injury, which is important for determining the need for further assessment and creation of an appropriate treatment plan. The timeline of the injury is important to clarify. Early treatment of soft tissue injuries is associated with optimal aesthetic outcomes and helps the surgeon estimate the resultant swelling of the wound that might make the identification of important landmarks challenging when performing the repair.[1]

Determining the mechanism of injury may identify special considerations for the surgeon when managing the wound(s). For example, crush injuries may result in a larger area of compromised tissue than appreciated on initial examination. Tissue that appears healthy initially may subsequently necrose, which may require management of the wound in a delayed fashion with serial debridement.[3]

Gunshot wounds are another example. The soft tissue damage created by a gunshot wound is

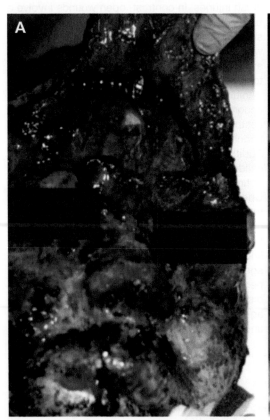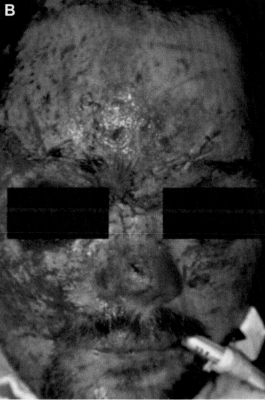

Fig. 1. (*A*) Complex facial laceration following motor vehicle crash. (*B*) Postoperative result following irrigation, debridement, and careful repositioning of remaining soft tissue. (*From* Wells MD, Skytta C. Craniofacial, Head and Neck Surgery; pediatric plastic surgery. In: Mueller RV. Plastic Surgery. 3rd edition. vol. 3. London: Elsevier Saunders; 2013. p. 32; with permission.)

largely determined by the velocity of the projectile, which is classified from low (<1000 fps) to high (>2000 fps) velocity. Wounds created by high-velocity weapons can exhibit significant secondary tissue damage that presents in a delayed fashion due to the concussion and cavitation of the projectile as it passes through the tissue.[4,5] In wounds created by high-velocity projectiles, the surgeon should have a high suspicion for tissue damage peripheral to the obvious wound and the potential need for serial debridement.

Finally, bite wounds also deserve special consideration. The type of bite and depth of injury, as well the offending animal are important to elucidate. Dog bites typically cause a crushing-type wound, whereas cat bites usually cause puncture wounds and/or lacerations. Human bites frequently cause crushing and/or tearing type injuries that also have an increased risk of infection compared with other bite wounds.[6–9]

Physical Examination

Once the history has been obtained, a thorough and systematic physical examination is performed. The site(s), depth, and nature of all wounds should be noted. In particular, the presence of nonviable tissue and/or the presence of gross contamination are important to discern. In some cases (ie, children, uncooperative patients), adequate inspection of the wound may not be possible until the area or the patient has been anesthetized. Palpation helps to identify the presence of bony injuries; however, the surgeon should have a low threshold for the use of imaging, which has greater sensitivity in identifying these injuries. It should be noted that the lack of a fracture does not eliminate the possibility of a severe soft tissue injury.

Each soft tissue wound can be classified according to its characteristics, which may help to guide treatment. Soft tissue wounds are frequently classified as described in the following sections.

Contusion

Typically caused by blunt trauma. There is extravasation of blood within the tissue that may or may not be accompanied by a hematoma. Most frequently, contusions are treated with conservative therapy even if a hematoma is present. In some instances, a hematoma may require evacuation and if neglected may lead to the accumulation of scar tissue.

Abrasion

Wounds created by friction can result in partial-thickness wounds without disruption of the deeper dermal layer. These wounds are treated conservatively but can result in abnormalities of pigment of the skin, especially in patients with Fitzpatrick Type IV skin type or higher.

Laceration

A laceration is a disruption of both the epidermis and dermis. The resultant wound may have clean edges that can be repaired with little manipulation or nonviable tissue that requires extensive debridement before closure.

Avulsion

An avulsion is the separation and subsequent loss of tissue. Avulsion injuries are the most challenging to repair and may require local or regional flaps. In extensive avulsion injuries, free tissue transfer may be required.

A complete neurologic examination of the head and neck should be performed noting any deficit(s) of the cranial nerves. In particular, the facial nerve should be evaluated for weakness and/or paralysis. The facial nerve has 4 primary branches that include the marginal mandibular, buccal, zygomatic, and frontal branches that supply motor innervation to the face. The fifth branch, the cervical, supplies the platysma muscle in the neck and is not of functional importance. Injuries to an isolated branch of the facial nerve will cause weakness or paralysis of the muscles innervated by that branch, whereas injury to the main trunk of the facial nerve will show deficits of all branches of the facial nerve distal to the injury. Although weakness of the facial nerve typically carries an excellent prognosis for recovery, paralysis of the facial nerve due to transection may require operative intervention. The location of the offending soft tissue injury is important to note, as injuries medial to the lateral canthus typically recover with an excellent functional outcome without intervention.[10]

Trauma to the periocular area requires careful evaluation. Although simple lacerations of the eyelid frequently occur without injury to deeper structures, the presence of chemosis, hyphema, pain in the globe, and absence of the pupillary light reflex may herald an injury to the globe that requires further evaluation by an ophthalmologist. Additionally, special attention should be paid to the tightness of the eyelid, especially the lower lid. Injuries to the medial or lateral canthus may lead to injury to the medial or lateral canthal tendon, which maintains apposition of the eyelid to the globe and could lead to ectropion if not identified and treated appropriately. Retraction of the lower lid with fingers should result in the lid snapping back against the globe; however, in the presence of injury to either tendon, the lid may no longer appose the globe or snap back into the appropriate position.

Injuries to the medial canthus carry the additional consideration of the lacrimal apparatus. If the surgeon suspects a lacrimal injury, a Jones test is performed. The Jones test involves instilling fluorescein eye drops in the affected eye. After a period of 5 to 10 minutes, an intranasal examination is performed looking for the presence of fluorescein in the nose. Alternatively, the patient can blow his or her nose and the presence or absence of fluorescein on the tissue noted. If fluorescein is not noted intranasally, the lacrimal duct should be probed to determine continuity. If the probe is visualized in the wound, the lacrimal duct has been disrupted.

INITIAL MANAGEMENT

The initial principles of management of soft tissue injuries include the control of blood loss, copious irrigation, debridement of devitalized tissue, and removal of foreign bodies before closure. Blood loss from facial soft tissue injuries can be significant secondary to the robust blood supply of the head and neck. Blood loss is minimized with local pressure while the wound is examined with suction, irrigation, and meticulous dissection to identify the offending vessel and avoid secondary damage to important structures of the head and neck region.[11] Copious irrigation serves to dilute the contamination present in a wound. All grossly contaminated wounds should be copiously irrigated with sterile saline as well as any clean wound in which repair occurs after 6 hours.[1] In addition to irrigation, broad-spectrum antibiotic prophylaxis is warranted in grossly contaminated wounds and bite wounds and in immunocompromised patients. Tetanus vaccination should be considered in patients with high-risk trauma. These risk factors include delayed presentation of more than 6 hours, depth of wound greater than 1 cm, gross contamination of the wound, and presence of vascular compromise.[11] Patients who have received the complete tetanus series but whose booster administration was more than 5 years ago also should receive the vaccine.[12]

Ideally, facial soft tissue injuries are closed as early as possible. Primary closure of a wound should be completed within 8 hours of injury when possible.[1] Early intervention and closure decreases the risk of infection as well as optimizes the functional and cosmetic result. There are many well-known suturing techniques; however, regardless of the type of repair performed, 3 important principles should be met: precise approximation and eversion of the skin edges,

avoidance of excessive tension, and a layered closure to prevent dead space and fluid accumulation.[13]

In certain circumstances, a delayed primary repair or repair via secondary intention may also be considered.[1] Delayed repair is a viable option in cases in which the viability of the tissue is compromised and full vascular demarcation is required before closure. It can also be considered in contaminated wounds after serial irrigation and debridement have been performed. Healing by secondary intention can be considered in concave areas of the head and neck such as those of the auricle, occiput, medial canthus, nasal alar crease, nasolabial fold, and temple. Scar revision can then be performed if necessary 6 to 12 months later.[3]

SOFT TISSUE RECONSTRUCTION BY SITE

There are multiple principles to be followed for optimal results following closure of all soft tissue wounds, such as precise approximation of wound edges, skin eversion of the skin edges, and the avoidance of excessive tension. However, there are specific considerations for each major subunit of the face, which are detailed as follows.

Scalp

The scalp possesses a rich vascular supply. The arterial supply to the scalp is from branches of the internal and external carotid arteries. These arterial branches form a dense network of vasculature that aides in healing but can also result in significant amount of blood loss, especially with degloving injuries. When presented with trauma to the scalp, life-threatening injuries, such as hemorrhage or intracranial injury, should be considered and treated as necessary before wound closure.

In cases of severe trauma to the scalp, blood loss can be a source of hypovolemic shock and fatality. Control of hemorrhage can be quickly achieved in an emergent setting via pressure dressing, suture ligature, and/or electrocautery. Pretensioned metal or plastic clips (ie, Raney clips) also can be placed along the edges of the scalp laceration to provide immediate hemostasis in emergent situations.[14]

The scalp covers and protects the underlying cranium and needs to be reconstructed. The goals of the repair of scalp wounds include obtaining a tension-free closure, maintaining the structure and function of the scalp, and restoring the protection of the underlying cranium.[11] Full-thickness defects less than 2 to 3 cm wide can typically be repaired primarily. A layered closure should be performed starting with the galea and subcutaneous tissue followed by the skin. Some defects require wide undermining in the subgaleal plane to allow for a tension-free closure. In addition to wide undermining, scoring the galea perpendicular to the direction of scalp movement further aids in tissue advancement and coverage of the defect.[15]

In situations in which there is tissue loss, local flaps, and in rare cases, tissue expansion or free tissue transfer may be necessary. Examples of local flaps useful in reconstruction of the scalp include the O to Z or "pinwheel" flap, which involves 2 to 4 axial-based full-thickness rotational flaps advanced to cover the defect. The flaps can be 4 to 6 times as long as the defect is wide (**Fig. 2**). For larger defects (>25 cm²), rotational flaps, such as the Orticochea flap, are useful to incorporate hair-bearing skin into the reconstruction. Similar to the O-Z and pinwheel flap, this flap involves 3 to 4 axial-based full-thickness rotation and advancement flaps to cover a larger defect. This type of technique requires the entire scalp be undermined.[16] Tissue expansion and

free-flap reconstruction are also options for large defects of the scalp (>25 cm²).[11]

Alopecia is a frequent complication of scalp wounds and results from injury to the hair follicles. Prevention of alopecia is best achieved by minimizing the use of monopolar cautery, as well as approximating the galea appropriately. Suturing the galea minimizes tension to the more superficial layers of the skin containing the hair follicles.[16] Alopecia also can result from shock loss of the hair, which may take months to return. In these cases, the authors have had excellent results with the use of bimatoprost (Latisse) off label.

FOREHEAD

Soft tissue injuries to the forehead are commonly encountered as isolated injuries or combined with other injuries to the face. The functional importance of the forehead lies in the frontalis muscle, which raises the eyebrow. The motor innervation of the frontalis muscle is supplied by the frontal branch of the facial nerve. The frontal

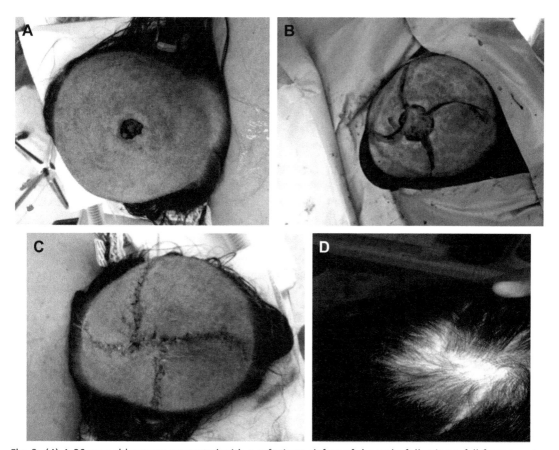

Fig. 2. (*A*) A 36-year-old woman presented with a soft tissue defect of the scalp following a fall from a motor vehicle 2 weeks prior. The same patient (*B*) intraoperatively and (*C*) immediately after closure of the defect using a pinwheel flap. (*D*) Same patient months after reconstruction. No revision performed.

branch of the facial nerve travels superficially in the temporoparietal fascia where it can be easily injured by even relatively superficial injuries to the lateral forehead. All patients with lateral forehead or temple injuries should be evaluated before the injection of local anesthetic by asking them to raise their eyebrows.

Principles of repair for the forehead are similar to the scalp. Primary repair is possible in most injuries with little functional or aesthetic sequelae. However, in cases of tissue loss, local flaps and/or tissue expansion may be necessary. Skin grafting is less preferable due to pigmentation mismatch.[15] When tissue rearrangement is necessary special attention is paid to not distorting the eyebrow, which may be permanently elevated leading to significant asymmetry and suboptimal aesthetic result.

When tissue rearrangement is necessary, there are multiple local flaps that are useful. Advancement flaps can be useful for defects of the eyebrow to restore the continuity of the hair-bearing skin. Bilateral advancement flaps can be used to move tissue in a horizontal manner to avoid the vertical displacement of the eyebrow. Alternatively, the O-Z flap also minimizes displacement of the eyebrow. The island pedicle flap can be useful for defects of the lateral eyebrow even when relatively large. The island pedicle flap takes advantage of the relatively redundant skin of the temple and lateral brow. Special care should be taken to avoid injury to the frontal branch of the facial nerve when performing the dissection. Defects of the medial eyebrow and glabella can be frequently repaired primarily in a vertical fashion. Any medial displacement of the eyebrow typically dissipates over time or is corrected with personal grooming.

PERIORBITAL

Appropriate management of eyelid lacerations and soft tissue injuries is vital to achieving optimal functional and aesthetic outcomes. There are 4 main areas of the periorbital region to be considered, which include the upper eyelid, lower eyelid, medial canthus, and lateral canthus. In addition to the region affected, periorbital injuries can also be classified according to whether they involve the full thickness of the eyelid or are partial thickness.

Similar to other sites in the head and neck, lacerations to the eyelid should be closed in layers; however, the layers to be closed in the eyelid differ from other regions. Full-thickness lacerations of the eyelid that can be closed primarily should include repair of conjunctiva, the tarsal plate, and skin in separate layers. Lacerations involving the

margin of the eyelid should be closed with appropriate eversion of the margin with a vertical mattress suture to avoid notching. Lacerations of the upper eyelid require further consideration for potential injury to the levator muscle, which would result in ptosis if not repaired.

Partial-thickness defects of the periorbital region can frequently be managed with local flaps or full-thickness skin grafts. Partial-thickness defects of less than 50% of the horizontal width of the eyelid can typically be managed with local advancement flaps or rotation advancement flaps recruiting skin from the laxity present in the temple. Partial-thickness defects involving more than 50% of the upper eyelid may require a full-thickness skin graft, whereas those of the lower eyelid are best repaired by using large cheek rotation flaps or full-thickness skin grafts where appropriate. It should be noted that partial-thickness defects of the lower eyelid repaired with full-thickness skin grafts can lead to ectropion, as the skin graft contracts over time. The surgeon should have a low threshold for performing a prophylactic lateral canthopexy or lateral tarsal strip procedure when repairing defects of the lower eyelid if concern for postoperative ectropion exists. Additionally, when using a full-thickness skin graft to repair the lower eyelid, a Frost suture is frequently necessary in the immediate postoperative setting.

Full-thickness defects of the upper or lower eyelid require reconstruction of all 3 layers of the eyelid. Defects involving less than 33% of the horizontal distance of the eyelid can typically be managed with advancement of the remaining tissue and a layered closure, as discussed previously.[17,18] In some cases, a lateral cantholysis can be performed to achieve closure of wider defects. Full-thickness defects involving 33% to 66% of the upper or lower eyelid require local flaps and/or composite flaps. The local flaps to reconstitute the skin are similar to those used to repair partial-thickness defects. These local flaps are combined with auricular cartilage grafts to recreate the tarsus in addition to mucosal grafts to replace the conjunctiva. In some cases, such as the Hughes flap and Cutler-Beard flap, the unaffected eyelid on that side can be used as a donor for multiple missing layers. However, both the Hughes flap and Cutler-Beard flap are multistage procedures.[17,18]

Defects of the eyelid 66% to 100% of the total horizontal distance of the eyelid are challenging to reconstruct. Central defects of the upper eyelid are frequently repaired with the Cutler-Beard flap. Total or near-total defects of the lower eyelid are reconstructed with a composite graft and cheek rotation flap. In some cases, total eyelid defect reconstruction can be accomplished with a regional flap such as the paramedian forehead flap or free tissue transfer using a radial forearm flap.

Injuries to the medial canthal region of the eyelid should alert the surgeon to a possible lacrimal system injury. Vertical lacerations of the eyelid, in particular, are more likely to involve the lacrimal system. Injuries to the lacrimal canaliculi should be repaired within 72 hours. There are multiple methods to repair lacrimal canalicular injuries, with most involving the repair of the lacrimal duct over a silicone stent that is left in place for multiple weeks[11,13] (**Fig. 3**). Specifics of these methods of repair are beyond the scope of this review.

CHEEK

The cheek represents the region of the face with the largest surface area and is frequently injured. The cheek subunit typically contains significant laxity, making primary repair of most small to moderate-sized defects possible. Healing by secondary intention is reasonable in small defects; however, the multitude of local and regional flaps available to repair wounds in this region make it a choice of last resort in most cases. Defects of the cheek not suitable for primary repair can frequently be repaired using advancement, rotation, and/or transposition flaps. Larger defects of the cheek may require regional flaps, such as the cervicofacial or cervicopectoral rotation advancement flaps. In severe soft tissue injuries, free tissue transfer may be necessary.

Facial Nerve Trauma

Soft tissue injuries to the cheek may injure the main trunk of the facial nerve and/or its branches. The plastic surgeon should thoroughly examine the patient before injection of anesthetic to determine if paresis or paralysis of the nerve exists. Weakness and injury to the facial nerve is graded on the House-Brackmann scale, with grade 1 being normal and grade 6 being complete paralysis.[19] Injuries of the facial nerve or its branches resulting in paresis can be managed conservatively, as even minimal distal function implies continuity of the nerve. Additionally, injuries to the nerve medial to the lateral canthus are typically also managed conservatively due to the extensive cross-innervation that exists in this area between branches.

The presence of complete paralysis portends a worse prognosis. Penetrating soft tissue injuries that result in complete paralysis of the facial nerve or its branches should be explored. Exploration should occur within 72 hours of the injury when possible to take advantage of the ability to use nerve stimulation to identify the distal nerve branches that may be very small and difficult to locate. Wallerian degeneration occurs after 72 hours, making distal nerve stimulation impossible after that time. Injuries to the facial nerve that result in discontinuity should be repaired. Microscopic primary repair with an 8-0 or smaller nonresorbable suture is preferred when possible. Dissection of both the proximal and distal nerve branches may be necessary to achieve a tension-free closure. An interpositional nerve graft may be necessary in nerve injuries in which

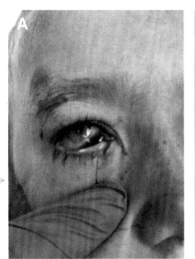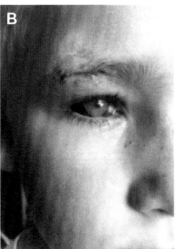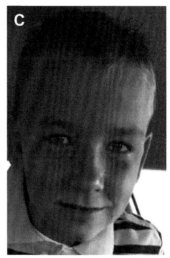

Fig. 3. (*A*) Eight-year-old boy with a laceration of the right lower eyelid involving the lacrimal apparatus. (*B*) Patient 2 days after dacryocystorhinostomy with nasolacrimal duct stenting. (*C*) Two months after repair with no evidence of epiphora. No revision surgery performed.

primary repair is not possible without significant tension or a portion of the nerve is missing or badly macerated. The great auricular nerve is an excellent donor source with minimal donor site morbidity. Commercially available nerve conduits are an alternative to interpositional nerve grafts.

Parotid Duct Trauma

Soft tissue injuries to the cheek may result in injury to the parenchyma of the parotid gland and/or the parotid duct (Stenson duct). It has been estimated that injuries to the parotid gland occur in 0.21% of soft tissue injuries to the face.[20] Although not common, injuries to either of these structures can lead to sialoadenitis and/or sialocele. In cases of sialocele, a draining fistula can form from the parotid gland to the skin. Identification and appropriate management of these injuries can prevent these complications and improve patient outcomes.

Injury to the parenchyma of the parotid gland can often be managed conservatively. If the capsule of the gland has been violated, the surgeon should be suspicious of a facial nerve injury in addition to the injury to the gland. In the absence of facial nerve injury, the capsule often can be oversewn, the wound closed, and a pressure dressing applied without sequela.

The plastic surgeon should be concerned about an injury to the parotid duct in soft tissue injuries to the cheek that lie behind the anterior border of the masseter muscle (**Fig. 4**). Initial evaluation can be performed by attempting to express saliva from the duct with massage and observing intraorally for its presence. If no saliva is observed, the surgeon can massage the gland and look for saliva in the wound. Alternatively, the duct can be cannulated intraorally with a probe and the wound observed for the presence of the probe.

If an injury is identified and the proximal portion of the duct can be identified, the duct should be repaired with nonresorbable suture over a silicone catheter. The catheter is typically left in place for 2 weeks, at which time it is removed intraorally. In some cases, the proximal portion of the duct cannot be identified and repair of the duct is not possible. In these cases, antisialogogues and pressure dressings can be used to try to prevent the occurrence of a sialocele. Additionally, botulinum toxin type A can be injected into the parenchyma of the gland, which will decrease saliva production, promoting atrophy and fibrosis of the gland over time.[21]

NOSE

Nasal soft tissue injuries are common due to their central location in the face. Nasal soft tissue

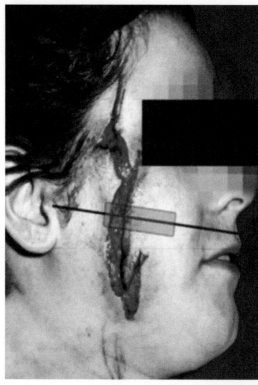

Fig. 4. The course of the parotid duct can be approximated by a line drawn from the tragus to the middle of the vertical height of the upper lip. Injury to the zygomatic or buccal branches of the facial nerve near the green-shaded area should raise suspicion of a parotid duct injury. (*From* Wells MD, Skytta C. Craniofacial, Head and Neck Surgery; pediatric plastic surgery. In: Mueller RV. Plastic Surgery. 3rd edition. vol. 3. London: Elsevier Saunders; 2013. p. 25; with permission.)

injuries are frequently associated with fractures, and the plastic surgeon should have a high degree of suspicion for associated bony injuries when evaluating nasal injuries. The presence of an external nasal injury also should arouse suspicion for the presence of intranasal injury and in particular a septal hematoma. A septal hematoma is a collection of blood under the mucoperichondrium of the septum. If untreated, a septal hematoma can result in cartilage loss, saddle nose deformity, abscess, and sepsis. A septal hematoma will appear as an ecchymotic bulge inside the nose on anterior rhinoscopy. Treatment consists of incision and drainage with appropriate antibiotic coverage. A small Penrose drain can be placed in the incision to prevent reaccumulation as well as light nasal packing.

External soft tissue injuries of the nose often can be repaired primarily. Full-thickness lacerations should be repaired in a multilayered fashion with the mucosa, lower lateral cartilages and skin being repaired in separate layers (**Fig. 5**). Lacerations involving the alar margin deserve special attention. These lacerations should be repaired with exaggerated eversion using vertical mattress sutures to prevent notching postoperatively.

Soft tissue injuries of the nose in which tissue has been avulsed or is missing are more challenging to repair. Small defects still may be able to be closed primarily using an elliptical excision of surrounding tissue. Defects in which primary closure is not possible may be repaired with local flaps that include the bilobe, dorsal nasal, and hatchet flaps, among others. Full-thickness skin grafts may be used in shallow defects, but frequently lead to unfavorable aesthetic outcomes when compared with local flaps in which the skin is a closer match for the sebaceous nature of nasal skin.

Large defects of the nose may require multistage procedures. Defects encompassing 50% or more of a convex aesthetic subunit of the nose are usually enlarged to involve the entire subunit where appropriate. The aesthetic result is typically more favorable when the entire subunit is reconstructed as a whole. Reconstruction of an entire or multiple subunits of the nose may require interpolated flaps. The melolabial flap is useful for repair of alar defects, whereas the paramedian forehead flap is useful for repair of large defects involving the nasal ala, tip, sidewalls, and dorsum. The paramedian forehead flap is particularly useful when multiple subunits of the nose must be reconstructed.[16]

Full-thickness defects of the nose require reconstruction of all 3 layers of the nose, including the mucosa, support structure, and the external covering of soft tissue and skin. Intranasal flaps, such as the bipedicled vestibular advancement flap, inferior turbinate flap, and septal hinge flaps, are useful for reconstituting the internal lining of the nose. Auricular and/or septal cartilage is used to reconstitute the support of the nasal sidewall and tip to prevent postoperative nasal collapse and obstruction. Surgeons should have a low threshold for the use of a columellar strut or other supportive cartilage grafting to prevent future nasal obstruction and tip ptosis. Finally, the external covering is recreated using the variety of local flaps described previously. In cases of near-total or total nasal defects, advances in prosthetics can offer excellent results or free tissue transfer may be considered.

PERIORAL

The lips represent the dynamic structure of the lower third of the face and contain unique anatomy. The perioral area has multiple landmarks that must be meticulously reconstructed, such as the philtral columns and Cupid bow; however, none is more important than the vermillion cutaneous border. The vermillion cutaneous border is the transition of the white lip to the red lip, and even minimal (<1 mm) misalignment can lead to noticeable cosmetic deformity.[11] The reconstructive surgeon should approach even minor lacerations of the vermillion cutaneous border with precise attention to detail. The adjacent landmarks in the perioral area, including the adjacent vermillion cutaneous borders should be marked before infiltration with local anesthesia, which can distort these important landmarks. The lacerations should be repaired in a layered fashion, including mucosa, muscle, subcutaneous, and finally the skin. In

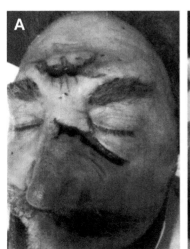
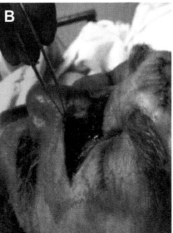
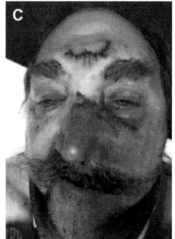

Fig. 5. (*A, B*) A 75-year-old man status post fall with a resultant full-thickness laceration of the nose with concomitant open fracture. (*C*) Same patient after repair of full-thickness laceration.

particular, the vermillion cutaneous border should be meticulously realigned with a vertical mattress suture to prevent notching and depression of the border (**Fig. 6**).

Injuries to the lip in which tissue is lost can frequently be repaired primarily when less than 33% of the width of lip is involved. In select cases, such as in elderly patients with significant laxity of the lower lip, primary closure can be considered for defects as large as 50% of the width of the lip. Partial-thickness defects involving the vermillion cutaneous border can be converted to full-thickness defects when less than 33% of the width of the lip is involved to achieve proper alignment of the vermillion cutaneous border.

Lip defects larger than 33% of the width usually require local flap reconstruction. Defects of the central lip not able to be closed primarily can be reconstructed with bilateral advancement flaps with crescentic alar excisions; however, this completely ablates the philtral columns as well as the Cupid bow. The Abbe, or lip-switch, flap represents a 2-stage alternative procedure that brings additional tissue into the reconstruction that helps to minimize microstomia and can be used in defects up to 50% of the width of the lip.[11,16] Defects involving the oral commissure can be reconstructed with the Estlander flap that uses adjacent tissue from the opposite lip that rotates around the commissure to reconstruct it. Defects of up to 66% of the upper lip and 75% of the lower lip can be reconstructed using the Karapandzic flap. The Karapandzic flap is an axial musculocutaneous flap that is based off of either the inferior or superior labial arteries. The innervation of the flap is maintained, making the resultant reconstruction sensate, which helps to maintain oral competence; however, microstomia is common. Large defects of the lower lip (up to 100%) can be reconstructed using the Bernard-Webster flap, which involves the excision of triangles of tissue along the bilateral nasolabial folds to allow for advancement of the remaining lower lip tissue; however, this can result in significant microstomia.[11,16] In total defects of the lip, free tissue transfer can be considered with the radial forearm flap being the most useful for reconstruction.

EAR

The auricle projects from the face, making it susceptible to injuries that may be as minor as simple lacerations or as complex as complete avulsions. Additionally, the thin skin, intricate cartilaginous structure, and tenuous blood supply present significant challenges to the reconstructive surgeon. Lacerations to the ear in which all tissue is present should be copiously irrigated, derided, and closed in a multilayered fashion. In particular, lacerations to the cartilage should be repaired with resorbable sutures before closure of the skin.

An auricular injury in which tissue is missing presents a greater reconstructive challenge due to the lack of laxity of the skin of the ear. Small defects of the posterior auricle, tragus, and lobule may be closed primarily. Primary closure is usually not possible with small defects of the remaining areas of the auricle. Small to medium defects of the

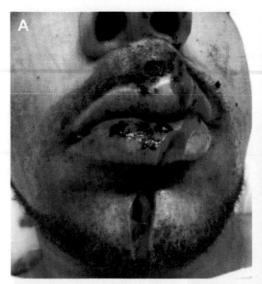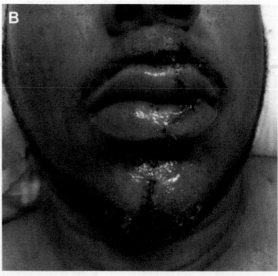

Fig. 6. (*A*) A 27-year-old man status post assault with resultant full-thickness lip and chin laceration involving the vermillion cutaneous border. (*B*) Immediately after repair and meticulous alignment of the vermillion cutaneous border.

antihelix, conchal bowl, and scapha can be reconstructed with full-thickness skin grafts if the perichondrium is intact. If the perichondrium is missing, the remaining cartilage can be resected before skin grafting.[22] Reconstruction of the helix of the ear in small to medium defects can be achieved with a wedge excision, helical advancement flap, or a composite graft from the opposite ear. Larger defects of the ear may require a staged procedure, such as a tubed postauricular flap or a postauricular advancement flap (**Fig. 7**).

Because of the projection of the ear from the head, partial and even complete avulsions are more common than other regions of the face. Small avulsions can be replanted with reasonable success if performed within 8 to 12 hours after injury. Larger avulsed segments may be placed in a postauricular pocket for 2 to 3 weeks to allow vascularization followed by transfer back to the ear. Unfortunately, the pocketed cartilage frequently resorbs and yields a poor cosmetic result. In cases of total or near-total avulsion of the ear, surgical replantation should be performed using microvascular techniques when donor and recipient vessels can be identified.

Severe injuries to the auricle, including near-total or complete avulsions in which replantation is not possible, have multiple options for reconstruction. The least invasive option is the use of a prosthesis. Others advocate for reconstruction using either autologous costal cartilage or porous polyethylene. Reconstruction with costal cartilage is a multistaged procedure but has the advantage of the use of autologous tissue, which does not present a significant risk of extrusion. The use of porous polyethylene provides excellent aesthetic results, but carries the risk of extrusion of the implant even years later secondary to even minimal trauma.[22]

Although lacerations to the ear are easily diagnosed, blunt trauma to the ear without laceration should not be dismissed without appropriate evaluation and treatment. An auricular hematoma can result from shearing or blunt trauma forces to the ear, leading to blood accumulation between the cartilage and perichondrium. The resultant hematoma can result in cartilage necrosis, infection, and/or deformity of the ear secondary to fibrosis of the remaining tissue. Treatment of an auricular hematoma consists of incision and drainage followed a compressive bolster dressing that can be removed in 5 to 7 days.[11]

Finally, lacerations of the external auditory canal pose the additional risk of scarring that leads to stenosis of the meatus and resultant difficulties with aural toilet, hearing aid fitting, and even

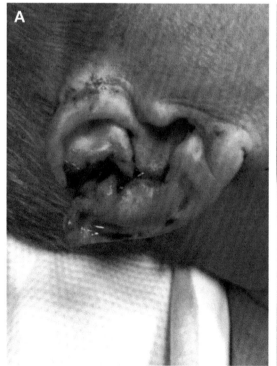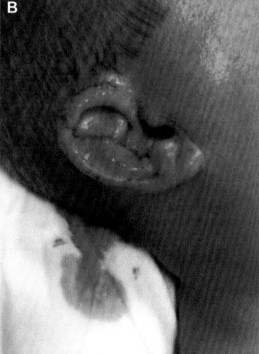

Fig. 7. (*A*) A 46-year-old man status post-rollover all-terrain vehicle accident with partial avulsion of the right auricle. (*B*) Same patient immediately after meticulous wound closure preserving the remaining tissue.

hearing in general when greater than 90% of the canal stenoses. Simple lacerations of the canal can be reapproximated, often in one layer due to the thin tissue present. Lacerations involving the cartilage and/or more than 50% of the circumference of the canal should be repaired in a layered fashion when possible and then consideration given for stenting of the external auditory canal while the laceration heals.[1] Although rare, if an avulsion of tissue from the canal occurs, a full-thickness skin graft or future meatoplasty may be necessary.

SUMMARY

Soft tissue injuries to the face are frequently encountered by the plastic surgeon and can have significant implications for patients both functionally and aesthetically. Management of soft tissue injuries to the face ranges from simple to very challenging based on the complexity of the injury and underlying structures that may be involved. A thorough evaluation and appropriate treatment plan are vital to ensuring the optimal aesthetic and functional outcome for each individual patient.

REFERENCES

1. Frodel JL, Holt GR, Larrabee WF Jr, et al. Facial plastic and reconstructive surgery. In: Papel ID, editor. 4th edition. New York: Thieme; 2016. p. 754–65.
2. Bullocks JM. Plastic surgery emergencies: principles and techniques, vol. 7. New York: Thieme; 2008. p. 54–5.
3. Diwan R, Tromovitch TA, Glogau RG, et al. Secondary intention healing. The primary approach for management of selected wounds. Arch Otolaryngol Head Neck Surg 1989;115(10):1248–9.
4. Vatsyayan A, Adhyapok AK, Debnath SC, et al. Reconstruction and rehabilitation of short-range gunshot injury to lower part of face: a systematic approach of three cases. Chin J Traumatol 2016; 19(4):239–43.
5. Hollerman JJ, Fackler ML, Coldwell DM, et al. Gunshot wounds: 1. Bullets, ballistics, and mechanisms of injury. AJR Am J Roentgenol 1990;155(4):685–90.
6. Talan DA, Citron DM, Abrahamian FM, et al. Bacteriologic analysis of infected dog and cat bites. N Engl J Med 1999;340(2):85–92.
7. Abrahamian FM. Dog bites: bacteriology, management, and prevention. Curr Infect Dis Rep 2000; 2(5):446–53.
8. Stevens DL, Bisno AL, Chambers HF, et al. Practice guidelines for the diagnosis and management of skin and soft-tissue infections. Clin Infect Dis 2005; 41(10):1373–406.
9. Kennedy SA, Stoll LE, Lauder AS. Human and other mammalian bite injuries of the hand: evaluation and management. J AM Acad Orthop Surg 2015;23(1): 47–57.
10. Alam DS. Facial trauma: evaluation and management. In: Chi JJ, editor. Cameron current surgical therapy. 11th edition. Elsevier Saunders; 2013. p. 1071.
11. Janis JE. Essentials of plastic surgery. 2nd edition. Boca Raton (FL): Quality Medical; 2014. p. 316–21, 382–5, 390, 480.
12. Kretsinger K, Broder KR, Cortese MM, et al. Preventing tetanus, diphtheria, and pertussis among adults: use of tetanus toxoid, reduced diphtheria toxoid and acellular pertussis vaccine recommendations of the Advisory Committee on Immunization Practices (ACIP) and recommendation of ACIP, supported by the Healthcare Infection Control Practices Advisory Committee (HICPAC), for use of Tdap among health-care personnel. MMWR Recomm Rep 2006; 55:1–37.
13. Thorne CH. Grabb and Smith's plastic surgery. 7th edition. Philadelphia: Lippincott Williams & Wilkins; 2014. p. 2.
14. Turnage B, Maull KI. Scalp laceration: an obvious occult cause of shock. South Med J 2000;90(3): 265–6.
15. Wells MD, Skytta C. Craniofacial, Head and Neck Surgery; pediatric plastic surgery. In: Mueller RV, editor. Plastic Surgery. 3rd edition. London: Elsevier Saunders; 2013. p. 24–8, 31–2, 34, 37, 39, 47, 109, 126.
16. Baker SR. Flap classification and design. In: Baker I, Shan R, editors. Baker local flaps in facial reconstruction. 3rd edition. Philadelphia: Elsevier Saunders; 2014. p. 75–6.
17. Murchison A, Bilyk J. Management of eyelid injuries. Facial Plast Surg 2010;26(06):464–81.
18. Morales M, Ghaiy R, Itani K. Eyelid reconstruction. Selected Readings in Plastic Surgery 2010;11(R2): 18–41.
19. Yen TL, Driscoll CL, Lalwani AK. Significance of House-Brackmann facial nerve grading global score in the setting of differential facial nerve function. Otol Neurotol 2003;24(1):118–22.
20. Lewis G, Knottenbelt JD. Parotid duct injury: is immediate surgical repair necessary? Injury 1991; 22(5):407–9.
21. Von Lindern JJ, Niederhagen B, Appel T, et al. New prospects in the treatment of traumatic and postoperative parotid fistulas with type A botulinum toxin. Plast Reconstr Surg 2002;109(7):2443–5.
22. Ha RY, Trovato MJ. Plastic surgery of the ear. Selected Readings in Plastic Surgery 2011;11(R3): 1–37.

Eyelid and Periorbital Soft Tissue Trauma

 CrossMark

Audrey C. Ko, MD[a], Kellie R. Satterfield, MD[a], Bobby S. Korn, MD, PhD[a,b],
Don O. Kikkawa, MD[a,b],*

KEYWORDS

- Ocular trauma • Periocular trauma • Facial trauma • Eyelid laceration • Canalicular laceration
- Facial degloving • Foreign bodies

KEY POINTS

- In periocular soft tissue injuries, the globe must be assessed for the possibility of rupture and conditions that are contraindications to periocular manipulation.
- Lacerations of the canaliculus must be repaired and stented to prevent tearing after injury.
- Lacerations of the eyelid margin must be repaired in a multilayered fashion to prevent eyelid malpositions and cosmetic defects after injury.

INTRODUCTION

Soft tissue trauma to the face is a common injury and comprises roughly 10% of all emergency room visits.[1–3] Because of the potential for post-traumatic functional and cosmetic sequelae, reconstructive expertise is required in the repair of any facial soft tissue injury, especially to the eyelids and periorbital soft tissues. Injuries to the periocular region are often complex and involve multiple anatomic structures. Soft tissue repair with optimal aesthetic and functional outcome can be achieved through meticulous planning and knowledge of facial reconstructive techniques. This article highlights key steps in patient evaluation and management of various types of injuries, and provides a review of current literature involving facial soft tissue trauma.

PATIENT ASSESSMENT

After stabilization of the patient, a detailed history of the mechanism of trauma and patient presentation is obtained. A full survey of the face and scalp is then performed, paying attention to signs of surface or penetrating wounds, foreign bodies, and avulsed or missing tissue. Often these wounds are difficult to visualize due to obscuration by debris and dried or coagulated blood, especially in areas that contain hair, such as the scalp and eyebrows. If present, cleaning the affected areas is indicated by irrigation with sterile saline and gentle debridement with gauze. If there is a marked amount of swelling, visualization can be aided by first applying ice to the affected area. If necessary, patient tolerance of the examination can also be helped by injection of lidocaine or moderate sedation in the emergency room. Photographs of the patient with multiple angles should be obtained for medical-legal documentation.

Ocular Assessment

A ruptured ocular globe is one of the few ophthalmic emergencies that warrant immediate surgery. Signs of a ruptured globe include

Disclosures: The authors have nothing to disclose.
[a] Division of Oculofacial Plastic and Reconstructive Surgery, UC San Diego Department of Ophthalmology, Shiley Eye Institute, 9415 Campus Point Drive, La Jolla, CA 92093, USA; [b] Division of Plastic Surgery, UC San Diego Department of Surgery, 9500 Gilman Drive, La Jolla, CA 92093, USA
* Corresponding author. 9415 Campus Point Drive, La Jolla, CA 92093.
E-mail address: dkikkawa@ucsd.edu

Facial Plast Surg Clin N Am 25 (2017) 605–616
http://dx.doi.org/10.1016/j.fsc.2017.06.011

decreased vision, focal bullous or 360° subconjunctival hemorrhage, an irregularly shaped pupil, ocular hypotony, and the presence of blood in the anterior chamber. If any of these signs are noted on the initial examination, prompt ocular protection by an eye shield and evaluation by an ophthalmologist is indicated.[4,5] Further periocular manipulation, such as examination of the eyelids or surrounding periorbital tissues, should be avoided or conducted with extreme caution to avoid pressure on the ocular globe that may lead to extrusion of intraocular contents.

In cases of significant injury to periorbital soft tissue and bony structures, the potential for concurrent eye damage should be assessed. A ruptured globe is an absolute contraindication to periocular and periorbital manipulation (Fig. 1). Additional ocular conditions that place the globe at high risk during periocular and periorbital manipulation, and possible future permanent decrease or complete loss of vision, include the following: hyphema, dislocated intraocular lens, intraocular foreign body, and retinal detachment. If any of these additional conditions exist, consultation should be obtained from the ophthalmology service to determine optimum time for surgical repair of other facial injuries.

Eyelid Assessment

In the initial assessment of the eyelids, any abrasions, ecchymosis, and lacerations should be noted. The presence of a traumatic ptosis can be assessed by looking for motility deficits while having the patient follow an object in upgaze and downgaze. Oftentimes swelling will limit the motility of the eyelid, and the eyelid motility will need to be reexamined at a future date.

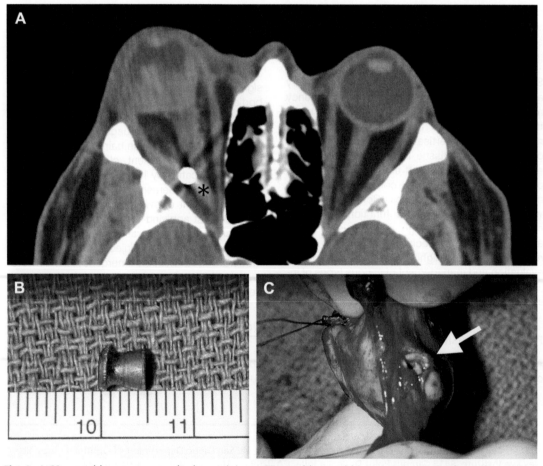

Fig. 1. A 60-year-old man was assaulted, sustaining a BB gun blast and blunt trauma to the face. The patient's vision was no light perception with a ruptured globe. The globe was found to be unsalvageable and was removed along with the pellet. This delayed treatment of his associated facial fractures. (*A*) CT-orbit demonstrating globe disruption and intraorbital foreign body (*asterisk*). (*B*) Removed pellet. (*C*) The ruptured globe and scleral exit wound (*arrow*).

Eyelid lacerations are categorized as partial or full-thickness lacerations. For reconstructive purposes, the eyelid is divided into anterior (skin and orbicularis muscle) and posterior (tarsus and conjunctiva) lamellae (**Fig. 2**). A full-thickness laceration involves the posterior lamella, and requires a more complex and layered closure. Involvement of the posterior lamella can be detected by examining the upper and lower eyelid margins for discontinuity or a notch. Some lid margin defects are difficult to appreciate on gross examination of the lid. Oftentimes an insignificant-appearing marginal discontinuity will have significant posterior extension; therefore, gentle eversion of the upper and lower eyelids is needed to assess for involvement of the tarsus. If not properly repaired at the time of injury, a large notch will be noted in the eyelid margin with separation of the eyelashes medially and laterally after it heals. This may subsequently affect blinking and the ocular surface interface. Failure to detect a marginal eyelid laceration may also result in a very noticeable aesthetic deformity that is bothersome and noticeable by patients.

The evaluation of eyelid lacerations also involves an assessment for avulsed or missing tissue. A full-thickness lid laceration frequently gives the appearance of missing tissue due to the wide gaping of the separated segments of the eyelid (**Fig. 3**). The eyelid is usually firmly opposed to the globe by the lateral canthal ligament laterally and medial canthal ligament medially; when split, the separated portions of the eyelid are widely pulled medially and laterally, mistakenly giving the appearance of missing tissue. If the eyelid tissues oppose easily with gentle reapproximation,

tissue avulsion is unlikely. If marked edema of the tissues hampers this determination, gentle application of ice for 20 minutes to decrease swelling is helpful.

Involvement of the lateral or medial canthal ligaments can occur with orbital fractures or downward distraction of the eyelid. Disinsertion of the lateral canthal ligament may manifest as rounding of the lateral canthal angle. Due to its insertion at the Whitnall tubercle, rounding of the lateral canthal angle may also be seen in fracture of the lateral orbital wall. In contrast, the medial canthal ligament has 2 attachments: anteriorly to the frontal process of the maxilla, and posteriorly to the thin lacrimal bone. Telecanthus and canthal rounding also can be seen with medial canthal ligament injuries. However, further investigation through imaging is needed to assess for bony involvement (**Table 1**), as reconstructive techniques vary depending on whether the ligament is solely involved, or if there is bony involvement as well.[6]

Lacrimal Assessment

Medial eyelid injuries may involve the medial canthus and violate of the integrity of the lacrimal system. Common mechanisms of injury differ in various patient populations; in the breast-fed infant, pediatric, adult, and elderly populations, the most common mechanisms are blouse hooks, dog bite, trauma, and falls, respectively.[7–9] Medial canthal lacerations are more commonly seen in children and young adults and more frequently involve the lower canaliculus. Interestingly, upper canalicular injuries are associated with globe

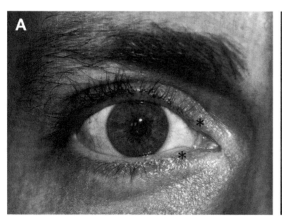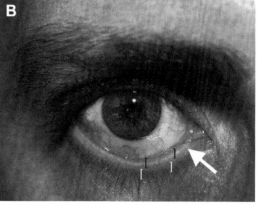

Fig. 2. Normal eyelid margins demonstrated (*A*) with black asterisks marking the locations of the upper and lower puncta. Note that the puncta are not normally visualized due to their anatomic position against the eyeball. (*B*) Everted right lower eyelid, showing the posterior lamella consisting of the conjunctiva and tarsus (*black brackets*) and anterior lamella consisting of the skin and orbicularis oculi muscle (*white brackets*). The punctum is visualized with eversion (*white arrow*).

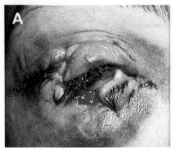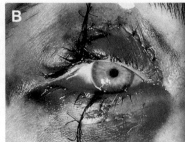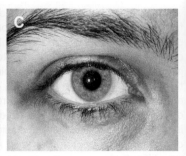

Fig. 3. A 22-year-old woman fell and hit her face on a clothing hook. (*A*) She presented with multiple full-thickness upper and lower eyelid lacerations with the suspicion of missing eyelid tissue. (*B*) Photograph of the patient immediately after repair. No tissue was noted to be missing. Note that the silk sutures were left long and secured away from the cornea to avoid mechanical abrasions. (*C*) Postoperative photograph showing a well-healed repair with minimal scarring. Note the smooth contour of the eyelid margin with absence of notching.

rupture in 20% to 25% of cases.[8,10] Therefore, if a canalicular injury is present, the index of suspicion for an injury to the globe should be heightened.

A thorough examination of the upper lacrimal drainage system is indicated with any injury involving the medial canthal region or medial upper and lower eyelid.[11] Any disruption of the tear drainage system that is not repaired initially may result in chronic epiphora. Superficially, the upper and lower puncta are visible as pinpoint openings along the medial eyelid (see **Fig. 2**), and run vertically for approximately 2 mm in length. The superior and inferior lacrimal drainage system then make a 90° turn medially for approximately 8 mm, and then join to form the common canaliculus, which then connects to the nasolacrimal duct that drains through the inferior meatus into the nose. Therefore, any laceration that occurs medial to the punctum requires probing (**Fig. 4**) and irrigation to assess for the integrity of the tear drainage system. A more subtle finding may show lateralization of the punctum, which usually also suggests disruption.

Orbital Assessment

Orbital involvement can occur with deep extension of superficial wounds. The orbital septum is a fibrous sheet that serves as the anterior orbital boundary. Deep to the septum lies the true orbital fat, which overlays the 2 elevators of the upper eyelid, the levator aponeurosis and Müller muscle. Visible fat in the preseptal orbicularis area warrants further exploration, as it signifies violation into the orbital space and possible deeper injury to the orbital soft tissues and/or to the eyelid elevators. If there is suspicion for a retained foreign body, imaging can be obtained.[5] Plain radiography and computed tomography (CT) scans are the recommended first line of imaging for most foreign body materials; MRI should be avoided due to risk of metallic foreign body.[12]

The integrity of the bony walls of the orbit and orbital soft tissue contents also may be affected. A detailed discussion of the evaluation and management of orbital fractures can be found in the article by (Scott E. Bevans and Kris. S. Moe's article, " Advances in the Reconstruction of

Table 1 Classification of nasoethmoidal fractures		
Type	**Description**	**Treatment**
I	Single-segment central fragment	Fixation of fragment to proper positioning
II	Comminuted central fragment with fractures remaining external to the medial canthal tendon insertion	Fixation of the fragment with adherence of the canthal ligament
III	Comminuted central fragment with fractures extending into bone bearing the canthal insertion	Fixation of the canthal ligament to fixed bone or periosteum

Data from Markowitz BL, Manson PN, Sargent L, et al. Management of the medial canthal tendon in nasoethmoid orbital fractures: the importance of the central fragment in classification and treatment. Plast Reconstr Surg 1991;87(5):843–53.

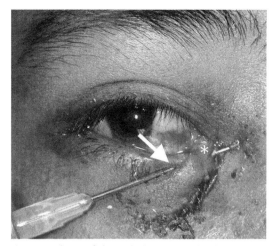

Fig. 4. Probing of the right lower canaliculus in a patient with medial canthal trauma. The white arrow denotes the entry point of probe into the punctum, and the white asterisk identifies the exit point through the lacerated canaliculus.

Orbital Fractures," elsewhere in this issue). With regard to the periocular examination in orbital fractures, the examiner can assess for the presence of bony step-offs and subcutaneous crepitus through palpation along the orbital rim. Hypesthesia in the maxillary (V2) division of the trigeminal nerve can occur secondary to bony impingement in orbital floor fractures, direct trauma, compression by soft tissue swelling, or irritation by localized inflammation. An assessment of the patient's vision is also required to detect optic neuropathy, which can occur in fractures of the optic canal. Last, extraocular muscle entrapment or impingement by bony fragments can be detected by observing ocular motility in upgaze, downgaze, and right and left gaze. Entrapment of extraocular muscles occurs most commonly in the pediatric population, but also can occur in the adult population. Upgaze limitation associated with inferior rectus impingement in orbital floor fractures is the most common, followed by lateral

gaze restriction associated with medial rectus entrapment in medial wall fractures. Enophthalmos or muscle contusion can masquerade as muscle entrapment, and can be differentiated from true entrapment through forced ductions testing. The presence of an ocular cardiac reflex, bradycardia secondary to increased vagal tone due to tension on an extraocular muscle, is an indication for emergent release of tissue and fracture repair.

Orbital hemorrhages in the orbital space may occur independently or in association with orbital fractures. Although small hemorrhages can be observed, accumulation of a large amount of blood in the retrobulbar space may lead to orbital compartment syndrome and permanently decreased or complete loss of vision through mechanical stretching of the optic nerve or blockage of ocular perfusion (**Fig. 5**). Proptosis secondary to posterior volume expansion by a retrobulbar hemorrhage can best be appreciated with a worm's eye view. To assess for possible optic nerve compromise, the examiner may check the visual acuity and color vision if the patient is alert and oriented. The presence of a relative afferent pupillary defect is also an objective indicator of optic nerve compression and can be assessed in nonresponsive patients. It is important to differentiate a retrobulbar hemorrhage from a preseptal hematoma, as both can present as nonspecific swelling of the eye externally. However, a preseptal hematoma is not typically vision threatening, as it is anterior to the orbital septum and thus does not cause a compartment syndrome resulting in optic nerve compression (**Fig. 6**).

MANAGEMENT OF INJURIES

After stabilization of the patient, soft tissue wounds should be repaired as soon as possible. Inasmuch as most facial soft tissue wounds are not life-threatening, urgent repair of these wounds is associated with improved postoperative

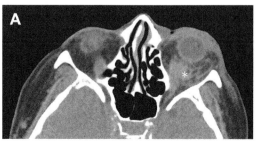
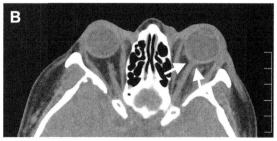

Fig. 5. A 69-year-old woman presented after a fall. (*A*) An axial CT of the orbits demonstrated a large left retrobulbar hemorrhage (*white asterisk*). (*B*) Cross-section showing posterior globe tenting and stretching of the optic nerve (*white arrows*).

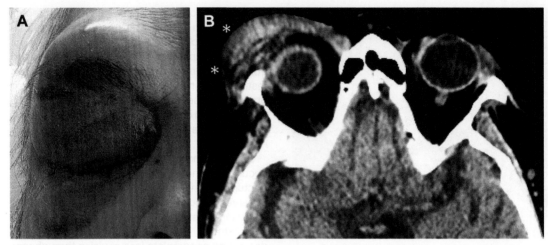

Fig. 6. An 82-year-old woman presented after a syncopal episode with loss of consciousness. (*A*) An external photograph shows significant swelling and ecchymosis. (*B*) Axial CT demonstrating a large preseptal hematoma (*white asterisks*) without intraorbital involvement.

aesthetic outcomes.[13,14] If repair must be delayed, application of antibiotic ointment and covering the wound with sterile nonstick dressing, such as Telfa Gauze (Kendall, Mansfield, MA) or Tegaderm dressing (3M Healthcare, Neuss, Germany), is recommended. To prevent corneal ulceration and exposure keratopathy, a moisture chamber should be placed on patients with eyelid defects with exposed cornea. These can be made by placing lubricating ophthalmic ointment over the cornea and sealing the periocular area with occlusive dressing.

Medications and Vaccination Status

Previous tetanus toxoid immunization history should be obtained and administered if warranted (**Table 2**).[15] Facial wounds tend to heal well and have a low risk of infection due to the significant amount of vascular supply and anastomoses present in the face.[16] Most patients do well with postoperative application of antibiotic ointment to the sutured wounds. Broad-spectrum ophthalmic antibiotic ointment should specifically be used for periocular injuries due to risk of ocular surface irritation and chemical conjunctivitis. However, systemic antibiotics should be considered if the patient is immune-compromised, diabetic, or a chronic smoker.[17] Penetrating and animal bite injuries require antibiotics due to higher risk of wound contamination compared with other types of injuries.[17] Commonly prescribed systemic antibiotics include amoxicillin/clavulanate 875 mg PO BID for 3 to 5 days due to its broad coverage of common offending organisms, including *P multocida* (often present with dog or cat bites), however local resistance patterns and severity of injury should be considered with antibiotic administration. Additionally, patients with animal bites may need vaccination with rabies vaccine (**Table 3**).[18,19]

Table 2 **Tetanus prophylaxis in routine wound management**				
Previous Doses of Tetanus Toxoid Vaccine	**Clean or Minor Wound**		**All Other Wounds[a]**	
	Tetanus Toxoid–Containing Vaccine	**Human Tetanus Immune Globulin**	**Tetanus Toxoid–Containing Vaccine**	**Human Tetanus Immune Globulin**
<3 doses	Yes	No	Yes	Yes
≥3 doses	Only if last dose ≥10 y previously	No	Only if last dose ≥5 y previously	No

[a] Including but not limited to wounds contaminated with soil, feces, saliva, or other debris; puncture wounds, other wounds caused by burns, frostbite, or crush injuries.

Data from Kim DK, Bridges CB, Harriman KH. Advisory Committee on immunization practices recommended immunization schedule for adults aged 19 years or older: United States, 2016. Ann Intern Med 2016;164:184.

Table 3
Rabies postexposure prophylaxis

Vaccination History	Prophylactic Treatment	
	Total Doses	Scheduling
Previously vaccinated persons	2	Day 0, 4
Vaccine naïve persons	4[a]	Day 0, 3, 7, 14

[a] Five doses should be given in any immune-compromised persons.

Data from Rupprecht CE, Briggs D, Brown CM, et al. Use of a reduced (4-dose) vaccine schedule for postexposure prophylaxis to prevent human rabies: recommendations of the advisory committee on immunization practices. MMWR Recomm Rep 2010;59:1; and Committee on Infectious Diseases. Rabies-prevention policy update: new reduced-dose schedule. Pediatrics 2011;127:785.

Irrigation and Debridement

Contaminated wounds or noncontaminated wounds more than 6 hours old should be copiously irrigated. Of note, noncontaminated wounds treated quickly have not been shown to benefit from irrigation.[20] The presence of contamination should not be a contraindication to urgent repair of tissues, as it has not been associated with an increase in complications.[21] Contaminated wounds should be irrigated with sterile saline. Surgical antiseptics are commonly used, but some reports show a possible association with delayed wound healing.[22] Debridement of devitalized tissue and clearance of debris should be performed before closure.

Abrasions

Small wounds that do not involve exposed vital structures may heal by secondary intention. However, this is not recommended if the wound is located in an area in which a scar would cause deformation and limitation of movement of natural creases or result in cicatricial displacement of structures with scar contracture (such as the upper eyelid crease or lower eyelid, **Fig. 7**). The patient should be educated on signs of cellulitis and followed closely. Application of a nonstick dressing, such as Telfa gauze, can help decrease pain with wound changes.

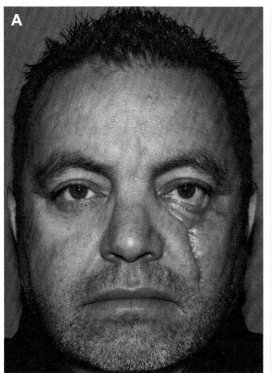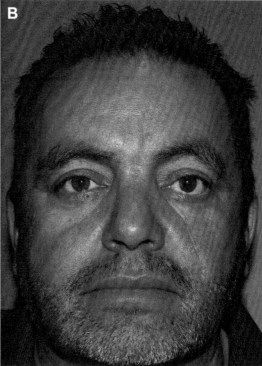

Fig. 7. A 45-year-old man developed (A) cicatricial ectropion and cosmetic deformity following an injury from an explosion at work. (B) Improvement of eyelid position after injection of 5-fluorouracil, scar revision, and cicatricial ectropion repair.

Lacerations of the Periorbital Area

The use of nonabsorbable polypropylene or nylon sutures are favored in contaminated wounds, as other types of suture may act as a nidus for infection. These types of sutures also minimize inflammation that can contribute to suboptimal outcomes in wound healing, such as postinflammatory hyperpigmentation or hypertrophic scarring. However, absorbable sutures may be considered in patients who have unreliable follow-up. Tissue adhesives are an alternative option for wound closure. In one study comparing tissue adhesives with standard closure, no difference in cosmetic outcome was appreciated, and patients reported decreased pain and redness; however, the rate of dehiscence was higher with adhesive as compared with standard wound closure.[23]

Periocular injuries call for close attention to the natural skin folds and skin creases around the eyelids and eyebrows. If relaxing incisions are necessary, they should be made within or parallel to skin tension lines and skin creases. If skin creases or tension lines are not readily apparent, visualization of more subtle lines can be highlighted by gently moving adjacent tissue to emphasize naturally existing skin creases. Defects that run parallel to the eyelid margin should be redirected to an angle perpendicular to the eyelid margin to maximize horizontal tension and minimize vertical tension to avoid eyelid distortion. Special attention should be paid to preserve symmetry of the medial brows, as this location is less forgiving in aesthetic outcome.[24] If primary closure is not possible, small defects in the brow or forehead can be repaired with flaps based off supraorbital and supratrochlear vascular circulations.

Lacerations of the Eyelid

In lacerations without missing tissue, reconstruction of the eyelid is more involved than simple approximation of the adjacent tissues. Careful alignment of the gray line and tarsal plate is necessary to prevent lid notching and to obtain a smooth eyelid margin contour. The upper and lower eyelid is divided into an anterior and posterior lamella (see **Fig. 2**), and the 2 layers are reconstructed separately.

With large soft tissue defects, it is likely that a secondary procedure will be necessary. Hence, it is best not to use any flaps in the primary closure that could compromise future reconstruction. In patients with missing eyelid tissue, the most important variable to consider in choosing a reconstruction method is the amount of tissue laxity. In older patients, the eyelid may have sufficient laxity for primary closure despite missing tissue. A lateral canthotomy and cantholysis also may create enough laxity to allow for primary closure. If a marked amount of tissue is missing, a semicircular flap from the lateral canthal area may allow for tissue to be shifted medially to be used for reconstruction. A complete loss of an upper or lower eyelid may require a lid-sharing procedure, such as a tarsoconjunctival pedicled flap.[25,26]

Lacerations of the Lacrimal System

A laceration of the upper and/or lower canaliculus requires prompt stenting to avoid canalicular obstruction leading to chronic epiphora. It is estimated that the lower and upper canaliculus performs 70% and 30% of the tear drainage, respectively.[27] Therefore, a nonpatent inferior canaliculus oftentimes leads to chronic epiphora and dermatitis. Monocanalicular laceration reconstructions should be considered in all cases, regardless of which canaliculus is involved.[28] Consideration should be given of repair in an operating room over a minor procedure room, as this has been shown to improve outcomes in some studies.[7,29] If there is difficulty visualizing the canaliculus for intubation, air (with the tissue submerged in fluid) or fluorescein can be injected into the opposite punctum. Viscoelastic can also be injected into the canalicular orifice to help tamponade the bleeding and identify the torn edges.[30]

There are various nasolacrimal stents that can be used in the repair of lacerations involving the lacrimal system. Common bicanalicular stents include the Ritleng (FCI Ophthalmics, Marshfield Hills, MA) and Crawford (Altomed, Boldon Colliery, UK); the most common monocanalicular stent is the Mini-Monoka (FCI Ophthalmics). Lacerations involving the upper and lower canaliculus can be stented with a bicanalicular stent, but these typically require retrieval through the nose and can be uncomfortable in a nonsedated patient. The use of 2 monocanalicular stents, or the Lacriflow bicanalicular stent (Kaneka, Osaka, Japan), may be a more comfortable option for a patient under local anesthetic only. Another option for avoiding nasal stent retrieval is the pigtail probe, which passes a stent through the canalicular system only and has the additional benefit of easy visualization of the cut end of the canaliculus. Care should be taken when using the pigtail probe, as excessive lateral traction may cause iatrogenic damage to the common canaliculus. Efficacy of stenting has not been shown to be significantly different between monocanalicular and bicanalicular stents.[29]

Secondary repair of the canaliculus is difficult; if unsuccessful, a complete bypass of the lacrimal drainage system with a Jones tube is required. Therefore, it is best to perform primary repair in the hands of a surgeon experienced in canalicular laceration repair if the lacrimal drainage system is involved.

Lateral and Medial Canthus Injuries

The medial and lateral canthal ligaments suspend and hold horizontal tension across the upper and lower eyelids. Injuries to the lateral and medical canthus are particularly bothersome to patients due to the cosmetically undesirable rounding of the involved canthus and shortening of the palpebral fissure, which is normally 28 to 30 mm.[31]

The lateral canthal ligament inserts at the Whitnall tubercle approximately 1.5 mm posterior to the lateral orbital rim and 10.6 mm inferior to the frontozygomatic suture.[32] The lateral canthal ligament then splits into a superior and inferior crus that attaches to the upper and lower eyelid, respectively. For injuries involving an isolated crus, its reinsertion to the remaining lateral canthal ligament complex is typically sufficient; however, if the entire lateral canthal complex is disinserted, reinsertion to the periosteum of the inner margin of the lateral orbital rim is required. During reinsertion, it is important to note that the normal anatomic position of insertion is posterior to the rim and 1 to 2 mm superior to the horizontal height of the medial canthus.[32] Failure to maintain this anatomic relationship can result in canthal dystopia. However, due to anatomic variations, it is best to align the canthal position with the opposite uninvolved side.

In contrast to the lateral canthal ligament, the medial canthal ligament is a more complex structure. There is an anterior and posterior tendinous portion with points of insertion at the anterior and posterior lacrimal crest, respectively. After these portions cross over the nasolacrimal sac, they fuse and divide into a superior and inferior arm that attach to the tarsal plate. Therefore, disruption to these structures also alters the normal blink dynamics and lacrimal pump mechanism, which may result in epiphora despite a patent lacrimal drainage system.

Repair of the medial canthal ligament consists of 2 parts. First, one must assess whether the anterior, posterior, or both portions of the ligament are disrupted. If only the anterior portion is disrupted, an eyelid malposition is unlikely and it can be directly reattached at its original point of insertion. However, if the entire ligament is avulsed, its point of reinsertion should be at the periosteum of the posterior lacrimal crest. Second, one must assess for the integrity of the bone (see **Table 1**) and repair fractures if necessary. If no periosteum is available for fixation, a miniplate or transnasal wiring may be needed to serve as an anchoring point of insertion.

Foreign Bodies

Foreign bodies that are superficial and not located near critical structures can be removed with irrigation, sterile cotton tip applicators, or sterile forceps. Organic material, graphite, or other pigmented material (such as lead) should be removed, as retention of the material may result in permanent skin pigmentation, granulomas, infections and inflammation. Deeper metallic foreign bodies may not require removal, as they pose a lower risk of infection and removal may cause greater harm to the patient rather than no intervention.[33] As demonstrated in **Fig. 8**, it is important to fully characterize the actual size and depth of the foreign body, as deeply embedded objects may appear small superficially. If there is any question regarding the depth or extent, radiologic studies can aid in further characterization of the foreign body.

In penetrating injuries, unwitnessed, or pediatric traumas in which the mechanism of injury is unknown, further investigation with imaging is required to assess for retained foreign body and damage to surrounding structures, particularly of vascular nature. CT scans are typically the first line of imaging for the identification of penetrating foreign bodies, characterization of their trajectory, and determining the extent of injuries. In cases of metallic foreign bodies in which imaging artifact may obstruct the surrounding tissue, plain-film radiographs in multiple views or 3-dimensional CT imaging can be used for better characterization of the anatomic location and involvement of surrounding tissues. In the scenario of high clinical suspicion but with negative imaging, surgical exploration is indicated for chronically draining wounds, persistent pain, or injury secondary to wood or other organic material.

Penetrating objects should be removed only in the controlled setting of an operating room. If preoperative angiography shows vascular involvement, intraoperative control of the vessel must be obtained before removal of the foreign body. Repeat angiography postoperatively is also recommended for reassessment of vascular flow.

Degloving Injuries

Degloving injuries are a subcategory of tissue avulsion injury that involves the separation of skin and

614

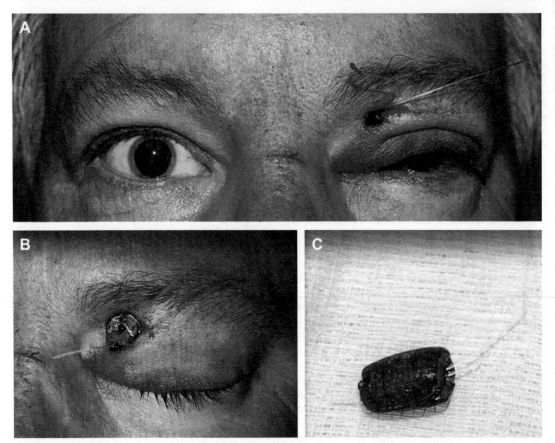

Fig. 8. A 57-year-old man presented after a fishing accident. The patient was reeling in his fishing line when the fishing weight caught and then snapped back, hitting him just inferior to his left medial brow. (*A*) The patient was found to have fishing line attached to a weight lodged into the left eyelid. (*B*) Further exploration showed a much larger and deeper foreign body. (*C*) The fishing weight after removal from the wound site.

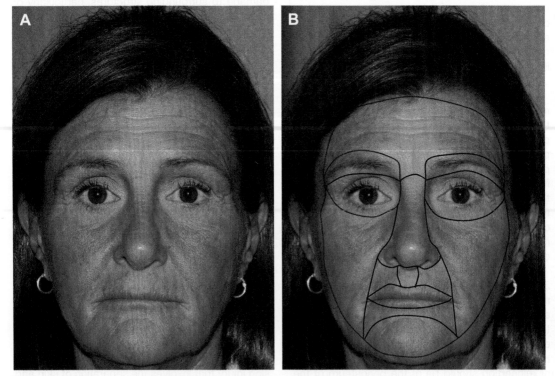

Fig. 9. Facial image of a female patient (*A*) with facial anesthetic units outlined (*B*).

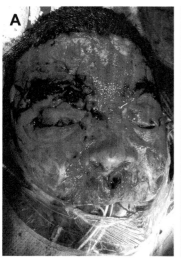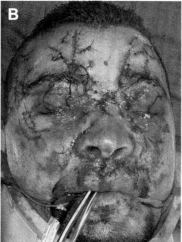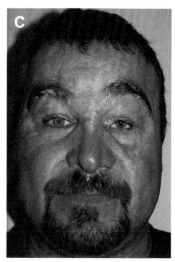

Fig. 10. A 35-year-old patient presented with multiple facial abrasions and lacerations (*A*) after being assaulted. (*B*) The patient immediately after initial reconstruction. The patient underwent numerous secondary reconstructions. (*C*) The patient at 12-year follow-up.

soft tissue from underlying bone and supporting structures. Vasculature is often compromised. Severe degloving injuries that involve an extensive area of skin, multiple anatomic structures, and vasculature are difficult to repair and can result in significant disfigurement and adverse functional outcomes. After an initial cleaning of the affected area with and debridement of devitalized tissues, the blood supply to each avulsed area of tissue is assessed. The integrity of larger vessels can be assessed with ultrasound; smaller vessels can be indirectly assessed by looking for areas of bleeding along the tissue flap edges.

If the degloved soft tissue flaps are viable, they are best replaced to their anatomic position. Preservation of facial aesthetic units (**Fig. 9**) can be achieved by aligning incisions, borders of flaps, and scars along preexisting creases or folds. In patients with missing tissue, it is preferable to use local advancement flaps or full-thickness skin grafts from other areas of the face (eg, upper eyelid skin, preauricular or postauricular skin) to avoid tissue discoloration and the appearance of a "stuck on" skin patch. Split-thickness skin grafts may be necessary to cover larger facial areas of deepithelialized tissue.

Due to the highly complex area of the medial canthus, medial canthal degloving injuries may present with multiple manifestations, including telecanthus, ptosis, and lacrimal involvement.[9] Severe degloving injuries may require additional revisions after the initial repair. Injection of antimetabolites, such as 5-fluorouracil, can help prevent hypertrophic scarring and scar contraction that can result in sequelae such as cicatricial eyelid malpositions (see **Fig. 7A**).[34,35]

SUMMARY

Patients with poor aesthetic and functional outcome wear facial stigmata of their injury, and it can have a profound effect on their self-esteem, ability to retain or perform their jobs, or allow them to move on emotionally from their trauma. However, even patients with severe facial soft tissue trauma can have an excellent long-term result (**Fig. 10**). Therefore, facial, eyelid, and periorbital soft tissue trauma should be repaired with thoughtful planning and expertise.

REFERENCES

1. Hussain K, Wijetunge DB, Grubnic S, et al. A comprehensive analysis of craniofacial trauma. J Trauma 1994;36:34–47.
2. Mitchener TA, Canham-Chervak M. Oral-maxillofacial injury surveillance in the Department of Defense, 1996-2005. Am J Prev Med 2010;38(1, Suppl):S86–93.
3. Ong TK, Dudley M. Craniofacial trauma presenting at an adult accident and emergency department with an emphasis on soft tissue injuries. Injury 1999;30:357–63.
4. Chazen JL, Lantos J, Gupta A, et al. Orbital soft-tissue trauma. Neuroimaging Clin N Am 2014; 24(3):425–37.
5. Betts AM, O'Brien WT, Davies BW, et al. A systematic approach to CT evaluation of orbital trauma. Emerg Radiol 2014;21(5):511–31.

6. Markowitz BL, Manson PN, Sargent L, et al. Management of the medial canthal tendon in nasoethmoid orbital fractures: the importance of the central fragment in classification and treatment. Plast Reconstr Surg 1991;87(5):843–53.

7. Murchison AP, Bilyk JR. Pediatric canalicular lacerations: epidemiology and variables affecting repair success. J Pediatr Ophthalmol Strabismus 2014; 51(4):242–8.

8. Naik MN, Kelapure A, Rath S, et al. Management of canalicular lacerations: epidemiological aspects and experience with mini-monoka monocanalicular stent. Am J Ophthalmol 2008;145(2):375–80.

9. Kennedy RH, May J, Daily J, et al. Canalicular laceration: an 11-year epidemiologic and clinical study. Ophthal Plast Reconstr Surg 1990;6(1):46–53.

10. Fayet B, Bernard JA, Ammar J, et al. Recent wounds of the lacrimal duct. Apropos of 262 cases treated as emergencies. J Fr Ophtalmol 1988;11:627–37.

11. Priel A, Leelapatranurak K, Oh SR, et al. Medial canthal degloving injuries: the triad of telecanthus, ptosis, and lacrimal trauma. Plast Reconstr Surg 2011; 128(4):300e–5e.

12. Wikner J, Riecke B, Gröbe A, et al. Imaging of the midfacial and orbital trauma. Facial Plast Surg 2014;30(5):528–36.

13. Benzil DL, Robotti E, Dagi TF, et al. Early single-stage repair of complex craniofacial trauma. Neurosurgery 1992;30:166–71 [discussion: 171–2].

14. Aveta A, Casati P. Soft tissue injuries of the face: early aesthetic reconstruction in polytrauma patients. Ann Ital Chir 2008;79:415–7.

15. Kim DK, Bridges CB, Harriman KH. Advisory committee on immunization practices recommended immunization schedule for adults aged 19 years or older: United States, 2016. Ann Intern Med 2016; 164:184.

16. Dickinson JT, Jaquiss GW, Thompson JN. Soft tissue trauma. Otolaryngol Clin North Am 1976;9:331–60.

17. Chhabra S, Chhabra N, Gaba S. Maxillofacial injuries due to animal bites. J Maxillofac Oral Surg 2015;14(2):142–53.

18. Rupprecht CE, Briggs D, Brown CM, et al. Use of a reduced (4-dose) vaccine schedule for postexposure prophylaxis to prevent human rabies: recommendations of the advisory committee on immunization practices. MMWR Recomm Rep 2010;59:1.

19. Committee on Infectious Diseases. Rabies-prevention policy update: new reduced-dose schedule. Pediatrics 2011;127:785.

20. Hollander JE, Richman PB, Werblud M, et al. Irrigation in facial and scalp lacerations: does it alter outcome? Ann Emerg Med 1998;31:73–7.

21. Stanley RB Jr, Schwartz MS. Immediate reconstruction of contaminated central craniofacial injuries with free autogenous grafts. Laryngoscope 1989;99(10 Pt 1):1011–5.

22. Krasner D. AHCPR Clinical practice guideline number 15, treatment of pressure ulcers: a pragmatist's critique for wound care providers. Ostomy Wound Manage 1995;41(7A suppl):97S–101S.

23. Beam JW. Tissue adhesives for simple traumatic lacerations. J Athl Train 2008;43(2):2224.

24. Hidalgo DA. Discussion: finesse in forehead and brow rejuvenation: modern concepts, including endoscopic methods. Plast Reconstr Surg 2014;134(6):1151–3.

25. Fischer T, Noever G, Langer M, et al. Experience in upper eyelid reconstruction with the Cutler-Beard technique. Ann Plast Surg 2001;47(3):338–42.

26. Hughes WL. A new method for rebuilding a lower lid: report of a case. Arch Ophthalmol 1937;17:1008–17.

27. Olver J, Cassidy L, Jutley G, et al. Ophthalmology at a glance. Chapter 28: lacrimation. West Sussex (UK): John Wiley & Sons; 2014.

28. Kalin-Hajdu E, Cadet N, Boulos PR. Controversies of the lacrimal system. Surv Ophthalmol 2016;61(3): 309–13.

29. Murchison AP, Bilyk JR. Canalicular laceration repair: an analysis of variables affecting success. Ophthal Plast Reconstr Surg 2014;30(5):410–4.

30. Örge FH, Dar SA. Canalicular laceration repair using a viscoelastic injection to locate and dilate the proximal torn edge. J AAPOS 2015;19(3):217–9.

31. Potter JK, Janis JE, Clark CP III. Blepharoplasty and browlift. Sel Readings Plast Surg 2005;10:1–35.

32. Gioia VM, Linberg JV, McCormick SA. The anatomy of the lateral canthal tendon. Arch Ophthalmol 1987; 105:529–32.

33. Halaas GW. Management of foreign bodies in the skin. Am Fam Physician 2007;76(5):683–8.

34. Monstrey S, Middelkoop E, Vranckx JJ, et al. Updated scar management practical guidelines: non-invasive and invasive measures. J Plast Reconstr Aesthet Surg 2014;67(8):1017–25.

35. Kummoona RK. Missile war injuries of the face. J Craniofac Surg 2011;22(6):2017–21.

Posttraumatic Laser Treatment of Soft Tissue Injury

Prem B. Tripathi, MD, MPH[a,b], J. Stuart Nelson, MD, PhD[a,c], Brian J. Wong, MD, PhD[a,b,c],*

KEYWORDS

- Laser • Scar • Ablative • Carbon dioxide • Erbium • Pulsed dye • Fractional
- Posttraumatic facial scar

KEY POINTS

- Lasers are a relatively safe and noninvasive modality in the management of posttraumatic facial scarring when used appropriately.
- Lasers exert their therapeutic effects through volumetric heating, selective photothermolysis, or frank ablation.
- Combining several lasers with or without surgical scar revision may continually improve the texture and appearance of facial scars.
- The literature regarding ideal dosimetry is mixed, and more randomized controlled trials and split scar studies may provide greater insight into the ideal management strategy based on scar type.

INTRODUCTION

Posttraumatic soft tissue injuries can result in complex, disfiguring, and often permanent scars, which may defy optimal restoration despite aggressive wound care, pharmacologic therapy, hyperbaric O_2, mechanical dermabrasion, and conventional surgery (scar revision). Whereas clean, straight lacerations may heal as well as a postoperative surgical incision, blast injuries, and penetrating and blunt trauma may result in crushed tissue, jagged wounds, and/or frank soft tissue loss leading to suboptimal closure, tension, and poor wound healing. Posttraumatic soft tissue injuries require thorough irrigation to reduce microbial burden, removal of debris to decrease risk of traumatic tattooing, proper selection of appropriate suture material, and meticulous skin closure without undue tension.[1,2] Several adjunctive measures after primary surgical management are known to reduce scar formation and improve appearance, including posttreatment dressings, silicone sheeting, isotretinoin, and dermabrasion. Although classic dermabrasion improves surface texture, contour, and, hence, the overall appearance of traumatic wounds, skin may bleed excessively during treatment, shear forces may disrupt the wound

The authors have nothing to disclose.

[a] Beckman Laser Institute and Medical Clinic, University of California Irvine, 1002 Health Sciences Road East, Irvine, CA 92612, USA; [b] Division of Facial Plastic Surgery, Department of Otolaryngology–Head and Neck Surgery, University of California Irvine, 101 The City Drive South, Building 56, Suite 500, Orange, CA 92868, USA; [c] Department of Biomedical Engineering, Henry Samueli School of Engineering, University of California, Irvine, 3120 Natural Sciences II, Irvine, CA 92697-2715, USA

* Corresponding author. Beckman Laser Institute and Medical Clinic, University Of California Irvine, 1002 Health Sciences Road East, Irvine, CA 92612.

E-mail address: bjwong@uci.edu

closure, and depth control is operator dependent, requiring skill and experience.[3]

Laser devices have revolutionized skin care and are used to treat fine rhytides, correct acne scars, manage dyschromia, eliminate vascular birthmarks, remove tattoos, and manage both surgical and posttraumatic injuries.[4–6] Lasers alter tissue based on the propagation of light through tissue, and subsequent absorption of photons with conversion to heat, photochemical interactions (photodynamic therapy), or generation of stress transients (photoacoustic waves). Clinicians have the ability to control the specific laser–tissue interaction by selecting dosimetry (pulse duration, energy density) and wavelength. Light propagates through tissue and is absorbed and scattered differentially depending on wavelength and, ultimately, this distribution of light dictates the tissue effect.[7] In the region of light distribution, if sufficient photons are absorbed, heat is generated, which may lead to a number effects, including (1) bulk volumetric heating with elevation of temperature (nonablative therapies), (2) selective photothermolysis,[5] (3) water vaporization (CO_2 or Erb:YAG resurfacing), (4) tissue pyrolysis, and (5) generation of photoacoustic transients (adiabatic heating causing stress waves as in laser lithotripsy). Photochemical modification (photodynamic therapy) and nonlinear multiphoton events, including plasma formation (keratorefractive eye surgery), also may occur, but generally have at present limited roles in the management of scars and soft tissue injury. In skin, the most widely used laser devices alter the skin via volumetric heating (nonablative techniques), selective photothermolysis (targeting of pigments such as hemoglobin or melanin), or frank ablation. Volumetric heating, such as that seen with the 1450-nm diode targets water resulting in localized heating in the upper dermis and subsequent tissue remodeling. Alternatively, lasers using selective photothermolysis, such as the pulsed-dye lasers (PDL) or Q-switched (QS) lasers work through selective chromophore targeting such as hemoglobin or exogenous pigments (ie, carbon particles), respectively, and are useful for treating cutaneous vascular malformations and tattoos.

The focus of the current review is on PDL, and ablative and nonablative resurfacing. Through the ablation process, heat generation incites inflammation and vascular permeability by inducing a pattern of thermal injury in the dermis, which stimulates complex tissue remodeling processes.[8] These treatments can be dramatic, with ablative resurfacing resulting in epidermal and superficial dermal vaporization, allowing later neocollagenesis and skin tightening. The unwanted side effects of ablative laser resurfacing (chiefly prolonged erythema and complete deepithelialization, but also third-degree burns) has been addressed through the development of alternative approaches, including nonablative and fractional laser devices.[2,8,9] Advances in fractional photothermolysis have revived the interest in both ablative and nonablative lasers in both treatment and prevention of posttraumatic scars by controlling the spatial extent of thermal injury in the upper dermis induced by the laser in both axial (in the direction of light propagation) and radial (lateral) directions. Because specifying dosimetry is the first step toward optimized therapy, controlling the spatial extent of laser-induced tissue modification has become equally as important.

Suffice it to say that many laser devices can be used to treat posttraumatic skin injuries, both acute and chronic, and there is much confusion with respect to developing a rational strategy for use. Herein we review lasers used for the management of posttraumatic facial scars and provide a flow chart (**Fig. 1**) to aid clinicians in optimizing therapy.

GENERAL TREATMENT CONSIDERATIONS

Posttraumatic skin injuries are challenging to manage, because patients may seek care either immediately after injury or even months later. Those seen acutely for example, after suture removal, may be amenable to laser treatments that may mitigate the acute inflammatory process and reduce scar formation. Patients who seek expert care long after the acute phases of wound healing may have erythematous, hypertrophic, or atrophic scars with discrete step offs, or in the case of the face, contractures compromising eyelid, nasal airway, or oral commissure function. The narrow laceration oriented along relaxed skin tension lines (RSTL) without contracture may heal well in a patient without keloid predisposition, and is generally well-suited for laser resurfacing, or no treatment at all. The challenge often lies in managing posttraumatic facial scars that were initially contaminated and insufficiently cleansed, have crushed or missing tissue, irregular wound edges, or were approximated under tension. These injuries may require classic scar revision surgery before or after laser resurfacing, because laser technology for the skin focuses primarily on optimizing surface texture, dermal remodeling, and pigmentation.

During initial scar evaluation, a thorough history should be obtained with particular attention to time

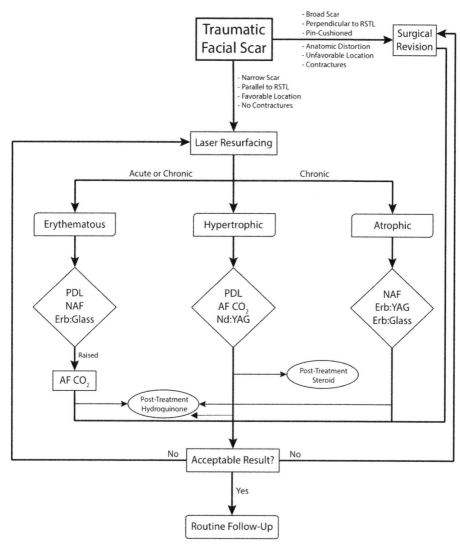

Fig. 1. Suggested algorithm for treating traumatic facial scars. Indications for surgical scar revision are outlined, and can be followed with laser resurfacing to achieve the desired outcome. Otherwise, resurfacing can commence based on scar characteristics. If acceptable clinical outcome is achieved, patients are followed. Otherwise, laser therapy continued or option for surgical revision provided. AF, ablative fractional; NAF, nonablative fractional; PDL, pulsed-dye laser; RSTL, relaxed skin tension lines.

course, history of keloids, immunodeficiency, connective tissue disorder, and previous trial of dermabrasion or laser resurfacing. The clinician should determine whether there is a personal or family history of vitiligo, and a recent or remote history of the use of isotretinoin (Accutane) or skin lightening agents such as hydroquinone, which may ultimately change the time course with which treatment may is initiated.[1] A detailed discussion with the patient should focus on expectations and goals, and explain that multiple procedures may be needed, or that recovery times will vary with specific devices. Before treatment, the clinician should consider the types of topical agents

used to promote wound healing, whether administration of prophylactic antibiotics is necessary, whether pretreatment with hydroquinone (for patients with Fitzpatrick type III or higher), analgesia, or antivirals are indicated.[6]

Scar Assessment

Several methods for assessing scars have been developed both from a patient and clinician perspective. The Vancouver Scar Scale is the most widely validated clinician survey used to assess scar pigmentation, pliability, vascularity and height.[10] Additionally, the Patient and

Observer Scar Assessment Scale allows for an observer determination, and goes one step further to assess patient perceptions of scar pain, pruritus, color, stiffness, thickness and irregularity. Proper evaluation before treatment requires detailed and consistent photography under appropriate lighting conditions. These assessments allow for consistent pretreatment and posttreatment assessment, and provide a useful tool for outcomes analysis as an adjunct to photodocumentation.

SCAR CLASSIFICATION

The characteristics of the posttraumatic scar in conjunction with patient preferences ultimately dictates the type of laser device and number of treatments required. Hypertrophic scars may benefit from multimodality therapy, such as laser resurfacing combined with intralesional steroids,[11] whereas combination resurfacing with multiple lasers may be needed to treat specific regions of a heterogeneous scar.

Hypertrophic Scars and Keloids

Within the first month of closure, hypertrophic scars may develop along the boundaries of the laceration and are characterized by pink or erythematous, raised, and firm areas within the scar boundary.[12] Closure under tensile deformation creates areas that are prone to slow healing, promoting unrestrained collagen proliferation,[3] increasing the propensity for an imbalance of stromal matrix collagen degradation and collagen biosynthesis in the setting of fibroblast proliferation.[13] Adjunct therapies for treating hypertrophic scarring include intralesional steroid and/or 5-flurouracil injections, compression therapy, and radiation, among others.[14,15] Several lasers have shown efficacy in reducing keloids and hypertrophic scar burden, which are discussed elsewhere in this article.

Keloids represent a unique process of continued fibroblast proliferation outside of the area of the scar that can continue to mature and grow. In addition to genetic or ethnic predisposition, wound closure under tension also predisposes the scar to keloid formation. In contrast with hypertrophic scars that may be pruritic or painful, keloids are generally asymptomatic.

Atrophic Scars

Whereas hypertrophic scars are the result of matrix imbalance and fibroblast proliferation, atrophic scars generally result from traumatic collagen loss.[16] Atrophic depressions in the dermis form as the inflammatory reaction results in collagen destruction, atrophy, dermal fibrosis, and scar contraction.[17] Before laser resurfacing, methods for treating scars were aimed at improving atrophic contour and included punch excision, hyaluronic acid fillers, and autologous fat transplant.[17,18] Although these have had variable success, laser resurfacing allows for the benefit of reproducible vaporization, neocollagenesis, and blending and contouring the scar with adjacent normal skin. Lasers have the added benefit of use at any time during the development of the scar given the lack of mechanical trauma to the skin.

Timing of Treatment

Precise control of dosimetry and, hence, tissue effect, has generated enthusiasm for using lasers earlier to treat posttraumatic injuries with the focus on altering the skin's inflammatory physiologic milieu during wound healing, and early application has shown promise in mitigating the development of scars and improved wound healing.[9] Classical wound care management dictates that early laser treatment would result in soft tissue destabilization and, therefore, should not be started before 1 year after complete scar maturation, after which time spontaneous resolution has been given ample opportunity, although dermabrasion is often performed as early as 8 weeks.[4] Over the past 15 years, the interval between injury and laser treatment as become shorter, such that resurfacing, PDL treatment, and nonablative therapy is initiated within the first 6 to 8 weeks, and even as early as the day of suture removal (personal communication with the late R. Fitzpatrick, MD, Encinitas, CA, 2004). Fractional and PDL have shown significant promise,[4] with the putative mechanisms being an alteration of the inflammatory cascade or reduction in local blood flow to the scar, respectively.[3] Fractional irradiation using Erb:Glass (nonablative), Erb:YAG,[19–21] CO_2,[22] and 810-nm diode lasers[23] has been performed as early as 10 days after surgical repair.[24] Although no specific protocol is currently established with respect to treatment initiation or laser type, energy density, or spot size, PDL at the time of suture removal and fractional therapy within 2 to 4 weeks are frequently used in the management of posttraumatic scars, and has proven successful in our experience.

Treatment Algorithm

Approaching the posttraumatic facial scar requires a thorough analysis of the scar's features, orientation, pattern, and relationship to surrounding tissue to determine both the type and extent of treatment. Our treatment algorithm (see **Fig. 1**) seeks to achieve a balance between repeated surgical revision and laser therapy. Do note, however, that the flow chart is fairly dynamic and going from relatively conservative approaches (ie, laser) to aggressive (surgery) is common. It is difficult to predict the response to laser treatment, but inasmuch as they are low morbidity treatments, laser therapy can be repeated multiple times. Failure of laser therapy to meet patient expectation would be a potential indication for surgical scar revision, which can always be optimized with more laser treatments. One may start with lasers first, particularly in regions of the face where surgical scar revision may have significant risk or if a patient is reluctant to proceed. In our practices, where we have access to a broad range of laser devices, treatment is always initiated first, except in cases where it is clinically obvious that scar revision is the first step. After the initial consultation, the surgeon must consider whether to initiate laser treatment first, or to begin with scar revision and appropriately time laser therapy. This decision should consider several scar characteristics, such as broadness, pliability, relationship to anatomically sensitive areas (ie, oral commissure, nasal ala, and medial and lateral canthi), presence or absence of scar contractures, and orientation along RSTL. A scar that is broad, thickened, and causing anatomic distortion of the oral philtrum may be unfavorable for initial laser therapy, and should undergo surgical scar revision, such as a Z-plasty, to assist in reorientation and reduce retraction of the upper lip. Laser therapy may commence soon after suture removal. In contrast, a patient with an acute, linear, and hyperemic scar parallel to cheek RSTL has a favorable scar amenable to early initiation of laser therapy soon after consultation.

When the decision to proceed with laser is made, the surgeon must consider the variety of options available and the effect desired. The descriptions of the lasers and suggested dosimetry are discussed elsewhere in this review. As an example, if a cheek scar on a 6-month-old is erythematous and raised, it is reasonable to begin combined treatment with PDL using an energy density of 7.5 to 8.0 J/cm^2, 6-ms pulse duration, with cryogen spray cooling. The hypertrophic component may then be addressed with ablative fractional Erb:YAG with a 250-μm ablation zone for 2 passes with postprocedure application of topical corticosteroids, performed every 3 to 5 weeks. If the scar continues to be raised, ablative fractional CO_2 laser can be used at 12.5 to 20 mJ

based on thickness. Conversely, a hypertrophic facial scar would benefit from PDL combined with early ablative fractional CO_2, followed by the administration of topical corticosteroids. Advocates for the use of topical corticosteroid immediately after fractional laser treatment cite improved penetration of the agent in the setting of microthermal injury zones. Likewise, much research has been focused on the delivery of these agents through these microchannels into the dermis. Last, tissue loss and necrosis can result in burdensome and unsightly atrophic facial scarring. Treatment of these scars may start with an Erbium-doped laser or nonablative fractional therapy such as 1550-diode Erb:Glass (Fraxel re:Store, Solta, Hayward, CA) using 8 mJ/cm^2 with a density of 100 MTZ/cm^2. In these 3 scenarios, posttreatment hydroquinone can be applied to prevent hyperpigmentation, particularly in patients with darker skin phototypes.

After either laser treatment(s) or surgical scar revision(s), the patient and surgeon must discuss whether improvements to the scar have been attained and what is realistically achievable. If after several laser treatments, a hypertrophic scar remains thickened, surgical revision may be considered. Similarly, if after surgical revision, there remains a significant erythematous area, repeat PDL treatment can be initiated. So long as the scar remains unacceptable to the patient and surgeon, a combination of treatments can continue until the surgeon and patient are in agreement regarding the realistic result; otherwise, routine follow-up is suggested. The different laser types and dosimetry are discussed elsewhere in this article.

LASER SELECTION

The selection of a laser for scar treatment is paramount in guiding treatment and predicting overall outcome, especially in the management of scars in their early healing phase. The appropriate wavelength is chosen based on desired effect, that is, volumetric heating (generally water) and ablation with CO_2 (10,600 nm), Erb:YAG (2940 nm), and Erb:glass (1550 nm), or targeting chromophores such as hemoglobin with potassium-titanyl-phosphate (532 nm) or PDL (595 nm). The scar type, that is, hypertrophic or atrophic, is a crucial consideration in determining the appropriate skin penetration depth required. For example, although PDL may be effective in modulating superficial scar progression by decreasing blood flow to tissue, its use for thicker or deeper scars is debatable.[25] Ablative lasers may be used for large, hypertrophic, or contracted scars, and nonablative lasers for atrophic and flat or mature scars.[4] The specific laser types and their applications are outlined elsewhere in this article and in our recommended treatment algorithm (see **Fig. 1**).

Ablative, Nonfractional

The initial enthusiasm over laser use for aesthetic surgery began with the development of CO_2 lasers to perform "laser skin resurfacing." CO_2 laser ablation removed the stratum corneum and papillary dermis to treat fine facial rhytides and scars. This process achieved similar outcomes and results to dermabrasion, albeit with notable differences including hemostasis and precise control over the depth of tissue removal. Unlike dermabrasion (or chemical peels), which require substantial skill, training, and experience, the degree of tissue removal by laser is purely governed by dosimetry; hence, this technology was rapidly adopted and widely used. Most ablative resurfacing relies primarily on water as the absorption target chromophore, with removal of the epidermis, and in part the papillary and upper reticular dermis. Collateral heating of deeper tissue layers results in modest tissue injury triggering reparative processes which include neocollagenesis.[6] Efficacy is a consequence of both tissue removal (with reepithelization from the preserved adnexa [hair follicles, glands, etc]) and thermal injury.

Carbon dioxide, 10,600 nm

The CO_2 laser was the first device used for laser skin resurfacing.[26] These lasers are still used to correct facial rhytides and atrophic scars, as well as elevated scars requiring contouring.[3] Light from this laser is absorbed within the most superficial 20 to 30 μm of the skin with a collateral axial thermal damage zone of up to 1 mm.[27] Heat generated during the ablation of tissue triggers neocollagenesis. Each subsequent pass of this laser removes additional tissue. Several studies showed efficacy of pulsed high-energy ablative CO_2 lasers for the treatment of atrophic acne scarring[10,28]; however, its use in posttraumatic scars has largely been replaced by fractional CO_2, Erb:YAG, and PDL, which are discussed elsewhere in this article. The superior result of this laser is directionally proportional to axial (into the plane of light propagation) tissue damage, and comes at the risk of hyperpigmentation, hypopigmentation, prolonged postoperative erythema, risk of infection, and scarring.[27,29] The dosimetry used for CO_2 laser skin resurfacing is broad, and can be used in a fractional form pulsed at 2 ms with an energy density of 40 J/cm² for

traumatic tattooing,[30] or pulsed at 200 ms at an energy of 102 mJ/pulse for posttraumatic facial scars[31]

Erb:YAG, 2940 nm

The side effect profile (chiefly prolonged erythema lasting months) of full facial resurfacing using CO_2 lasers led engineers to develop Erb:YAG ablative lasers. The Erb:YAG emitting at a wavelength of 2940 nm is absorbed by tissue water by a factor of 12 to 18 times higher as compared with the CO_2 laser. The depth of penetration is much more superficial, depending on the energy density applied, as compared with the CO_2 laser.[32] The consequence of this decreased skin penetration depth is decreased focal damage axially,[26] less collagen regeneration, and reduced postoperative erythema. The Erb:YAG laser is useful for depressed or atrophic scars, although it is considered by some to be less efficacious than CO_2 lasers for cosmetic applications. Energy density selection is variable with 4 J/cm² indicated for delicate tissue areas and superficial lesions, or higher (12–15 J/cm²) with multiple passes indicated for complex scars.[16,32] The depth of penetration can also range up to 200 μm, with 50 μm sequential coagulation for atrophic scars[28] or no coagulation for hypertrophic scars. The Erb:YAG laser can be used in patients with Fitzpatrick skin phototypes III or higher.[33] Pulsed Erb:YAG has value in treating several types of scars,[34] and fractional Erb:YAG lasers may result in improvement of color, stiffness, thickness, irregularity, and overall patient satisfaction as compared with fully ablative Erb:YAG resurfacing.[35]

Pulsed-dye Laser, 595 nm

The PDL targets hemoglobin as its chromophore and relies on selective photothermolysis for efficacy, because 595-nm light is highly absorbed by hemoglobin and poorly absorbed by water and other dermal matrix proteins.[3,5,36,37] Primarily used to treat vascular lesions (ie, the port wine stain), the PDL has value in treating the hyperemic components of posttraumatic scars,[38] hypertrophic scars, and keloids,[12] and may lead to improvement in skin color, texture, and pliability while reducing dyspigmentation, scar bulk, and vascularity. PDLs are increasingly being used to treat early, immature scars to prevent hypertrophy in the remodeling phase,[39] potentially obviating the need for surgical scar revision for posttraumatic scarring.[40,41] Literature regarding dosimetry is adjustable, and varies from 4.0 to 8.0 J/cm² based on spot size, with short pulse durations of 0.45 to 3.0 ms with treatments repeated every 3 weeks to 2 months depending on surgeon and patient preference and expectations.[4,38]

Combining PDL with adjunct therapy has also shown promise in small studies.[36,38] Depth of penetration for the PDL is about 1 to 2 mm and can be combined with corticosteroids for keloid management.[36] Combination PDL followed by fractional Erb:glass or 1450-nm diode has been found valuable in small studies evaluating post-traumatic scars.[38,42] Here the hyperproliferative vascular component is treated with PDL, and a fractional laser is used to induce dermal remodeling to recreate a more uniform skin appearance.

Keloids present a unique challenge given their location in areas under tension, thickness, and resistance to intralesional steroid injections. Systematic reviews suggest that PDL treatment significantly improves Vancouver Scar Scale scores in patients with keloids with respect to scar pigmentation.[12] It is equivocal whether scar thickness or erythema decreases, although the PDL has demonstrated some promising results. Outcomes have proven superior in patients with lighter skin phototypes and adverse events are minimized when lower energy densities (eg, 4 J/cm^2) are used. Keloids have been treated by PDL using energy densities of 3.5 to 9.0 J/cm^2 with a pulse duration of 0.45 to 1.5 m, every 4 to 8 weeks for 2 to 12 treatments, used in conjunction with intralesional triamcinolone, 5-flurouralcil, or erbium lasers.[12]

Fractional Ablation

Fractional skin resurfacing involves the selective ablation of specific regions of tissue using micro-laser spots distributed with a user-defined density across the skin surface. Fractional laser devices intersperse healthy tissue between ablation sites and these pristine regions remain as potent nutrient reservoirs and as a source for keratinocytes to repopulate ablated tissue.[6,8] This process, collectively referred to as "focal destruction with islands of spared tissue," results in collagen remodeling and elastic tissue formation, which leads to more rapid wound healing, less downtime, and reduced postoperative erythema.[11] These devices (chiefly CO_2 and Erb:YAG) can be used to debulk fibrotic scars and, in each microspot, incite new collagen formation.[43] They are valuable to treat posttraumatic[44,45] and postsurgical facial scarring,[46–48] hypertrophic facial scarring,[35] and posttraumatic extremity scarring.[49] Innumerable fractional ablation devices have been developed and differ in terms of which specific laser used, and parameters that govern microlaser spot size and density.

Nonablative, Nonfractional

By selectively heating the dermis while sparing the epidermis from thermal injury, nonablative laser devices possess a lower side effect profile

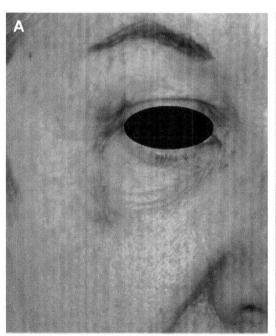
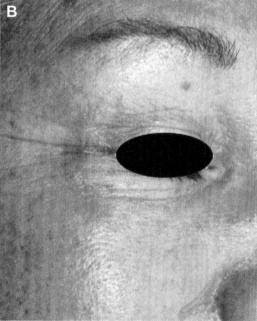

Fig. 2. A 57-year-old female patient with a traumatic scar lateral to the right lateral canthus with vertical extension at (A) 2 weeks posttrauma and (B) 6 month after 5 treatments of pulsed-dye and Erb:YAG laser. There was significant reduction in scar erythema and thickness.

with respect to erythema, infection, and risk of herpetic reactivation. Accordingly, outcomes are modest[1,28] when compared with ablative modalities. Several nonablative lasers have been developed including 1319-nm pulsed energy (Sciton, Palo Alto, CA) for rhytides and acne pulsed at 5 to 200 ms for 30 J/cm^2, 1.320-nm Nd:YAG (Cool-Touch CT3Plus, Alma Harmony XL, Syneron, Roseville, CA) pulsed at 450-μs for the same purposes,[17,50] and 1450-nm diode for posttraumatic facial scars.[51] For atrophic and hypertrophic scarring alike, the 1450-nm diode has been safely used with an energy density of' 12 J/cm^2 with a 6-mm spot size, and combined with PDL.[42,52] These devices have been used primarily for the treatment of postacne scarring and facial rejuvenation; however, small nonrandomized trials have shown some benefit for posttraumatic scars.[53]

Nonablative, Fractional

Nonablative fractional lasers can be used to safely treat darker skinned (Fitzpatrick III and above) individuals and may have value for posttraumatic scar resurfacing.[26] Originally developed for use in rejuvenation procedures, they have largely been replaced by ablative fractional lasers because the effects are modest. The fractionated nonablative Erb:Glass laser 1550-nm (Solta Fraxel re:store) may improve the texture and appearance of posttraumatic scars. This can be combined with PDL treatments,[38] using an energy density of 6 J/cm^2, spot size of 6 mm, and 3 a ms-pulse duration for the PDL, and energy density of 8 mJ/cm^2 and density of 100 MTZ/cm^2 for the fractional laser at 3-week intervals. This efficacy may be enhanced with greater energy densities, but requires further investigation.[24] Additionally, when combined with traditional CO_2 laser, fractional Erb:glass results in significant reduction in Vancouver Scar Scale scores, with more improvement in scar pliability and pigmentation.[37]

TRAUMATIC TATTOO

Traumatic tattoos are the result of pigmented deposition from lodged foreign debris in the dermis owing to abrasions, explosive forces, "road rash," and inadequate wound irrigation before closure.[3,54] Optimal treatment requires the use of a QS laser. These devices release high energy in extremely short pulse durations, on the order of nanoseconds or picoseconds, leading to high temperature gradients and induced acoustic waves within the particle. The pigmented particles

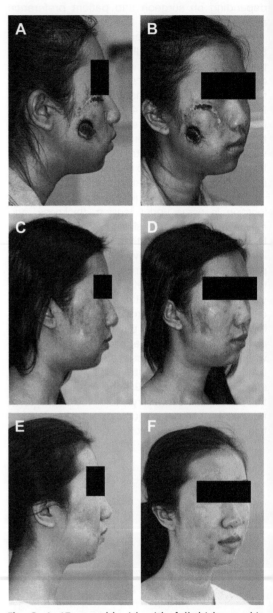

Fig. 3. A 17-year-old girl with full-thickness skin necrosis secondary to embolization of vascular arteriovenous malformation. (*A, B*) The lesion extends from her malar eminence inferiorly toward the mandibular body. (*C, D*) Significant improvement at 18 months in overall erythema and atrophic scarring after multiple treatments with a pulsed-dye laser using an energy density of 8 J/cm^2, 10-ms pulse duration, and fractional 1550 erbium/1927 thulium treatment (Fraxel Dual) using an energy of 45 mJ deposited at a depth of 1176 μm for the middle cheek, and 70 mJ at 1359 depth for the upper and lateral cheek. (*E, F*) Continued improvement at 30 months after surgical scar revision of lower broad scar and continued 1550 erbium/1927 thulium.

fragment and eventually undergo macrophage-mediated phagocytosis. Currently, QS ruby, QS Nd:YAG, and QS alexandrite are used for traumatic tattoo removal, although fractional CO_2 has shown some benefit.[30] QS ruby initiated at energy densities of 3 to 4 J/cm^2 repeated at 6-week intervals can very effectively reduce pigment from traumatic tattoos.

Clinical Examples

In our practice, we have had excellent results with combination treatment laser therapy to treat specific components of posttraumatic scars as per our algorithm. The patient in **Fig. 2** had sustained blunt force trauma lateral to the right eye, resulting in atrophic surrounding skin and a raised and erythematous scar perpendicular to the RSTL. She opted for laser resurfacing alone, and underwent combination PDL at 7.5 to 8 J/cm^2, 6-m pulse duration for the hyperemic portion and fractional Erb:YAG, at 150 to 200 μm depth to treat the hypertrophic portions. After 5 treatments, the scar was noted to be smoother, with a dramatic reduction in erythema and hypertrophy. The patient self-reported improvement based on a 50% improvement in her overall Patient and Observer Scar Assessment Scale score, with a reduction in pain and itching, and improvement in color, stiffness, thickness, and overall appearance. Similarly, our patient in **Fig. 3** had

right facial skin necrosis, resulting in significant skin fibrosis, retraction, and atrophy along the right cheek with erythema inferior to the right orbital rim. She was initially managed conservatively with local wound care as the wound began to declare. She eventually underwent combined PDL and Fraxel Dual (Solta) using energies of 45 to 70 mJ deposited at a depth of 1176 to 1359 μm, over 10 treatments, over 2 years. She underwent surgical scar revision with excision of the inferior hypertrophic scar followed but continued combination laser treatment resulting in near-total resolution of the superior hyperemia and overall reduction in the atrophy and evening of the scar with respect to her native skin. Last, our patient in **Fig. 4** demonstrates the dramatic effects of surgical scar revision and tincture of time. She was injured in a dog mauling, which resulted in a straight left cheek laceration that extended on the left lateral nasal sidewall and was closed primarily in the operating room. She subsequently underwent 2 major surgical scar revisions over 4 years, resulting in dramatic improvement in overall scar characteristics, resolution of hypertrophy and erythema, and thinning of the scar overall.

POSTTREATMENT COMPLICATIONS

As mentioned, laser treatments for scars are generally well-tolerated, but complications can

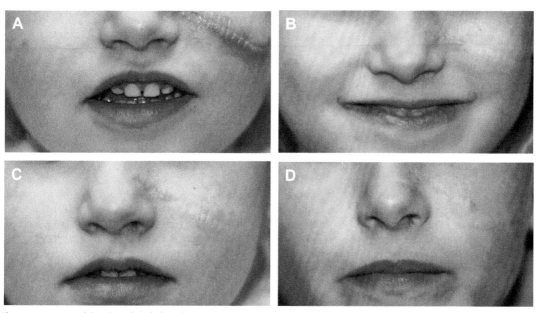

Fig. 4. A 3-year-old girl with left facial trauma secondary to dog bite injury after multiple surgical scar revisions. (*A*) Laceration extending from left nasal sidewall to malar eminence 14 days after closure. (*B*) Follow-up at 19 months shows improvement in hypertrophic scar over the nasal sidewall after surgical scar revision 2 months previously. (*C*) Follow-up at 22 months showing continued improvement in scar erythema and texture. (*D*) Follow-up at 4 years after second scar revision.

occur. Immediate posttreatment erythema is considered a normal part of the dermal remodeling process; however, it may persist. Generally, erythema persisting for 4 days is common for nonablative treatment, and 1 month for ablative. In 12.5% of patients treated with ablative lasers,[6] erythema can persist for up to 6 months. Pinpoint bleeding is also worse with fractionated CO_2 compared with Erb:YAG given the increase in zone of coagulation with the former.[4] Significant thermal damage can also result in hypertrophic scarring and skin weeping, and although these complications can be mitigated with compresses, analgesia, and steroids, they can increase patient downtime. Local skin irritation can also result in significant dermatitis, bacterial or fungal superinfection, or viral reactivation; therefore, judicious follow-up and discussion of prophylactic antimicrobial and antiviral therapy is warranted. Posttreatment scarring can also result from conventional ablative lasers, and is also seen with patients receiving ablative fractional therapy.[9] The most feared complication is postinflammatory hyperpigmentation, which is more common in patients with darker Fitzpatrick skin phototypes. This hyperpigmentation can be managed through rigorous patient and laser selection, as well as preprocedural bleaching agents, such as compounded tretinoin, hydrocortisone, or hydroquinone[3] and strict sun avoidance after the laser procedure for a minimum of 3 months.

SUMMARY

Although initially applied to the treatment of postacne scarring and deep facial rhytides, laser technology has undergone a dramatic shift in clinical application and is an effective method for reducing the appearance and thickness of posttraumatic facial scars. Laser resurfacing for facial scars offers the facial plastic surgeon a variety of options for reducing the appearance of posttraumatic atrophy, hypertrophy, and dyspigmentation. This technology has equipped the clinician to intervene early with a modality that mediates the inflammatory effects of tissue healing soon after traumatic laceration, while offering an adjunct therapy to surgical scar revision. The surgeon must paint a realistic picture of what is attainable before delving into a goal-directed laser selection based on scar characteristics, patient skin type, risk of posttreatment complications, and consideration of patient downtime. Although the results of these treatments are promising, ideal dosimetry remains an ongoing challenge as the literature emphasizes experience-based rather than evidence-based practice; large-scale, randomized, controlled trials and split-scar studies are lacking, especially with combination modalities. Nevertheless, the variety of lasers, variable time with which to initiate therapy, and countless combinations offer the clinician a stocked armamentarium from which treatment algorithms may be tailored and designed.

REFERENCES

1. Mobley SR, Sjogren PP. Soft tissue trauma and scar revision. Facial Plast Surg Clin North Am 2014;22(4): 639–51.
2. Oliaei S, Nelson JS, Fitzpatrick R, et al. Use of lasers in acute management of surgical and traumatic incisions on the face. Facial Plast Surg Clin North Am 2011;19(3):543–50.
3. Oliaei S, Nelson JS, Fitzpatrick R, et al. Laser treatment of scars. Facial Plast Surg 2012;28(5):518–24.
4. Anderson RR, Donelan MB, Hivnor C, et al. Laser treatment of traumatic scars with an emphasis on ablative fractional laser resurfacing: consensus report. JAMA Dermatol 2014;150(2):187–93.
5. Anderson R, Parrish J. Selective photothermolysis: precise microsurgery by selective absorption of pulsed radiation. Science 1983;220(4596):524–7.
6. Saedi N, Petelin A, Zachary C. Fractionation: a new era in laser resurfacing. Clin Plast Surg 2011;38(3): 449–61, vii.
7. Jacques SL. Role of tissue optics and pulse duration on tissue effects during high-power laser irradiation. Appl Opt 1993;32(13):2447–54.
8. Manstein D, Herron GS, Sink RK, et al. Fractional photothermolysis: a new concept for cutaneous remodeling using microscopic patterns of thermal injury. Lasers Surg Med 2004;34(5):426–38.
9. Avram MM, Tope WD, Yu T, et al. Hypertrophic scarring of the neck following ablative fractional carbon dioxide laser resurfacing. Lasers Surg Med 2009; 41(3):185–8.
10. Baryza MJ, Baryza GA. The Vancouver Scar Scale: an administration tool and its interrater reliability. J Burn Care Rehabil 1995;16(5):535–8.
11. Waibel JS, Wulkan AJ, Shumaker PR. Treatment of hypertrophic scars using laser and laser assisted corticosteroid delivery. Lasers Surg Med 2013; 45(3):135–40.
12. de las Alas JM, Siripunvarapon AH, Dofitas BL. Pulsed dye laser for the treatment of keloid and hypertrophic scars: a systematic review. Expert Rev Med Devices 2012;9(6):641–50.
13. Jin R, Huang X, Li H, et al. Laser therapy for prevention and treatment of pathologic excessive scars. Plast Reconstr Surg 2013;132(6):1747–58.
14. Alster TS, Tanzi EL. Hypertrophic scars and keloids: etiology and management. Am J Clin Dermatol 2003;4(4):235–43.

15. Leclere FM, Mordon SR. Twenty-five years of active laser prevention of scars: what have we learned? J Cosmet Laser Ther 2010;12(5):227–34.

16. Alster TS, Tanzi EL, Lazarus M. The use of fractional laser photothermolysis for the treatment of atrophic scars. Dermatol Surg 2007;33(3):295–9.

17. Rogachefsky AS, Hussain M, Goldberg DJ. Atrophic and a mixed pattern of acne scars improved with a 1320-nm Nd:YAG laser. Dermatol Surg 2003;29(9): 904–8.

18. Alster TS, West TB. Resurfacing of atrophic facial acne scars with a high-energy, pulsed carbon dioxide laser. Dermatol Surg 1996;22(2):151–4 [discussion: 154–5].

19. Kim HS, Lee JH, Park YM, et al. Comparison of the effectiveness of nonablative fractional laser versus ablative fractional laser in thyroidectomy scar prevention: a pilot study. J Cosmet Laser Ther 2012; 14(2):89–93.

20. Choe JH, Park YL, Kim BJ, et al. Prevention of thyroidectomy scar using a new 1,550-nm fractional erbium-glass laser. Dermatol Surg 2009;35(8):1199–205.

21. Park KY, Oh IY, Seo SJ, et al. Appropriate timing for thyroidectomy scar treatment using a 1,550-nm fractional erbium-glass laser. Dermatol Surg 2013; 39(12):1827–34.

22. Jung JY, Jeong JJ, Roh HJ, et al. Early postoperative treatment of thyroidectomy scars using a fractional carbon dioxide laser. Dermatol Surg 2011;37(2): 217–23.

23. Capon A, Iarmarcovai G, Gonnelli D, et al. Scar prevention using Laser-Assisted Skin Healing (LASH) in plastic surgery. Aesthetic Plast Surg 2010;34(4): 438–46.

24. Shim HS, Jun DW, Kim SW, et al. Low versus high fluence parameters in the treatment of facial laceration scars with a 1,550 nm fractional erbium-glass laser. Biomed Research Int 2015;2015:825309.

25. Bouzari N, Davis SC, Nouri K. Laser treatment of keloids and hypertrophic scars. Int J Dermatol 2007; 46(1):80–8.

26. Preissig J, Hamilton K, Markus R. Current laser resurfacing technologies: a review that delves beneath the surface. Semin Plast Surg 2012;26(3):109–16.

27. Green HA, Domankevitz Y, Nishioka NS. Pulsed carbon dioxide laser ablation of burned skin: in vitro and in vivo analysis. Lasers Surg Med 1990;10(5): 476–84.

28. You HJ, Kim DW, Yoon ES, et al. Comparison of four different lasers for acne scars: resurfacing and fractional lasers. J Plast Reconstr Aesthet Surg 2016; 69(4):e87–95.

29. Ward PD, Baker SR. Long-term results of carbon dioxide laser resurfacing of the face. Arch Facial Plast Surg 2008;10(4):238–43 [discussion: 244–35].

30. Seitz AT, Grunewald S, Wagner JA, et al. Fractional CO2 laser is as effective as Q-switched ruby laser for the initial treatment of a traumatic tattoo. J Cosmet Laser Ther 2014;16(6):303–5.

31. Lapidoth M, Halachmi S, Cohen S, et al. Fractional CO2 laser in the treatment of facial scars in children. Lasers Med Sci 2014;29(2):855–7.

32. Alster TS, Lupton JR. Erbium:YAG cutaneous laser resurfacing. Dermatol Clin 2001;19(3):453–66.

33. Polnikorn N, Goldberg DJ, Suwanchinda A, et al. Erbium:YAG laser resurfacing in Asians. Dermatol Surg 1998;24(12):1303–7.

34. Kwon SD, Kye YC. Treatment of Scars with a pulsed Er:YAG laser. J Cutan Laser Ther 2000; 2(1):27–31.

35. Tidwell WJ, Owen CE, Kulp-Shorten C, et al. Fractionated Er:YAG laser versus fully ablative Er:YAG laser for scar revision: results of a split scar, double blinded, prospective trial. Lasers Surg Med 2016; 48(9):837–43.

36. Khansa I, Harrison B, Janis JE. Evidence-based scar management: how to improve results with technique and technology. Plast Reconstr Surg 2016; 138(3 Suppl):165s–78s.

37. Ibrahim SM, Elsaie ML, Kamel MI, et al. Successful treatment of traumatic scars with combined nonablative fractional laser and pinpoint technique of standard CO2 laser. Dermatol Ther 2016;29(1): 52–7.

38. Park KY, Hyun MY, Moon NJ, et al. Combined treatment with 595-nm pulsed dye laser and 1550-nm erbium-glass fractional laser for traumatic scars. J Cosmet Laser Ther 2016;18:387–8.

39. Brewin MP, Lister TS. Prevention or treatment of hypertrophic burn scarring: a review of when and how to treat with the pulsed dye laser. Burns 2014;40(5): 797–804.

40. Donelan MB, Parrett BM, Sheridan RL. Pulsed dye laser therapy and z-plasty for facial burn scars: the alternative to excision. Ann Plast Surg 2008;60(5): 480–6.

41. Gold MH, McGuire M, Mustoe TA, et al. Updated international clinical recommendations on scar management: part 2–algorithms for scar prevention and treatment. Dermatol Surg 2014;40(8):825–31.

42. Katz TM, Glaich AS, Goldberg LH, et al. 595-nm long pulsed dye laser and 1450-nm diode laser in combination with intralesional triamcinolone/5-fluorouracil for hypertrophic scarring following a phenol peel. J Am Acad Dermatol 2010;62(6): 1045–9.

43. Qu L, Liu A, Zhou L, et al. Clinical and molecular effects on mature burn scars after treatment with a fractional CO(2) laser. Lasers Surg Med 2012; 44(7):517–24.

44. Cervelli V, Gentile P, Spallone D, et al. Ultrapulsed fractional CO2 laser for the treatment of posttraumatic and pathological scars. J Drugs Dermatol 2010;9(11):1328–31.

45. Uebelhoer NS, Ross EV, Shumaker PR. Ablative fractional resurfacing for the treatment of traumatic scars and contractures. Semin Cutan Med Surg 2012;31(2):110–20.

46. Sobanko JF, Vachiramon V, Rattanaumpawan P, et al. Early postoperative single treatment ablative fractional lasing of Mohs micrographic surgery facial scars: a split-scar, evaluator-blinded study. Lasers Surg Med 2015;47(1):1–5.

47. Lee SH, Zheng Z, Roh MR. Early postoperative treatment of surgical scars using a fractional carbon dioxide laser: a split-scar, evaluator-blinded study. Dermatol Surg 2013;39(8):1190–6.

48. Jared Christophel J, Elm C, Endrizzi BT, et al. A randomized controlled trial of fractional laser therapy and dermabrasion for scar resurfacing. Dermatol Surg 2012;38(4):595–602.

49. Shumaker PR, Kwan JM, Badiavas EV, et al. Rapid healing of scar-associated chronic wounds after ablative fractional resurfacing. Arch Dermatol 2012;148(11):1289–93.

50. Tanzi EL, Alster TS. Comparison of a 1450-nm diode laser and a 1320-nm Nd:YAG laser in the treatment of atrophic facial scars: a prospective clinical and histologic study. Dermatol Surg 2004;30(2 Pt 1): 152–7.

51. Jih MH, Friedman PM, Kimyai-Asadi A, et al. Successful treatment of a chronic atrophic dog-bite scar with the 1450-nm diode laser. Dermatol Surg 2004;30(8):1161–3.

52. Wada T, Kawada A, Hirao A, et al. Efficacy and safety of a low-energy double-pass 1450-nm diode laser for the treatment of acne scars. Photomed Laser Surg 2012;30(2):107–11.

53. Al-Mohamady Ael S, Ibrahim SM, Muhammad MM. Pulsed dye laser versus long-pulsed Nd:YAG laser in the treatment of hypertrophic scars and keloid: a comparative randomized split-scar trial. J Cosmet Laser Ther 2016;18(4):208–12.

54. Kent KM, Graber EM. Laser tattoo removal: a review. Dermatol Surg 2012;38(1):1–13.

Evidence-Based Medicine in Facial Trauma

William M. Dougherty, MD, John Jared Christophel, MD, Stephen S. Park, MD*

KEYWORDS

- Facial fractures • Facial trauma • Evidence-based medicine • Mandible fractures
- Midface fractures

KEY POINTS

- There is a relative paucity of high-quality evidence in facial trauma and most published studies are retrospective in nature.
- Antimicrobial prophylaxis is indicated for fractures of the dentate mandible, but no more than 24 to 48 hours postoperatively.
- Antimicrobial prophylaxis is not indicated for skull base fractures with cerebrospinal fluid leak.
- A 2-plate approach for open reduction and internal fixation (ORIF) of mandibular angle fractures does not appear to offer an advantage over a single superior border plate (Champy plate or lateral superior border plate).
- Lag screw fixation for anterior mandible fractures is superior to ORIF using 2 miniplates.

INTRODUCTION

Nearly 25 years have passed since the introduction of a "new paradigm"[1] in clinical practice: *evidence-based medicine*. This shift from tradition, theoretic reasoning, and expert opinion as the basis for clinical decision-making toward *evidence* backed by high-level, prospective, randomized, controlled trials (RCTs) has affected every medical specialty. This emphasis generally results in delivery of more consistent, cost-effective care in a contemporary medical environment. Large medical specialties with common diseases established the first high-level trials with large gains in management of peptic ulcer disease (triple therapy)[2] and human immunodeficiency virus (antiretroviral therapy),[3] among many others. There are unique challenges to practitioners of smaller medical fields, such as the facial traumatologist, as many of the diseases treated are relatively rare, resulting in a paucity of high-level evidence. Cost, recruitment, inconsistent follow-up, and concomitant injuries (affecting timing of treatments) lend additional challenge to large prospective trials in facial trauma. Nevertheless, this type of evidence must be sought. Our goal in formulating this article was to provide the reader with both a comprehensive review of high-level evidence-based medicine in facial trauma and to highlight areas in our field devoid of high-level evidence, that these might be explored in the future. The article is organized in the order one might approach a clinical problem: starting with the workup, followed by treatment considerations, operative decisions, and postoperative treatments. Individual injuries are discussed within each section, with an overview of the available high-level clinical evidence. We methodically searched available evidence-based databases for high-level trials and have cited the level of evidence for each topic, according to the Oxford Center for Evidence-Based Guidelines.[4]

Disclosure Statement: The authors have nothing to disclose.
Department of Otolaryngology–Head and Neck Surgery, Division of Facial Plastic and Reconstructive Surgery, University of Virginia, 1215 Lee Street, Charlottesville, VA 22903, USA
* Corresponding author. UVA Health System, Box 800713, Charlottesville, VA 22908.
E-mail address: SSP8A@hscmail.mcc.virginia.edu

Facial Plast Surg Clin N Am 25 (2017) 629–643
http://dx.doi.org/10.1016/j.fsc.2017.06.013
1064-7406/17/© 2017 Elsevier Inc. All rights reserved.

The vast majority of facial trauma publications are retrospective and based on small study populations. We searched a broad range of topics regarding patient evaluation, the timing of repair, method for repair, and postoperative management, generally limiting our discussion to topics for which there existed level 2 or higher evidence. This article will not only provide a quick reference for the facial traumatologist, but also allow the reader to identify areas of our practice that lack high-level evidence, perhaps motivating future endeavors. Previous investigators have also reviewed evidence-based management of facial fractures[5] and readers are directed toward this quality review.

Despite emphasis on evidence-based medicine, tacit knowledge derived from clinical experience must not be disregarded. There are editorialized sections of this article, where the authors insert their preferences and these sections are clearly marked for the reader.

IMAGING
Ultrasonography for Diagnosis of Facial Fractures, Level 2a

Historically, plain film series were used for evaluation of facial bony injuries. Today, this has been supplanted by computed tomography (CT) with high-resolution, 3-dimensional (3D) images providing unparalleled accuracy of bony anatomy, particularly for operative planning. Ultrasound represents a relatively simple, noninvasive modality for evaluating bony facial trauma, without the radiation exposure of CT. With advances in high-resolution ultrasound,[6] imaging of deeper bony structures is possible. Limitations of ultrasound include the need for probe placement, which can be painful in the acute setting, and limited use in the setting of massive soft tissue edema.

Adeyemo and Akadiri[7] conducted a systematic review of the use of ultrasound in facial fracture diagnosis. Included were 17 articles; all but 1 are prospective in nature and included use of ultrasound in orbital (9 articles), midface (3 articles), nasal (3 articles), and mandible fractures (3 articles). Pooled analysis showed a high sensitivity and specificity for diagnosis of nasal fractures, orbital fractures, anterior maxillary wall fractures, and zygomatic arch fractures. Limitations of ultrasound were noted, including poor ability to image orbital floor fractures extending more than 4 cm from the orbital margin, inability to delineate multiple complex fractures, difficulty differentiating new fractures from old, and difficulty in detecting nondisplaced fractures. No strong evidence exists currently for the use of ultrasound in diagnosing mandible fractures, although the authors suggest that the use of ultrasound in detection of subcondylar fractures remains a promising area of investigation.

This demonstrated utility of ultrasound in facial fracture imaging not only has implications in diagnosis, but also in intraoperative assessment where the small footprint of the ultrasonography equipment represents an advantage over other imaging modalities.

Intraoperative Imaging for Facial Fracture Management, Level 2a

The possibilities of limiting postoperative imaging and reoperation, as well as the ability to assess unexposed buttresses, have led many facial traumatologists to use intraoperative imaging, particularly in complex and pan-facial fractures. There is, however, a lack of scientific evidence proving the superiority of intraoperative imaging. One must also consider cost and availability ($200,000–$850,000 for a portable CT scanner[8]), as well as the potential additional radiation exposure to the patient.

Among isolated facial fractures, zygomaticomaxillary complex (ZMC) fractures are uniquely challenging to the facial traumatologist. As 4 bony articulations are affected, the clinician must decide which, and how many, to expose in an effort to achieve appropriate reduction, balancing the potential increased morbidity associated with additional approaches. Van Hout and colleagues[9] reviewed intraoperative imaging (CT or ultrasound) for ZMC and orbital floor fractures, with 6 studies meeting inclusion criteria. The outcome measure of all studies was the frequency of additional reduction after the initial reduction was assessed intraoperatively. The pooled revision rates for zygoma fractures and orbital floor fractures were 18% (0%–54%) and 9% (0%–15%), respectively. The investigators note that the revision rate in the lone study using ultrasound for assessment of zygoma reduction was 54%, and if this study was omitted from analysis as an outlier, the remainder of the studies, using CT, had a revision rate of 11% (0%–20%). The investigators conclude that intraoperative imaging often affected surgical treatment, but none of the available studies evaluated functional and aesthetic outcomes related to the use of intraoperative imaging.

Further investigation is necessary to determine whether intraoperative imaging improves clinical outcomes in patients with facial trauma, but early experience is certainly promising.

PATIENT PREPARATION
Wound Cleansing, Level 1a

Wound cleansing is an integral part in appropriately managing facial soft tissue trauma. Cleansing is traditionally performed with sterile normal saline, presumed to be advantageous, as it is sterile and isotonic to tissue. Some advocate for the addition of antiseptics, such as iodine, although clinical trials show mixed results and in vitro studies[7] show cellular toxicity related to iodine, prompting concerns of an effect on wound healing.[10] Others manage wound cleansing with tap water, which is advantageous in terms of accessibility, low cost, and ease of application. Fernandez and Griffiths[11] performed a systematic review and meta-analysis of 11 included studies, demonstrating no difference in the rate of infections when wounds are cleansed with tap water versus normal saline. Moscati and colleagues[12] included many head and neck injuries in their similar comparison, again noting no difference in infections, and additionally estimated a cost savings of $65 million per year if all wounds in the emergency room were irrigated with tap water rather than normal saline. These investigations demonstrate that the most important factor in wound cleansing is likely the volume and pressure of irrigation to adequately remove debris and decrease bacterial contaminant, rather than which particular solution is used.

Local Versus General Anesthesia for Closed Nasal Reduction, Level 1a

Nasal bone fractures are the most commonly encountered fracture of the facial skeleton. Given the central location on the face and role in respiration, inadequate treatment of nasal bone fractures has significant aesthetic and functional consequences. Treatment of nasal bone fractures involves either manipulation of the nasal bones (closed nasal reduction) or open approaches for more severe fractures, particularly with a significant septal fracture. Closed nasal reduction can be performed with the patient awake and a local anesthetic, or under general anesthesia, but there is ongoing debate over which approach is superior. Proponents of a local anesthetic approach claim equivalent results while avoiding the cost and risk of general anesthesia. Proponents of general anesthesia argue improved accuracy of reduction and greater patient satisfaction. Al-Moraissi and Ellis[13] published a systematic review and meta-analysis of trials investigating local anesthetic versus general anesthetic for closed nasal reduction. Eight studies were included in their analysis and the investigators conclude that general anesthetic is superior. Cited are statistically significant differences in the patient satisfaction in the appearance of the nose and the need for subsequent septoplasty. Nonsignificant differences were demonstrated for functional improvement, patient satisfaction with anesthetic, need for subsequent septorhinoplasty or rhinoplasty, or preference of anesthesia if the nose were fractured again. The investigators conclude that, regardless of cost and risk of general anesthetic, closed nasal reduction under general anesthesia is superior to reduction under local anesthesia.

Authors' Preference

Although the preceding review is the highest-level evidence available comparing anesthetic techniques for closed nasal reduction, there are several limitations. The authors conclude superiority of general anesthetic, citing a trend toward better outcomes, however only 2 of these (patient satisfaction with appearance and need for subsequent septoplasty) were significant differences. Our preference is to close most nasal bone fractures under local anesthetic in the clinic. In our experience, this allows for satisfactory results with lower cost and risk to the patient. Another advantage is greater surgeon control over the timing of repair, as operating room time may be challenging to acquire within the optimal time to perform closed nasal reduction. Additionally, if a patient is unable to tolerate the procedure or the reduction is not satisfactory, reduction under general anesthesia can be subsequently arranged.

ANTIMICROBIAL PROPHYLAXIS

Antibiotic use, and overuse, are associated with increasing bacterial resistance, increased rates of Clostridium difficile colitis (as many as 3 million cases per year[14]), and is even suspected to increase the risk for the subsequent development of inflammatory bowel disease in children.[15] Despite relatively low rates of wound infections in the head and neck (due to the robust vascularity of the region), the facial traumatologist often prescribes prophylactic antibiotics. Despite common use, there is controversy about antimicrobial prophylaxis use in facial trauma and quality evidence is challenging to obtain due to varying fracture patterns and degrees of wound contamination. In this section, we evaluate evidence for antimicrobial prophylaxis for site-specific facial injuries, including soft tissue injuries, facial fractures, and skull base fractures.

Antimicrobial Prophylaxis in Facial Lacerations, Level 2a

There is lack of high-level investigation regarding antimicrobial prophylaxis for simple facial lacerations that do not cross a mucocutaneous junction. Mark and Granquist[16] analyzed the available literature pertaining to intraoral lacerations and the need for prophylactic antibiotics. Included were 4 trials, but only 1 was a placebo-controlled double-blinded RCT, and this trial had low study size (n = 76). The other trials were not blinded, or were observational in nature. No study was able to show a significant decrease in infection rate with the administration of prophylactic antibiotics.

Authors' Preference

The face carries great cosmetic importance relative to other areas of the body. Infection and poor wound healing are distressing for the patient and may lead to additional procedures and scarring. We generally have a low threshold for administering prophylactic antibiotics for facial lacerations in the setting of a grossly contaminated wound, delayed closure, or mucosal violation. However, antibiotics are not provided routinely for noncontaminated wounds, closed under sterile technique, in a timely fashion.

Antimicrobial Prophylaxis for Bites, Level 1a

Animal, including occasionally human, bites of the face are a common clinical problem for facial traumatologists. Primary closure of facial bite wounds is proven effective and safe following formal wound cleansing,[17] and prevention of tetanus and rabies are universally accepted measures; however, there is debate regarding the need for antibiotic administration. Medeiros and Saconato[18] reviewed antibiotic administration in mammalian bites (not exclusive to the face), including and analyzing 8 randomized trials. There was no significant difference in the rate of infection between antibiotic and control groups in dog or cat bites. As the investigators point out, only 1 study included cat bites, and only 1 study included human bites. In the study examining human bites, there was a statistically significant lower rate of infection in the antibiotic group (0%) than the control (47%). It is classically taught that the puncture-type wound from a cat bite is *more* prone to infection than a bite from a dog; however, the investigators did not find any difference in the infection rate for different wound types. As bite wounds tend to be polymicrobial, the investigators do cite the antibiotic selection of some of the studies as a potential weakness, as some of the antibiotic

selection may have been inappropriate. The investigators state that there are insufficient data to draw conclusions regarding the impact of prophylactic antibiotics in dog bites, as the studies included were all small and methodologically deficient, and there is weak evidence supporting the use of antibiotics with human bites.

Authors' Preference

Our practice provides a broad-spectrum beta-lactam associated with beta lactamase (amoxicillin/clavulanic acid) for all animal bites to the face, after cleansing and closure. Because of the cosmetic importance of the face and often severe nature of bite wounds, it is important to create an optimal environment for wound healing free of infection.

Antimicrobial Prophylaxis in Facial Fractures, Level 2a

Antibiotic use in the preoperative and postoperative setting for facial fractures remains a controversial area. There is little agreement on when, and for what duration, prophylaxis is indicated. This was demonstrated by Brooke and colleagues,[19] who surveyed 205 facial traumatologists, demonstrating that 85% always provide prophylaxis and 15% "sometimes" do. Also, 60% of respondents provide 3 to 7 days of antibiotic prophylaxis, but the duration was variable among respondents. Due to heterogeneity of fracture pattern and severity, investigators have difficulty demonstrating clear clinical benefit with prophylactic antibiotics.

In 2006, Andreasen and colleagues[20] conducted a systematic review of antibiotic prophylaxis for facial fractures, identifying 4 randomized studies. The individual studies had weaknesses, including inadequately described method of randomization and, in some, poor documentation of antibiotic choice and regimen. Overall, the infection rates for zygoma, maxillary, and mandibular condyle fractures were similarly very low (nonexistent) in the antibiotic and control groups. For fractures of the dentate mandible, the investigators found a nearly fourfold decrease in the rate of infection with administration of 24 to 48 hours of antibiotics, particularly when the fracture undergoes open treatment. Kyzas[21] systematically reviewed antibiotic use in mandible fractures in 2011, including 9 prospective RCTs and 22 retrospective studies. The investigator stated that it is not possible to draw any conclusion on the use of antibiotics in mandible fractures based on the current literature, which is limited, as discussed previously. Although there was variability in the class of antibiotic between studies, many included first-generation cephalosporins, which may not be sufficient for addressing intraoral contamination in open mandible fractures.

Miles and colleagues[22] conducted a prospective, randomized trial of 181 included patients investigating the efficacy of postoperative antibiotic regimens in mandibular fractures. All patients received preoperative and intraoperative antibiotics, with patients in the antibiotic group (81) receiving 5 to 7 days of clindamycin postoperatively and patients in the nonantibiotic group (100) receiving no antibiotic postoperatively. There were 22 patients with postoperative infections, 8 in the antibiotic group and 14 in the nonantibiotic group, a nonsignificant difference ($P = .0399$). A similar lack of benefit for extended postoperative antibiotic regimens was demonstrated in other prospective studies for mandible fractures,[23] as well as zygoma/maxillary fractures[24] and orbital fractures.[25] Generally, the infection rate for nonmandibular fractures is very low,[26] even when a transoral approach is used.

Certainly, there is not a consensus on the use of prophylactic antibiotics in facial fractures; however, the infection rate is demonstrably lower for fractures of the midface, orbit, and mandibular condyle as compared with the dentate mandible. In addition, open treatment of fractures may increase the risk of infection versus closed treatment. Although acknowledging that larger randomized clinical trials are needed to make definitive recommendations, Morris and Kellman[27] conclude that the current literature supports the use of prophylactic antibiotics in mandibular fractures, probably from the time of injury until after the surgery, but no more than 24 to 48 hours postoperatively; however, there is not enough evidence currently to make a recommendation regarding prophylactic antibiotics in other facial fractures, save that extended postoperative prophylactic antibiotics do not appear to be indicated for any fracture.

Antimicrobial Prophylaxis for Skull Base Fractures, Level 1a

The use of prophylactic antibiotics in skull base fractures with cerebrospinal fluid (CSF) leak is a controversial topic. Intuitively, one would assume that skull base fractures expose the central nervous system to contamination with upper autodigestive tract bacteria, thereby predisposing the patient to developing meningitis. The reported incidence of meningitis following a skull base fracture is 9.2% to 17.8%,[28] with some proposing that the risk is higher in severe head trauma, when the patient is predisposed to bacteremia through a

relative state of immunosuppression, and in cases in which the CSF leak persists beyond 7 days. There are studies to suggest there is a decrease in the rate of infection with administration of prophylactic antibiotics in patients with skull base fractures and CSF leaks,[29] but others have demonstrated no statistical difference in patients with skull base fractures, independent of the presence of CSF leak.[28,30] Ratilal and colleagues[31] published a systematic review and meta-analysis of 5 included RCTs regarding the use of prophylactic antibiotics in skull base fractures, comprising a total of 208 patients with skull base fractures, 109 of who had a CSF leak. They found no significant differences between the rate of meningitis in the antibiotic and nonantibiotic groups, even when subgroup analysis was performed only on patients with CSF leaks. Although there are limitations in the available literature, currently evidence does not support the routine use of prophylactic antibiotics in skull base fractures, including those with CSF leak.[32]

TIMING OF REPAIR

Broadly speaking, there are benefits and consequences of delaying treatment of traumatic facial fractures. In some cases, delay is advised before recommending surgery, as the final functional or aesthetic outcome may not be readily apparent in the acutely injured face. In most cases, delay also will allow some of the edema to subside, possibly improving surgical exposure, allowing for safer surgery. At the same time, there are concerns that delay in treatment may lead to higher rates of infection and nonunion/malunion in the case of fractures. Additionally, there is often granulation tissue that forms in a fracture line during the acute healing phase, increasing the difficulty of reducing bony fragments to preinjury alignment. This section reviews the available high-level literature investigating the effect of immediate or delayed repair on final outcome in facial traumatic injuries.

Facial Lacerations, Level 2b

Delayed treatment of facial soft tissue injuries is rarely indicated, unless the patient is clinically unstable or repair of another injury takes precedence. However, delayed treatment may occur in severely injured trauma patients, or in the patient who delayed seeking treatment. Waseem and colleagues[33] published a prospective, observational study in 2012 for patients presenting to a single emergency department, including 297 lacerations of all sites, none of whom received antibiotics. Ten patients developed wound infections, including 1 on the face. Median wound closure time in the infected group was 867 minutes, versus 330 minutes in the noninfected group, a difference the investigators conclude is statistically significant. There are obvious limitations to this study, namely the number of confounding factors possible in an observational study; however, the results suggest that timely closure lowers the risk of infection, and that there may be consideration for prophylactic antibiotics if wound closure is greatly delayed.

Mandible Fractures, Level 2a

Although mandible fractures rarely require urgent treatment, many pioneers in the open treatment of mandible fractures advocated for repair within 24 to 72 hours. Still, treatment must occasionally be delayed until the patient is stabilized or other concomitant injuries are treated. However, there are other times when treatment may be delayed for logistical reasons. For example, for patients with isolated mandible fractures referred from outside hospitals, it is often more convenient if the patient can be seen in the outpatient clinic, with surgery scheduled within 1 week of the injury. This does raise concern about whether a delay in treatment affects the ultimate outcome, and whether efforts should be made to treat these patients more urgently. In addition to patient discomfort and increased risk for contamination and infection, delayed treatment also results in inflammation and early healing at the fracture site with deposition of fibrinous tissue that may contribute to technical difficulties during surgery.

Hurrell and Batstone[34] published a systematic review in 2014 evaluating the effect of delay in treatment on *all* facial fractures. Included were 30 studies; however, 28 were case series, with only 1 RCT. The lone RCT was actually randomized prospectively for antibiotic treatment, and evaluated only the effect of delayed treatment retrospectively. Twenty-one of the studies were regarding mandible fractures, 1 study for ZMC fractures, and 8 studies involved multiple fractures. The analysis demonstrated inconsistent results with 18 studies finding no effect of delayed treatment on the outcome, 8 studies finding a worse outcome with delay, and the remainder of the studies with conflicting results. Thus, no reasonable conclusions can be drawn from the conflicting, low-level studies that are available. Interestingly, a single retrospective study by Czerwinski and colleagues[35] found no increase in infection rate with delay, but did associate increased infection rate with substance abuse.

Although a large high-quality RCT may resolve the inconsistencies in the current literature, such a trial would be challenging to achieve, as treatment delays in this population are frequently unavoidable, whether due to the nature of the concomitant injuries, or a delay in seeking treatment. In addition, it would be difficult to satisfy the principle of clinical equipoise in randomizing some patients to delay repair.

Orbital Floor Fractures, Level 2a

Isolated orbital floor fracture presents a challenging problem for the facial traumatologist, particularly when deciding the need for open repair. Clearly, if there is an imminent threat to vision from the fracture, such as extraocular muscle entrapment or bony impingement on the optic nerve, or if there is indication of an oculocardiac reflex, then immediate decompression and orbital floor reconstruction is indicated. Early, nonurgent, repair is indicated when there is evidence of early enophthalmos greater than 2 mm, as this will almost certainly worsen as edema resolves. There have been several other proposed indications for repair to prevent late enophthalmos, such as a defect larger than 2 cm² (or >50% of the floor), more than 2 mm soft tissue prolapse into the maxillary sinus,[36] and rounding of the inferior rectus muscle to a height-to-width ratio greater than 1 on coronal CT.[37] The conundrum faced by surgeons is when to consider repair of fractures on an elective basis when there are no definite or relative indications present, specifically when the patient should be evaluated for repair and if there are adverse effects of delaying such repair.

Traditional teaching is that orbital floor fractures should be treated within 14 days postinjury, because it is proposed that further delay will result in fibrosis that will complicate the reconstruction.[38] Enophthalmos, however, may not occur conveniently within a 14-day window, leaving the physician to use criteria, such as those listed previously, when deciding which patients need surgical reconstruction. Thus, there may be a role for delayed (>14 days) repair, but is this approach safe and efficacious?

One retrospective study,[39] published in 2008, evaluated 58 patients who underwent orbital floor and medial wall repairs for prevention of late enophthalmos. Thirty-six patients underwent early repair (<14 days) and 22 underwent late repair (15–29 days). Diplopia rates were similar in both groups preoperatively and postoperatively. Additional retrospective studies have similarly showed no difference in early or late repair,[40,41] including in the improvement in degree of enophthalmos.

However, other studies contradict these findings, suggesting delayed repair is associated with higher postoperative motility disturbance and degree of enophthalmos.[42,43]

Dubois and colleagues[44] published a 2015 systematic review of timing for repair of orbital floor fractures, identifying 17 studies, of which 2 were prospective (but none in which timing of repair was randomized) and 15 retrospective studies. The investigators conclude that there is currently insufficient evidence for providing guidelines on the timing of repair in orbital floor fractures (excluding those that are recommended to undergo repair immediately), as the available evidence is predominately retrospective in nature and there is no agreement in published conclusions.

METHOD OF REPAIR
Open Versus Closed Treatment of Mandibular Condyle Fractures, Level 2a

The mandibular condyle is an inherently weak area and prone to fracture. The goals in treatment of a condyle fracture include restoration of occlusion, symmetry, and normal range of motion. Although nondisplaced fractures of the condyle are treated with short periods of intermaxillary fixation or with only a soft diet, there is debate over which displaced fractures can be treated conservatively, and which require open reduction and internal fixation (ORIF). Although ORIF is generally favored in treatment of fractures at other sites, open approaches to the condyle carry more significant morbidity. The condyle is generally approached transcutaneously, either pre-auricular or retromandibular, resulting in a scar and placing the facial nerve at risk. Closed treatment of the mandibular condyle is generally easier and less invasive, but potentially subject to long-term complications, such as chronic pain, deviation of chin/facial asymmetry, malocclusion, arthritis, and limited range of motion due to joint ankylosis. Due to the inherent challenges of treating condylar fractures, the current literature is limited, and it is impossible to make definitive conclusions. In this section, we present the highest-quality articles, many of which do suggest superiority of one treatment over another, but all studies are methodologically limited.

A Cochrane review in 2010[45] summarized that there were no high-quality trials evaluating outcomes with closed or open treatment of mandibular condyle fractures. The investigators reviewed a randomized controlled multicenter trial published in 2008 by Schneider and colleagues,[46] which was excluded from the Cochrane review

because of a 25% dropout rate with no intention-to-treat analysis. This trial demonstrated superiority of an open approach to the mandibular condyle as measured by a significant difference in range of motion and pain at 6-month follow-up.

Al-Moraissi and Ellis[47] reviewed 23 studies, including 5 RCTs, 16 prospective cohort studies, and 2 retrospective studies, concluding that open treatment for condylar fractures is superior in terms of long-term joint mobility and pain. The investigators do acknowledge the limitations of the included studies, as they are low level, prone to bias, used various approaches, and many included other mandibular or facial fractures treated concomitantly with the condylar fracture. Other meta-analyses[48,49] have similarly reported that ORIF may be superior and appears to carry low morbidity.

In the past decade, intraoral approaches using endoscopic equipment have grown in popularity, and may allow more fractures to undergo open treatment without the potential morbidity of a transcutaneous approach. A small RCT comparing endoscopic versus open approaches for condyle fractures demonstrated no difference in functional outcome or rate of facial paresis between the 2 groups, but the endoscopic group had a significantly longer operative time.[50] In addition to the need for specialized equipment and the technical challenge of the procedure, endoscopic approaches are generally feasible only for a fracture pattern with a laterally displaced proximal segment.

When closed treatment is preferred over ORIF, various techniques may be used, including Erich arch bars, intermaxillary fixation (IMF) screws, and interdental wiring. Van den Bergh and colleagues[51] published an RCT comparing arch bars versus IMF screw placement for fractures of the mandibular condyle, with or without other concomitant mandible fractures. Fifty patients were randomized to either arch bar placement or IMF screws, which were both removed at 6 weeks postoperatively. The primary outcome, pain, was demonstrated to be significantly lower in the IMF screw cohort in both the early postoperative period, and with removal, which for both groups was performed under local anesthesia at 6 weeks. Both groups had favorable occlusal results, but the IMF screws were associated with significantly fewer needle stick injuries and shorter operative time. There are reports of tooth root penetration with placement of IMF screws, ranging from 0% to 14%,[51–53] but these are almost always asymptomatic. A separate RCT[52] reported improved hygiene and lower complication rates with IMF screws, but suggested that arch bars may be superior for long-term maxillomandibular fixation (MMF), as the IMF screws had propensity to loosen at approximately 5 to 6 weeks, requiring replacement.

Condylar fractures represent a significant challenge for the facial traumatologist and there remains a lack of high-level evidence to support one therapeutic approach over another. Although it is agreed that nondisplaced fractures can be treated conservatively and intracapsular fractures should be treated with closed techniques, the debate over when and how to perform ORIF remains. The evidence presented suggests better long-term outcomes with ORIF of displaced condylar fractures and that there are comparable outcomes with endoscopic approaches to the condyle. For closed treatment, IMF screws are an appropriate option and result in less pain for the patient and decreased operative time. However, the results may not be reproducible at all centers, as many of these studies are from high-volume centers with surgeons who perform open approaches to the condyle frequently and with low morbidity.

Method of Fixation for Angle Fractures, Level 1a

The lack of cross-sectional bony support and possible presence of third mandibular molars contributes to the inherent weakness of the mandibular angle, making it the most common site of mandible fracture,[54] and traditional treatment methods are associated with high complication rates,[55] thought to be related to the posterior position and the biomechanical stress placed on this region during mastication. Traditional open approaches to the mandible involve both an intraoral approach to the superior border and a transcutaneous, submandibular, approach to the lower border. However, many surgeons prefer to use only a single plate placed transorally at the superior border external oblique ridge (Champy plate) or superior lateral border via a transbuccal incision and percutaneous trocar. The theoretic advantage to the 2-plate approach is that the lower border plate bears the compressive forces along the lower mandible, at the cost of a visible scar, increased exposure, increased operative time, and risk to the marginal mandibular branch of the facial nerve. Intuitively, a single-plate approach would decrease cost, operative time, risk of neurosensory disturbance, and periosteal stripping (which interrupts blood supply and is considered a risk factor predisposing to infection). A survey of 110 surgeons demonstrated that most prefer a single Champy plate with or without MMF for angle

fractures.[56] But, is there evidence that a single-plate method is superior, or even equivalent to a 2-plate approach?

Ellis[57] prospectively compared 185 patients with isolated angle fractures repair by using 1 of 3 methods:

1. Nonrigid internal wire fixation with 5 to 6 weeks of MMF (60 patients)
2. Champy plate with no postoperative MMF (62 patients)
3. Two-plate fixation (63 patients)

The placement of a single Champy plate was shown to have a significantly shorter operating time and significantly fewer wound complications relative to the other groups, supporting it as a superior technique.

Siddiqui and colleagues[58] published an RCT in 2007 comparing 1-plate versus 2-plate fixation of angle fractures. There were a total of 62 patients included in the final analysis. Overall, most patients experienced some complication, but there was no difference in complication rates between the 2 groups. The investigators concluded that the second miniplate does not seem to confer additional benefit. It should be noted that the patients in this study had other mandibular and facial fractures in addition the angle fracture. Two additional small RCTs[59,60] similarly demonstrated that there is no additional benefit to a second plate.

Al-Moraissi and Ellis[61] published a systematic review and meta-analysis of both prospective and retrospective studies comparing methods of fixation for angle fractures, which included 20 studies: 9 RCTs, 3 non-RCTs, and 8 retrospective studies. Ten of the studies compared 1-plate versus 2-plate fixation. Five studies compared a single Champy plate versus a single lateral superior border plate placed through the buccal mucosa and secured with a transcutaneous trocar. Six studies compared 3D plates with conventional miniplates. The meta-analysis revealed a statistical difference between complication rates in single versus double miniplate fixation, favoring single-plate fixation. However, only hardware failure (plate exposure, loosening of screws) and scarring were significantly different between the groups, whereas malunion, nonunion, and infection were not. When comparing the Champy plate versus the lateral superior border plate, the lateral border plate was superior when comparing overall complications. A significant difference was noted for infection, wound dehiscence, and hardware failure, but not malocclusion, paresthesia, or nonunion. There was also a lower complication rate with the use of a single 3D plate, versus 2 miniplates. Again, although this analysis includes a large number of patients, the retrospective nature and biases of many of the individual studies should not be discounted when interpreting the conclusions.

A final consideration in the treatment of some angle fractures is whether to remove a tooth that lies within the fracture line. Impacted third molars are thought to contribute to the high frequency of angle fractures, and are frequently found in the fracture line. Generally speaking, dental experts advocate for maintaining healthy teeth that are involved in a mandibular fracture, provided the teeth do not show mobility or pathologic alteration.[62] A 2013 systematic review[63] investigated the impact of tooth involvement in angle fractures, including 10 retrospective and 3 prospective studies in their meta-analysis. The investigators concluded that there is no significant difference in infection rate whether a tooth is left in place or removed when treating an angle fracture. The retrospective nature of most studies should be noted, as many teeth considered nonviable at initial assessment were likely removed.

Although there remains a lack of high-level evidence for management of angle fractures, there is an abundance of investigation. Currently, literature supports use of single-plate fixation for mandible fractures, and may favor a lateral superior border plate over the Champy plate. Clearly, patient and fracture factors, for example, severe commination, may mandate additional fixation. As with other areas in facial trauma, physicians must draw on their own experience and expertise, as well as the available literature, to guide treatment decisions in managing angle fractures.

Method of Treatment for Anterior Mandible Fractures, Level 1a

Anterior mandible fractures, including both symphyseal and parasymphyseal fractures, are the second most common site of fracture in the mandible,[54] and perhaps the region of the mandible most consistently treated with open reduction and fixation. Champy[64] originally described the use of 2 miniplates for anterior mandible fractures, one at the inferior border and another 5 mm above. More recently, alternative techniques have been favored by some, including lag screw fixation, single inferior border plate with arch bar placement, and the use of 3D plates. Potential complications of ORIF of anterior mandible fractures include damage to tooth roots, mental nerve injury, infection, wound dehiscence, and the need for hardware removal.

Al-Moraissi and Ellis[65] published a systematic review and meta-analysis in 2014 evaluating the various treatments for anterior mandible fractures, including 13 studies in the analysis: 8 randomized controlled trials, 3 controlled clinical trials, and 2 retrospective studies. Four studies compared lag screws and 2 miniplates, 7 studies compared a 3D plate with 2 miniplates, and 2 studies compared 1 miniplate with arch bar placement versus 2 miniplates.

Lag screws were demonstrated to have a 30% decrease in complications compared with 2 miniplates, specifically with regard to infection, wound dehiscence, and hardware failure. Lag screw placement also had significantly shorter operative times in the 2 studies that reported this outcome. The use of a single miniplate with arch bars was associated with lower complication rates then 2 miniplates, whereas the use of a 3D plate had no statistical difference from 2-miniplate fixation in complication rates, but the 3D plate did result in a shorter operative time.

Although surgeon experience and fracture pattern may influence the method of treatments for anterior mandible fractures, the literature favors other techniques over 2 miniplates for fixation. In particular, lag screw fixation reduces both the operating time and the rates of complications.

Authors' Preference

Lag screw fixation is an excellent choice for appropriate mandible fractures, as the compressive forces across the fracture line result in more primary bone healing than miniplate fixation (in which bone heals predominately secondarily with callus formation). However, the screw placement must be perpendicular to the fracture line, which requires significant periosteal stripping and may be technically challenging in fractures that are not close to midline. Lag screws are also useful in very oblique fractures, as may be seen in the mandibular body.

Management of Zygomatico-Maxillary Complex Fractures, Level 1b

ZMC fractures are commonly encountered by the facial traumatologist and typically must be treated with ORIF to restore appropriate facial symmetry, cheek height, and facial width. The tetrapod zygoma meets the maxilla at the lateral buttress and inferior orbital rim, the temporal bone at the zygomatic arch, the frontal bone at the lateral orbital rim, and the sphenoid bone at the lateral orbital wall. Because of this unique structure, ZMC fractures require reduction with an appreciation of the 3D orientation of the zygoma. Each suture line may be approached and reduced in the treatment of a ZMC fracture and all, save the zygomatico-sphenoid suture, may be plated. But, each approach carries additional patient morbidity; so how many sutures, and which specific ones, need to undergo fixation? This question has been debated for decades, yet most of the evidence supporting various approaches is based on expert opinion and retrospective studies, rather than high-quality RCTs. Some advocate for 3-point fixation, and others argue only 2-point, or even 1-point, fixation are necessary. The lack of RCTs is likely related to the variability of these fractures, including the level of comminution and difficulty of reduction, making comparison difficult.

Rana and colleagues[66] randomized 100 patients with ZMC fractures to undergo ORIF with either 2-point or 3-point fixation. All fractures were reduced with either an intraoral or temporal approach. The 2-point fixation group underwent fixation at the zygomaticofrontal (ZF) suture and the zygomaticomaxillary (ZM) suture, whereas patients in the 3-point fixation group had the previously described points plated in addition to the inferior orbital rim. No patients had comminuted fractures. Patients were followed to 6 weeks postoperatively, with measurements of malar height and vertical dystopia at the first, third, and sixth weeks postoperatively. When evaluating malar height, they found no difference between the 2 groups at the first and third weeks; however, at week 6, the malar height was maintained in the 3-point fixation group, whereas the 2-point fixation group had a statistically significant decrease in malar height of approximately 3 mm. Vertical dystopia was found to be statistically different between the 2 groups at the third and sixth week postoperatively, again favoring the 3-point fixation group. It is interesting that the advantage of 3-point fixation in this study was not seen immediately in the postoperative period, but rather with follow-up at 6 weeks suggesting, as the investigators conclude, that the advantage of a 3-point fixation technique is in resisting the forces of the muscles of mastication on displacing the reduced ZMC fracture.

The previously described results suggest that 3-point fixation is superior as measured by postoperative maintenance of malar height and prevention of vertical dystopia. However, the differences between the 2 groups are not necessarily clinically relevant. Additionally, some fractures may be more amenable to lesser fixation than others. Still, the results suggest that facial traumatologists should be mindful of the forces that the muscles of mastication may have in the postoperative period resulting in movement of ZMC fractures that were deemed appropriately reduced intraoperatively.

POSTOPERATIVE MANAGEMENT
Postoperative Management of Facial Lacerations

The ultimate cosmetic outcome of a facial laceration repair may be influenced as much by postoperative care as it is by a meticulous, tension-free closure. A moist environment and prevention of a scab are paramount to ideal healing, as demonstrated in animal studies,[67] and appreciated clinically. However, questions remain regarding the need for topical antibiotic ointment, or whether a petroleum-alone ointment is sufficient. Although generally safe, topical antibiotics are associated with variable rates of contact dermatitis, up to 10% for neomycin[68] and 9.2% for bacitracin.[16] Schauerhamer and colleagues[69] inoculated guinea pig wounds, finding that infection occurred only when wounds were exposed within the first 48 hours postoperatively, suggesting that the epithelial barrier is restored after this period. These results suggest that topical antibiotics may not be useful after 48 hours; however, the results of this study are not necessarily translatable to humans, especially if the wound is cleanly cared for in the postoperative period. Physicians treating facial lacerations may choose to use antibiotic ointments sparingly (only for 48 hours), or not at all, provided there is no demonstrated benefit by high-level investigation, and there is potential for development of contact dermatitis. Medel and colleagues[70] published an excellent review of postoperative care for facial lacerations, and the reader is directed to this article. Medel and colleagues[70] also cite several publications demonstrating no increased rates of infection with early showering after laceration repair, including randomized trials and meta-analyses.[71,72]

Time to Mobilization After Fractures of the Mandible, Level 2b

The advent of ORIF for treatment of mandible fractures in the latter half of the twentieth century sparked a revolutionary change in management, as patients previously requiring long periods of MMF were able to return to normal activity earlier. However, variable rates of postoperative MMF have been used following successful ORIF. Although most facial traumatologists commonly use MMF intraoperatively to aid in appropriate reduction, some have abandoned postoperative MMF in certain cases. Kaplan and colleagues[73] designed a randomized, prospective study to evaluate immediate postoperative release versus 2 weeks of postoperative MMF in 29 patients with angle, body, or parasymphyseal fractures. All patients were examined postoperatively by a surgeon who was blinded to the method of treatment. No statistical differences were found for any of the evaluated outcomes, including nonunion, malunion, infection, wound breakdown, trismus, pain, dental hygiene, and weight loss. A retrospective study[74] of 118 patients similarly found no difference in patients who underwent immediate release of MMF. Higher-level studies are required to better elucidate which fractures are most amenable to immediate postoperative release; however, these findings suggest it is an appropriate option in many patients.

SUMMARY

The facial trauma literature contains high-level evidence for some clinical entities, particularly mandible fractures, but most of the data are limited by a retrospective nature and small study size. Despite the challenges of acquiring high-level evidence, it is imperative that we strive to support our treatment decisions with well-designed randomized trials, basing less on anecdotal evidence and tradition. These large trials may necessarily be coordinated between multiple large centers, given the relative rarity of many facial injuries.

REFERENCES

1. Evidence-Based Medicine Working Group. Evidence-based medicine. A new approach to teaching the practice of medicine. JAMA 1992;268(17):2420–5. Available at: http://ovidsp.ovid.com/ovidweb.cgi?T=JS&CSC=Y&NEWS=N&PAGE=fulltext&D=med3&AN=1404801. Accessed 19921125.

2. Veldhuyzen van Zanten SJ, Sherman PM. Indications for treatment of *Helicobacter pylori* infection: a systematic overview. CMAJ 1994; 150(2):189–98. Available at: http://ovidsp.ovid.com/ovidweb.cgi?T=JS&CSC=Y&NEWS=N&PAGE=fulltext&D=med3&AN=8287341. Accessed 19940218.

3. Fischl MA, Richman DD, Grieco MH, et al. The efficacy of azidothymidine (AZT) in the treatment of patients with AIDS and AIDS-related complex. A double-blind, placebo-controlled trial. N Engl J Med 1987;317(4):185–91.

4. Available at: www.CEBM.net.

5. Doerr TD. Evidence-based facial fracture management. Facial Plast Surg Clin North Am 2015;23(3): 335–45. Available at: http://ovidsp.ovid.com/ovidweb.cgi?T=JS&CSC=Y&NEWS=N&PAGE=fulltext&D=medl&AN=26208771. Accessed 20150725.

6. Harvey CJ, Pilcher JM, Eckersley RJ, et al. Advances in ultrasound. Clin Radiol 2002;57(3):157–77. Available at: http://ovidsp.ovid.com/ovidweb.cgi?T=JS&CSC=Y&NEWS=N&PAGE=fulltext&D=med4&AN=11952309. Accessed 20020415.

7. Adeyemo WL, Akadiri OA. A systematic review of the diagnostic role of ultrasonography in maxillofacial fractures. Int J Oral Maxillofac Surg 2011;40(7):655–61. Available at: http://ovidsp.ovid.com/ovidweb.cgi?T=JS&CSC=Y&NEWS=N&PAGE=fulltext&D=med5&AN=21377837. Accessed 20110725.

8. Strong EB, Tollefson TT. Intraoperative use of CT imaging. Otolaryngol Clin North Am 2013;46(5):719–32. Available at: http://ovidsp.ovid.com/ovidweb.cgi?T=JS&CSC=Y&NEWS=N&PAGE=fulltext&D=medl&AN=24138733. Accessed 20131021.

9. van Hout WM, Van Cann EM, Muradin MS, et al. Intraoperative imaging for the repair of zygomaticomaxillary complex fractures: a comprehensive review of the literature. J Craniomaxillofac Surg 2014;42(8):1918–23. Available at: http://ovidsp.ovid.com/ovidweb.cgi?T=JS&CSC=Y&NEWS=N&PAGE=fulltext&D=medl&AN=25213198. Accessed 20141209.

10. Khan MN, Naqvi AH. Antiseptics, iodine, povidone iodine and traumatic wound cleansing. J Tissue Viability 2006;16(4):6–10. Available at: http://ovidsp.ovid.com/ovidweb.cgi?T=JS&CSC=Y&NEWS=N&PAGE=fulltext&D=med5&AN=17153117. Accessed 20061208.

11. Fernandez R, Griffiths R. Water for wound cleansing. Cochrane Database Syst Rev 2012;2:003861. Available at: http://ovidsp.ovid.com/ovidweb.cgi?T=JS&CSC=Y&NEWS=N&PAGE=fulltext&D=medl&AN=22336796. Accessed 20120216.

12. Moscati RM, Mayrose J, Reardon RF, et al. A multicenter comparison of tap water versus sterile saline for wound irrigation. Acad Emerg Med 2007; 14(5):404–9. Available at: http://ovidsp.ovid.com/ovidweb.cgi?T=JS&CSC=Y&NEWS=N&PAGE=fulltext&D=med5&AN=17456554. Accessed 20070425.

13. Al-Moraissi EA, Ellis E 3rd. Local versus general anesthesia for the management of nasal bone fractures: a systematic review and meta-analysis. J Oral Maxillofac Surg 2015;73(4):606–15. Available at: http://ovidsp.ovid.com/ovidweb.cgi?T=JS&CSC=Y&NEWS=N&PAGE=fulltext&D=medl&AN=25577456. Accessed 20150321.

14. Available at: http://www.cdc.gov/VitalSigns/Hai/StoppingCdifficile/. Accessed 20120306.

15. Blaser M. Antibiotic overuse: stop the killing of beneficial bacteria. Nature 2011;476(7361):393–4. Available at: http://ovidsp.ovid.com/ovidweb.cgi?T=JS&CSC=Y&NEWS=N&PAGE=fulltext&D=med5&AN=21866137. Accessed 20110825.

16. Mark DG, Granquist EJ. Are prophylactic oral antibiotics indicated for the treatment of intraoral wounds? Ann Emerg Med 2008;52(4):368–72. Available at: http://ovidsp.ovid.com/ovidweb.cgi?T=JS&CSC=Y&NEWS=N&PAGE=fulltext&D=med5&AN=18819178. Accessed 20080925.

17. Rui-feng C, Li-song H, Ji-bo Z, et al. Emergency treatment on facial laceration of dog bite wounds with immediate primary closure: a prospective randomized trial study. BMC Emerg Med 2013;13(Suppl 1):S2. Available at: http://ovidsp.ovid.com/ovidweb.cgi?T=JS&CSC=Y&NEWS=N&PAGE=fulltext&D=medl&AN=23902527. Accessed 20130801.

18. Medeiros I, Saconato H. Antibiotic prophylaxis for mammalian bites. Cochrane Database Syst Rev 2001;(2). CD001738. Available at: http://ovidsp.ovid.com/ovidweb.cgi?T=JS&CSC=Y&NEWS=N&PAGE=fulltext&D=med4&AN=11406003. Accessed 20010614.

19. Brooke SM, Goyal N, Michelotti BF, et al. A multidisciplinary evaluation of prescribing practices for prophylactic antibiotics in operative and nonoperative facial fractures. J Craniofac Surg 2015;26(8):2299–303. Available at: http://ovidsp.ovid.com/ovidweb.cgi?T=JS&CSC=Y&NEWS=N&PAGE=fulltext&D=prem&AN=26517453. Accessed 20151124.

20. Andreasen JO, Jensen SS, Schwartz O, et al. A systematic review of prophylactic antibiotics in the surgical treatment of maxillofacial fractures. J Oral Maxillofac Surg 2006;64(11):1664–8. Available at: http://ovidsp.ovid.com/ovidweb.cgi?T=JS&CSC=Y&NEWS=N&PAGE=fulltext&D=med5&AN=17052593. Accessed 20061020.

21. Kyzas PA. Use of antibiotics in the treatment of mandible fractures: a systematic review. J Oral Maxillofac Surg 2011;69(4):1129–45. Available at: http://ovidsp.ovid.com/ovidweb.cgi?T=JS&CSC=Y&NEWS=N&PAGE=fulltext&D=med5&AN=20727642. Accessed 20110328.

22. Miles BA, Potter JK, Ellis E 3rd. The efficacy of postoperative antibiotic regimens in the open treatment of mandibular fractures: a prospective randomized trial. J Oral Maxillofac Surg 2006;64(4):576–82. Available at: http://ovidsp.ovid.com/ovidweb.cgi?T=JS&CSC=Y&NEWS=N&PAGE=fulltext&D=med5&AN=16546635. Accessed 20060320.

23. Schaller B, Soong PL, Zix J, et al. The role of postoperative prophylactic antibiotics in the treatment of facial fractures: a randomized, double-blind, placebo-controlled pilot clinical study. Part 2: Mandibular fractures in 59 patients. Br J Oral Maxillofac Surg 2013;51(8):803–7. Available at: http://ovidsp.ovid.com/ovidweb.cgi?T=JS&CSC=Y&NEWS=N&PAGE=fulltext&D=medl&AN=24012053. Accessed 20131127.

24. Soong PL, Schaller B, Zix J, et al. The role of postoperative prophylactic antibiotics in the treatment of facial fractures: a randomised, double-blind, placebo-controlled pilot clinical study. Part 3: Le fort and zygomatic fractures in 94 patients. Br J Oral Maxillofac Surg 2014;52(4):329–33. Available at: http://ovidsp.ovid.com/ovidweb.cgi?T=JS&CSC=Y&NEWS=N&PAGE=fulltext&D=medl&AN=24602602. Accessed 20140324.

25. Zix J, Schaller B, Iizuka T, et al. The role of postoperative prophylactic antibiotics in the treatment of facial fractures: a randomised, double-blind, placebo-controlled pilot clinical study. Part 1: orbital fractures in 62 patients. Br J Oral Maxillofac Surg 2013;51(4):332–6. Available at: http://ovidsp.ovid.com/ovidweb.cgi?T=JS&CSC=Y&NEWS=N&PAGE=fulltext&D=medl&AN=22981342. Accessed 20130506.

26. Knepil GJ, Loukota RA. Outcomes of prophylactic antibiotics following surgery for zygomatic bone fractures. J Craniomaxillofac Surg 2010;38(2):131–3. Available at: http://ovidsp.ovid.com/ovidweb.cgi?T=JS&CSC=Y&NEWS=N&PAGE=fulltext&D=med5&AN=19447637. Accessed 20100226.

27. Morris LM, Kellman RM. Are prophylactic antibiotics useful in the management of facial fractures? Laryngoscope 2014;124(6):1282–4. Available at: http://ovidsp.ovid.com/ovidweb.cgi?T=JS&CSC=Y&NEWS=N&PAGE=fulltext&D=medl&AN=24105690. Accessed 20140528.

28. Eftekhar B, Ghodsi M, Nejat F, et al. Prophylactic administration of ceftriaxone for the prevention of meningitis after traumatic pneumocephalus: results of a clinical trial. J Neurosurg 2004;101(5):757–61. Available at: http://ovidsp.ovid.com/ovidweb.cgi?T=JS&CSC=Y&NEWS=N&PAGE=fulltext&D=med5&AN=15540912. Accessed 20041115.

29. Brodie HA. Prophylactic antibiotics for posttraumatic cerebrospinal fluid fistulae. A meta-analysis. Arch Otolaryngol Head Neck Surg 1997;123(7):749–52. Available at: http://ovidsp.ovid.com/ovidweb.cgi?T=JS&CSC=Y&NEWS=N&PAGE=fulltext&D=med4&AN=9236597. Accessed 19970814.

30. Villalobos T, Arango C, Kubilis P, et al. Antibiotic prophylaxis after basilar skull fractures: a meta-analysis. Clin Infect Dis 1998;27(2):364–9. Available at: http://ovidsp.ovid.com/ovidweb.cgi?T=JS&CSC=Y&NEWS=N&PAGE=fulltext&D=med4&AN=9709888. Accessed 19981027.

31. Ratilal BO, Costa J, Pappamikail L, et al. Antibiotic prophylaxis for preventing meningitis in patients with basilar skull fractures. Cochrane Database Syst Rev 2015;4:004884. Available at: http://ovidsp.ovid.com/ovidweb.cgi?T=JS&CSC=Y&NEWS=N&PAGE=fulltext&D=medl&AN=25918919. Accessed 20150501.

32. Nellis JC, Kesser BW, Park SS. What is the efficacy of prophylactic antibiotics in basilar skull fractures? Laryngoscope 2014;124(1):8–9. Available at: http://ovidsp.ovid.com/ovidweb.cgi?T=JS&CSC=Y&NEWS=N&PAGE=fulltext&D=medl&AN=24122671. Accessed 20131230.

33. Waseem M, Lakdawala V, Patel R, et al. Is there a relationship between wound infections and

laceration closure times? Int J Emerg Med 2012; 5(1):32. Available at: http://ovidsp.ovid.com/ovid web.cgi?T=JS&CSC=Y&NEWS=N&PAGE=full text&D=prem&AN=22835090. Accessed 20120810.

34. Hurrell MJL, Batstone MD. The effect of treatment timing on the management of facial fractures: a systematic review. Int J Oral Maxillofac Surg 2014; 43(8):944–50. Available at: http://ovidsp.ovid.com/ ovidweb.cgi?T=JS&CSC=Y&NEWS=N&PAGE=full-text&D=medl&AN=24703494. Accessed 20140707.

35. Czerwinski M, Parker WL, Correa JA, et al. Effect of treatment delay on mandibular fracture infection rate. Plast Reconstr Surg 2008;122(3):881–5. Available at: http://ovidsp.ovid.com/ovidweb.cgi?T=JS&CSC=Y&-NEWS=N&PAGE=fulltext&D=med5&AN=18766054. Accessed 20080903.

36. Belli E, Matteini C, Mazzone N. Evolution in diagnosis and repairing of orbital medial wall fractures. J Craniofac Surg 2009;20(1):191–3. Available at: http://ovidsp.ovid.com/ovidweb.cgi?T=JS&CSC=Y&-NEWS=N&PAGE=fulltext&D=med5&AN=19165024. Accessed 20090123.

37. Matic DB, Tse R, Banerjee A, et al. Rounding of the inferior rectus muscle as a predictor of enophthalmos in orbital floor fractures. J Craniofac Surg 2007;18(1):127–32. Available at: http://ovidsp.ovid.com/ovidweb.cgi?T=JS&CSC=Y&NEWS=N&PAGE=fulltext&D=med5&AN=17251850. Accessed 20070125.

38. Harris GJ. Orbital blow-out fractures: surgical timing and technique. Eye 2006;20(10):1207–12. Available at: http://ovidsp.ovid.com/ovidweb.cgi?T=JS&CSC=Y&NEWS=N&PAGE=fulltext&D=me-d5&AN=17019420. Accessed 20061004.

39. Dal Canto AJ, Linberg JV. Comparison of orbital fracture repair performed within 14 days versus 15 to 29 days after trauma. Ophthal Plast Reconstr Surg 2008;24(6):437–43. Available at: http://ovidsp.ovid.com/ovidweb.cgi?T=JS&CSC=Y&NEWS=N&-PAGE=fulltext&D=med5&AN=19033838. Accessed 20081126.

40. Shin KH, Baek SH, Chi M. Comparison of the outcomes of non-trapdoor-type blowout fracture repair according to the time of surgery. J Craniofac Surg 2011;22(4):1426–9. Available at: http://ovidsp.ovid.com/ovidweb.cgi?T=JS&CSC=Y&NEWS=N&PA-GE=fulltext&D=med5&AN=21772172. Accessed 20110722.

41. Simon GJB, Syed HM, McCann JD, et al. Early versus late repair of orbital blowout fractures. Ophthalmic Surg Lasers Imaging 2009;40(2):141–8. Available at: http://ovidsp.ovid.com/ovidweb.cgi?T=JS&CSC=Y&NEWS=N&PAGE=fulltext&D=me-d5&AN=19320303. Accessed 20090326.

42. Verhoeff K, Grootendorst RJ, Wijngaarde R, et al. Surgical repair of orbital fractures: how soon after trauma? Strabismus 1998;6(2):77–80.

43. Brucoli M, Arcuri F, Cavenaghi R, et al. Analysis of complications after surgical repair of orbital fractures. J Craniofac Surg 2011;22(4):1387–90. Available at: http://ovidsp.ovid.com/ovidweb.cgi?T=JS&CSC=Y&NEWS=N&PAGE=fulltext&D=me-d5&AN=21772169. Accessed 20110722.

44. Dubois L, Steenen SA, Gooris PJJ, et al. Controversies in orbital reconstruction–II. Timing of post-traumatic orbital reconstruction: a systematic review. Int J Oral Maxillofac Surg 2015;44(4):433–40. Available at: http://ovidsp.ovid.com/ovidweb.cgi?T=JS&CSC=Y&NEWS=N&PAGE=fulltext&D=med-l&AN=25543904. Accessed 20150313.

45. Sharif MO, Fedorowicz Z, Drews P, et al. Interventions for the treatment of fractures of the mandibular condyle. Cochrane Database Syst Rev 2010;(4): CD006538.

46. Schneider M, Erasmus F, Gerlach KL, et al. Open reduction and internal fixation versus closed treatment and mandibulomaxillary fixation of fractures of the mandibular condylar process: a randomized, prospective, multicenter study with special evaluation of fracture level. J Oral Maxillofac Surg 2008; 66(12):2537–44. Available at: http://ovidsp.ovid.com/ovidweb.cgi?T=JS&CSC=Y&NEWS=N&PA-GE=fulltext&D=med5&AN=19022134. Accessed 20081121.

47. Al-Moraissi EA, Ellis E 3rd. Surgical treatment of adult mandibular condylar fractures provides better outcomes than closed treatment: a systematic review and meta-analysis. J Oral Maxillofac Surg 2015;73(3):482–93. Available at: http://ovidsp.ovid.com/ovidweb.cgi?T=JS&CSC=Y&NEWS=N&PA-GE=fulltext&D=medl&AN=25577459. Accessed 20150216.

48. Kyzas PA, Saeed A, Tabbenor O. The treatment of mandibular condyle fractures: a meta-analysis. J Craniomaxillofac Surg 2012;40(8):e438–52. Available at: http://ovidsp.ovid.com/ovidweb.cgi?T=JS&CSC=Y&NEWS=N&PAGE=fulltext&D=med-l&AN=22503083. Accessed 20121119.

49. Liu Y, Bai N, Song G, et al. Open versus closed treatment of unilateral moderately displaced mandibular condylar fractures: a meta-analysis of randomized controlled trials. Oral Surg Oral Med Oral Pathol Oral Radiol 2013;116(2):169–73. Available at: http://ovidsp.ovid.com/ovidweb.cgi?T=JS&CSC=Y&NEWS=N&PAGE=fulltext&D=med-l&AN=23663989. Accessed 20130715.

50. Schmelzeisen R, Cienfuegos-Monroy R, Schön R, et al. Patient benefit from endoscopically assisted fixation of condylar neck fractures–a randomized controlled trial. J Oral Maxillofac Surg 2009;67(1): 147–58.

51. van den Bergh B, Blankestijn J, van der Ploeg T, et al. Conservative treatment of a mandibular condyle fracture: comparing intermaxillary fixation with screws or

arch bar. A randomised clinical trial. J Craniomaxillofac Surg 2015;43(5):671–6. Available at: http://ovidsp.ovid.com/ovidweb.cgi?T=JS&CSC=Y&NEWS=N&PAGE=fulltext&D=prem&AN=25911121. Accessed 20150601.

52. Rai A, Datarkar A, Borle RM. Are maxillomandibular fixation screws a better option than Erich arch bars in achieving maxillomandibular fixation? A randomized clinical study. J Oral Maxillofac Surg 2011; 69(12):3015–8.

53. West GH, Griggs JA, Chandran R, et al. Treatment outcomes with the use of maxillomandibular fixation screws in the management of mandible fractures. J Oral Maxillofac Surg 2014;72(1): 112–20.

54. Paza AO, Abuabara A, Passeri LA. Analysis of 115 mandibular angle fractures. J Oral Maxillofac Surg 2008;66(1):73–6. Available at: http://ovidsp.ovid.com/ovidweb.cgi?T=JS&CSC=Y&NEWS=N&PAGE=fulltext&D=med5&AN=18083418. Accessed 20071217.

55. Ellis E 3rd. Treatment methods for fractures of the mandibular angle. Int J Oral Maxillofac Surg 1999; 28(4):243–52.

56. Gear AJL, Apasova E, Schmitz JP, et al. Treatment modalities for mandibular angle fractures. J Oral Maxillofac Surg 2005;63(5):655–63. Available at: http://ovidsp.ovid.com/ovidweb.cgi?T=JS&CSC=Y&NEWS=N&PAGE=fulltext&D=med5&AN=15883941. Accessed 20050510.

57. Ellis E 3rd. A prospective study of 3 treatment methods for isolated fractures of the mandibular angle. J Oral Maxillofac Surg 2010;68(11):2743–54. Available at: http://ovidsp.ovid.com/ovidweb.cgi?T=JS&CSC=Y&NEWS=N&PAGE=fulltext&D=med5&AN=20869149. Accessed 20101025.

58. Siddiqui A, Markose G, Moos KF, et al. One miniplate versus two in the management of mandibular angle fractures: a prospective randomised study. Br J Oral Maxillofac Surg 2007;45(3):223–5. Available at: http://ovidsp.ovid.com/ovidweb.cgi?T=JS&CSC=Y&NEWS=N&PAGE=fulltext&D=med5&AN=17110006. Accessed 20070302.

59. Danda AK. Comparison of a single noncompression miniplate versus 2 noncompression miniplates in the treatment of mandibular angle fractures: a prospective, randomized clinical trial. J Oral Maxillofac Surg 2010;68(7):1565–7. Available at: http://ovidsp.ovid.com/ovidweb.cgi?T=JS&CSC=Y&NEWS=N&PAGE=fulltext&D=med5&AN=20430504. Accessed 20100621.

60. Schierle HP, Schmelzeisen R, Rahn B, et al. One- or two-plate fixation of mandibular angle fractures? J Craniomaxillofac Surg 1997;25(3):162–8. Available at: http://ovidsp.ovid.com/ovidweb.cgi?T=JS&CSC=Y&NEWS=N&PAGE=fulltext&D=med4&AN=9234097. Accessed 19970812.

61. Al-Moraissi EA, Ellis E 3rd. What method for management of unilateral mandibular angle fractures has the lowest rate of postoperative complications? A systematic review and meta-analysis. J Oral Maxillofac Surg 2014;72(11):2197–211. Available at: http://ovidsp.ovid.com/ovidweb.cgi?T=JS&CSC=Y&NEWS=N&PAGE=fulltext&D=medl&AN=25236822. Accessed 20141202.

62. Shetty V, Freymiller E. Teeth in the line of fracture: a review. J Oral Maxillofac Surg 1989;47(12):1303–6. Available at: http://ovidsp.ovid.com/ovidweb.cgi?T=JS&CSC=Y&NEWS=N&PAGE=fulltext&D=med3&AN=2685211. Accessed 19900105.

63. Bobrowski AN, Sonego CL, Chagas Junior OL. Postoperative infection associated with mandibular angle fracture treatment in the presence of teeth on the fracture line: a systematic review and meta-analysis. Int J Oral Maxillofac Surg 2013;42(9):1041–8. Available at: http://ovidsp.ovid.com/ovidweb.cgi?T=JS&CSC=Y&NEWS=N&PAGE=fulltext&D=medl&AN=23623782. Accessed 20130812.

64. Champy M, Lodde JP, Schmitt R, et al. Mandibular osteosynthesis by miniature screwed plates via a buccal approach. J Maxillofac Surg 1978; 6(1):14–21. Available at: http://ovidsp.ovid.com/ovidweb.cgi?T=JS&CSC=Y&NEWS=N&PAGE=fulltext&D=med1&AN=274501. Accessed 19780715.

65. Al-Moraissi EA, Ellis E. Surgical management of anterior mandibular fractures: a systematic review and meta-analysis. J Oral Maxillofac Surg 2014; 72(12):2507.e1-11. Available at: http://ovidsp.ovid.com/ovidweb.cgi?T=JS&CSC=Y&NEWS=N&PAGE=fulltext&D=medl&AN=25315317. Accessed 20141203.

66. Rana M, Warraich R, Tahir S, et al. Surgical treatment of zygomatic bone fracture using two points fixation versus three point fixation–a randomised prospective clinical trial. Trials 2012;13:36. Available at: http://ovidsp.ovid.com/ovidweb.cgi?T=JS&CSC=Y&NEWS=N&PAGE=fulltext&D=medl&AN=22497773. Accessed 20120509.

67. Winter GD. Formation of the scab and the rate of epithelization of superficial wounds in the skin of the young domestic pig. Nature 1962;193:293–4. Available at: http://ovidsp.ovid.com/ovidweb.cgi?T=JS&CSC=Y&NEWS=N&PAGE=fulltext&D=med1&AN=14007593. Accessed 19621201.

68. Zug KA, Warshaw EM, Fowler JFJ, et al. Patch-test results of the North American contact dermatitis group 2005-2006. Dermatitis 2009;20(3):149–60. Available at: http://ovidsp.ovid.com/ovidweb.cgi?T=JS&CSC=Y&NEWS=N&PAGE=fulltext&D=med5&AN=19470301. Accessed 20090527.

69. Schauerhamer RA, Edlich RF, Panek P, et al. Studies in the management of the contaminated wound. VII. Susceptibility of surgical wounds to postoperative surface contamination. Am J Surg 1971;

122(1):74–7. Available at: http://ovidsp.ovid.com/ovidweb.cgi?T=JS&CSC=Y&NEWS=N&PAGE=fulltext&D=med1&AN=4933377. Accessed 19710821.

70. Medel N, Panchal N, Ellis E. Postoperative care of the facial laceration. Craniomaxillofac Trauma Reconstr 2010;3(4):189–200. Available at: http://ovidsp.ovid.com/ovidweb.cgi?T=JS&CSC=Y&NEWS=N&PAGE=fulltext&D=prem&AN=22132257. Accessed 20111201.

71. Goldberg HM, Rosenthal SA, Nemetz JC. Effect of washing closed head and neck wounds on wound healing and infection. Am J Surg 1981;141(3):358–9. Available at: http://ovidsp.ovid.com/ovidweb.cgi?T=JS&CSC=Y&NEWS=N&PAGE=fulltext&D=med2&AN=7212184. Accessed 19810513.

72. Heal C, Buettner P, Raasch B, et al. Can sutures get wet? Prospective randomised controlled trial of wound management in general practice. BMJ 2006;332(7549):1053–6. Available at: http://ovidsp.ovid.com/ovidweb.cgi?T=JS&CSC=Y&NEWS=N&PAGE=fulltext&D=med5&AN=16636023. Accessed 20060505.

73. Kaplan BA, Hoard MA, Park SS. Immediate mobilization following fixation of mandible fractures: a prospective, randomized study. Laryngoscope 2001;111(9):1520–4. Available at: http://ovidsp.ovid.com/ovidweb.cgi?T=JS&CSC=Y&NEWS=N&PAGE=fulltext&D=med4&AN=11572207. Accessed 20010925.

74. Kumar I, Singh V, Bhagol A, et al. Supplemental maxillomandibular fixation with miniplate osteosynthesis-required or not? Oral Maxillofac Surg 2011;15(1):27–30.

UNITED STATES POSTAL SERVICE ®

Statement of Ownership, Management, and Circulation
(All Periodicals Publications Except Requester Publications)

1. Publication Title	2. Publication Number	3. Filing Date
FACIAL PLASTIC SURGERY CLINICS OF NORTH AMERICA	013 – 122	9/18/2017

4. Issue Frequency	5. Number of Issues Published Annually	6. Annual Subscription Price
FEB, MAY, AUG, NOV	4	$390.00

7. Complete Mailing Address of Known Office of Publication (Not printer) (Street, city, county, state, and ZIP+4®)

ELSEVIER INC.
230 Park Avenue, Suite 800
New York, NY 10169

Contact Person
STEPHEN R. BUSHING

Telephone (Include area code)
215-239-3688

8. Complete Mailing Address of Headquarters or General Business Office of Publisher (Not printer)

ELSEVIER INC.
230 Park Avenue, Suite 800
New York, NY 10169

9. Full Names and Complete Mailing Addresses of Publisher, Editor, and Managing Editor (Do not leave blank)

Publisher (Name and complete mailing address)

ADRIANNE BRIGIDO, ELSEVIER INC.
1600 JOHN F KENNEDY BLVD. SUITE 1800
PHILADELPHIA, PA 19103-2899

Editor (Name and complete mailing address)

JESSICA MCCOOL, ELSEVIER INC.
1600 JOHN F KENNEDY BLVD. SUITE 1800
PHILADELPHIA, PA 19103-2899

Managing Editor (Name and complete mailing address)

PATRICK MANLEY, ELSEVIER INC.
1600 JOHN F KENNEDY BLVD. SUITE 1800
PHILADELPHIA, PA 19103-2899

10. Owner (Do not leave blank. If the publication is owned by a corporation, give the name and address of the corporation immediately followed by the names and addresses of all stockholders owning or holding 1 percent or more of the total amount of stock. If not owned by a corporation, give the names and addresses of the individual owners. If owned by a partnership or other unincorporated firm, give its name and address as well as those of each individual owner. If the publication is published by a nonprofit organization, give its name and address.)

Full Name	Complete Mailing Address
WHOLLY OWNED SUBSIDIARY OF REED/ELSEVIER, US HOLDINGS	1600 JOHN F KENNEDY BLVD, SUITE 1800 PHILADELPHIA, PA 19103-2899

11. Known Bondholders, Mortgagees, and Other Security Holders Owning or Holding 1 Percent or More of Total Amount of Bonds, Mortgages, or Other Securities. If none, check box ► ☐ None

Full Name	Complete Mailing Address
N/A	

12. Tax Status (For completion by nonprofit organizations authorized to mail at nonprofit rates) (Check one)
The purpose, function, and nonprofit status of this organization and the exempt status for federal income tax purposes:
☒ Has Not Changed During Preceding 12 Months
☐ Has Changed During Preceding 12 Months (Publisher must submit explanation of change with this statement)

PS Form 3526, July 2014 [Page 1 of 4 (see instructions page 4)] PSN: 7530-01-000-9931   PRIVACY NOTICE: See our privacy policy on www.usps.com

---

13. Publication Title	14. Issue Date for Circulation Data Below
FACIAL PLASTIC SURGERY CLINICS OF NORTH AMERICA	AUGUST 2017

15. Extent and Nature of Circulation		Average No. Copies Each Issue During Preceding 12 Months	No. Copies of Single Issue Published Nearest to Filing Date
a. Total Number of Copies (Net press run)		332	287
b. Paid Circulation (By Mail and Outside the Mail)	(1) Mailed Outside-County Paid Subscriptions Stated on PS Form 3541 (Include paid distribution above nominal rate, advertiser's proof copies, and exchange copies)	184	172
	(2) Mailed In-County Paid Subscriptions Stated on PS Form 3541 (Include paid distribution above nominal rate, advertiser's proof copies, and exchange copies)	0	0
	(3) Paid Distribution Outside the Mails Including Sales Through Dealers and Carriers, Street Vendors, Counter Sales, and Other Paid Distribution Outside USPS®	36	36
	(4) Paid Distribution by Other Classes of Mail Through the USPS (e.g. First-Class Mail®)	0	0
c. Total Paid Distribution (Sum of 15b (1), (2), (3), and (4))		220	208
d. Free or Nominal Rate Distribution (By Mail and Outside the Mail)	(1) Free or Nominal Rate Outside-County Copies Included on PS Form 3541	50	79
	(2) Free or Nominal Rate In-County Copies Included on PS Form 3541	0	0
	(3) Free or Nominal Rate Copies Mailed at Other Classes Through the USPS (e.g. First-Class Mail)	0	0
	(4) Free or Nominal Rate Distribution Outside the Mail (Carriers or other means)	0	0
e. Total Free or Nominal Rate Distribution (Sum of 15d (1), (2), (3) and (4))		50	79
f. Total Distribution (Sum of 15c and 15e)		270	287
g. Copies not Distributed (See instructions to Publishers #4 (page #3))		62	0
h. Total (Sum of 15f and g)		332	287
i. Percent Paid (15c divided by 15f times 100)		81.48%	72.47%

* If you are claiming electronic copies, go to line 16 on page 3. If you are not claiming electronic copies, skip to line 17 on page 3.

16. Electronic Copy Circulation	Average No. Copies Each Issue During Preceding 12 Months	No. Copies of Single Issue Published Nearest to Filing Date
a. Paid Electronic Copies ►	0	0
b. Total Paid Print Copies (Line 15c) + Paid Electronic Copies (Line 16a) ►	220	208
c. Total Print Distribution (Line 15f) + Paid Electronic Copies (Line 16a) ►	270	287
d. Percent Paid (Both Print & Electronic Copies) (16b divided by 16c × 100) ►	81.48%	72.47%

☒ I certify that 50% of all my distributed copies (electronic and print) are paid above a nominal price.

17. Publication of Statement of Ownership
☒ If the publication is a general publication, publication of this statement is required. Will be printed in the NOVEMBER 2017 issue of this publication.   ☐ Publication not required.

18. Signature and Title of Editor, Publisher, Business Manager, or Owner

STEPHEN R. BUSHING - INVENTORY DISTRIBUTION CONTROL MANAGER

Date 9/18/2017

I certify that all information furnished on this form is true and complete. I understand that anyone who furnishes false or misleading information on this form or who omits material or information requested on the form may be subject to criminal sanctions (including fines and imprisonment) and/or civil sanctions (including civil penalties).

PS Form 3526, July 2014 (Page 3 of 4)   PRIVACY NOTICE: See our privacy policy on www.usps.com

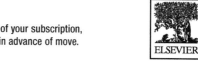
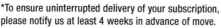

Printed and bound by CPI Group (UK) Ltd, Croydon, CR0 4YY

08/05/2025

01864703-0019